TOTAL

HEALTH

FOR WOMEN

TOTAL HEALTH FOR WOMEN

From Allergies and Back Pain
to Overweight and PMS,
the Best Preventive and Curative Advice
for More Than 100 Women's Health Problems

BY ELLEN MICHAUD, ELISABETH TORG
AND THE EDITORS OF *PREVENTION* MAGAZINE HEALTH BOOKS

Rodale Press, Inc.
Emmaus, Pennsylvania

Library of Congress Cataloging-in-Publication Data

Michaud, Ellen.
    Total health for women: from allergies and back pain to
overweight and PMS, the best preventive and curative advice for over
100 women's health problems / by Ellen Michaud, Elisabeth Torg and
the editors of Prevention Magazine Health Books.
        p.   cm.
    Includes index.
    ISBN 0–87596–271–8   hardcover
    1. Women–Health and hygiene. 2. Medicine, Popular. 3. Women–
Mental health. 4. Women–Diseases. I. Torg, Elisabeth.
II. Prevention Magazine Health Books. III. Title.
RA778.M493   1995
613′.04244–dc20

Distributed in the book trade by St. Martin's Press

2 4 6 8 10 9 7 5 3 1   hardcover

Total Health for Women Editorial Staff

Editor: Patricia Fisher
Staff Writers: Ellen Michaud and Elisabeth Torg, with Jennifer Haigh, Sarí Harrar and Barbara Loecher
Contributing Writers: Toni Donina, Sheila Anne Feeney, JoAnn Greco, Doreen Mangan, Gail North, Kathy Perlmutter, Deborah Quilter
Associate Art Director: Faith Hague
Interior Designer: Elizabeth Youngblood
Cover Designer: Clare Donohue
Studio Manager: Joe Golden
Supervising Technical Artist: Kristen Morgan Downey
Technical Artists: Liz Reap, Bernie Siegle
Cover Illustrator: Sandra Bruce
Researchers and Fact-Checkers: Susan E. Burdick, Carlotta Cuerdon, Christine Dreisbach, Valerie Edwards-Paulik, Jan Eickmeier, Theresa Fogarty, Carol J. Gilmore, Deborah Pedron, Sally A. Reith, Sandra Salera-Lloyd, Anita Small, Bernadette Sukley, Carol Svec, Michelle M. Szulborski, John Waldron
Senior Copy Editor: Jane Sherman
Production Manager: Helen Clogston
Manufacturing Coordinator: Melinda B. Rizzo
Office Staff: Roberta Mulliner, Julie Kehs, Bernadette Sauerwine, Mary Lou Stephen

Rodale Health and Fitness Books

Vice-President and Editorial Director: Debora T. Yost
Art Director: Jane Colby Knutila
Research Manager: Ann Gossy Yermish
Copy Manager: Lisa D. Andruscavage
Senior Vice-President and Editor-in-Chief, Rodale Books: Bill Gottlieb

JUDITH N. WASSERHEIT, M.D.
Director of the Division of STD/HIV Prevention at the Centers for Disease Control and Prevention in Atlanta

ANNE COLSTON WENTZ, M.D.
Special assistant in the contraceptive development branch in the Center for Population Research at the National Institute of Child Health and Human Development at the National Institutes of Health in Bethesda, Maryland

Contents

Contents

Foreword

Every woman knows what a challenge it is to find an informative, straightforward discussion of her health concerns, expressed in language free of medical jargon and gender bias.

Total Health for Women is a book that offers timely information on the causes and treatments of a wide variety of health problems commonly experienced by women. It's a reader-friendly, informative reference on conditions and diseases that affect the health and well-being of women from menarche to menopause and the years beyond.

In today's world, knowledge is power. This book helps women not only become more knowledgeable about ways to preserve and protect their health but also become better-informed consumers of health-care services. *Total Health for Women* will empower you to improve your health through self-education and self-knowledge.

Many women today have concerns about the risks, benefits and possible consequences of such medical interventions as hysterectomy, mastectomy and postmenopausal hormone replacement therapy. Unfortunately, hard, scientific data about both the progression of and optimum treatments for many diseases and conditions in women are lacking.

In the past, medical research often studied diseases and treatments that affect both men and women but used primarily men as research subjects. As a result, there are many gaps in our knowledge of women's health. In fact, we have not yet acquired a complete understanding of what constitutes normal growth, development and aging in girls and women throughout their lives.

In many areas where knowledge of women's health is incomplete, this book reflects the issues currently being debated and studied by the medical community. *Total Health for Women* summarizes much of the research done to date, and the writers discuss the advantages and disadvantages of various interventions.

Under "Hysterectomy," for example, you'll find an important list of specific questions to ask your doctor about this procedure—which is the second most frequently performed major surgery in the United States. Or turn to the section on "Breast Cancer" to find out about the natural changes that occur in breasts as women age and how these changes can affect the diagnostic accuracy of mammograms.

This book discusses at length the significance of the ratio between HDL ("good") and LDL ("bad") cholesterol and the need for further research to establish guidelines on HDL cholesterol levels for women. These are important issues for women. Cardiovascular disease has long been the number one killer of women in the United States: Heart disease is the leading cause of death, and stroke accounts for a higher percentage of deaths among women than among men at all stages of life.

Yet this is one area in which women have traditionally received less attention than men, both in the frequency of medical treatment and in the forms of intervention that are used. The neglect of women's heart health has been compounded by the fact that, until recently, women have often not been adequately represented in some of the major clinical research studies of cardiovascular disease, nor in studies of drugs to treat it.

Fortunately, the medical community has begun to discover answers to many of the still-unanswered questions concerning women's health. In 1990, the Office of Research on Women's Health (ORWH) was established at the National Institutes of Health (NIH) to foster basic and clinical research aimed at providing the scientific knowledge base that is needed to develop gender-appropriate techniques. The ORWH seeks efficacious treatments and interventions to improve the health of women across their life span.

As part of its legislative mandate, the office has the responsibility for establishing the NIH's agenda for research on women's health and for setting priorities for such research. Through its comprehensive research agenda on diseases and conditions exclusive to women, as well as those common to both women and men, the ORWH has helped to sensitize the medical and scientific community to women's health issues and broadened the traditional definition of women's health to encompass far more than women's reproductive capacity and reproductive years.

The ORWH's research agenda emphasizes the fact that women's health is not the exclusive concern of gynecologists and obstetricians. We must engage the talents and efforts of researchers and practitioners across the entire spectrum of medical specialties and scientific disciplines if the fragmentation of women's health research and health care is to be remedied.

The agenda for research at ORWH addresses the full spectrum of diseases and conditions that affect women from birth and childhood through menopause and the later years of life. Our concern is not only conditions unique to women but also diseases and conditions that may affect both men and women. If interventions have been defined using men as the research model, we want to know how effective those interventions are for women.

Another important element of the ORWH's mandate is to ensure the fulfillment of an NIH policy stipulating that women be included in all NIH clinical research studies of conditions and diseases that affect them. This NIH policy has been strengthened and given the force of law in the NIH Revitalization Act, passed by Congress in 1993. In addition to monitoring progress toward including women in research studies, the ORWH has the mandate to increase opportunities for women's participation and advancement in biomedical careers.

The mandate and efforts of the ORWH are complemented by another NIH program, the Women's Health Initiative. Since the turn of the century, women's average life expectancy has increased by almost 30 years, which means that about one-third of a woman's life span follows menopause. It is imperative that the medical community provide guidance and treatments to keep women healthy during those years.

The Women's Health Initiative, a 15-year clinical study that will involve some 160,000 women nationwide, is designed to answer questions concerning the major diseases and conditions that affect women following menopause, including heart disease, cancer and osteoporosis. This initiative is looking at the benefits and risks associated with hormone replacement therapy, the effect of a low-fat diet on the prevention of breast and colon cancer and coronary heart disease, the effect of hormone replacement therapy on the prevention of coronary heart disease and osteoporotic fractures, and the effect of calcium and vitamin D supplementation on the prevention of osteoporotic fractures and colon cancer.

In view of new policies, programs and medical advances, women now enjoy unprecedented opportunities for improving their health. While the federal government and the health-care community work to provide sound scientific data and appropriate interventions to improve women's health, women themselves can and must take steps to protect their own health by making use of the information and resources currently available to them.

Total Health for Women is one such resource. In every chapter you'll find advice from leading experts in medicine, providing practical guidance to help you prevent disease and preserve good health. This book draws you into the experiences of women who have coped successfully with a wide array of health problems. With *Total Health for Women* you can gain the knowledge necessary to make the right choices—to enjoy improved health and a better quality of life.

VIVIAN W. PINN, M.D.
ASSOCIATE DIRECTOR FOR RESEARCH ON WOMEN'S HEALTH
DIRECTOR, OFFICE OF RESEARCH ON WOMEN'S HEALTH
NATIONAL INSTITUTES OF HEALTH

FOREWORD

Introduction

Taking Control of Your Health

A woman feels a lump in her breast. Doctors say it's nothing. She insists on a closer look. They find cancer. She survives.

A woman with fibroid tumors is told she needs a hysterectomy. But she wants children, so she searches for a less invasive treatment. She finds it. A few years later, she gives birth to a healthy baby.

Two different women with one important connection: Both took control of their health. They trusted their instincts and invested time and energy to get the health care they wanted. So can you.

How? By being informed about how your body functions and what your health-care options are.

"Women need to become more aware," says Judith LaRosa, Ph.D., clinical professor of public health at the Tulane University School of Public Health and Tropical Medicine and former deputy director of the Office of Research on Women's Health at the National Institutes of Health. "They need to gather information. To ask questions of their doctors. To be assertive."

Separate and Unequal

But there aren't always answers to our questions. For decades, in fact, there has been a deep and dangerous silence surrounding some of women's physical and emotional health needs.

The silence has meant unequal, and some say inadequate, health care for many of the 127 million American women who make up more than 51 percent of the population.

"Women's health has never been taken seriously in medicine," says Karen Johnson, M.D., clinical scholar in women's health at Stanford University, author of the book *Trusting Ourselves* and a sponsor of the movement to develop a women's health specialty in medical education. "And that has led to the unnecessary death and disability of hundreds of thousands of women." It's an issue that requires women to be vigilant about what they believe they need, says Dr. LaRosa.

"Because we don't always understand what is going on medically in women," Dr. LaRosa says, "a woman sometimes has to be very insistent that, yes, her symptoms are real and not just in her head."

A Void of Information

Sometimes it seems that the only people talking about women's health are women themselves: mothers and daughters, friends and co-workers. But even then, communication can break down. For some of us, menstruation was marked by an embarrassed visit from Mom, a small pink pamphlet and a box of sanitary pads. Menopause got barely a comment from older relatives and friends.

But even when women take the leap to discuss their bodies and their health, hard facts are often difficult to come by.

"My impression is, women talk a lot to each other about what's going on," notes Dr. Johnson. "But our institutions are not providing us with scientifically grounded information so that we can make informed decisions."

What are the major questions about women's health that cry out for answers?

"The area that's been neglected the most is how the menstrual cycle and pregnancy affect diseases, drugs, drug absorption and alcohol absorption," says Janice Werbinski, M.D., medical director of the Center for Women's Health of Bronson Methodist Hospital in Kalamazoo, Michigan, and clinical professor of obstetrics and gynecology at the College of Human Medicine at Michigan State University in Ann Arbor. "Just about every chronic disease, for example, can get worse right before menstruation begins. But nobody knows why."

In fact, doctors and researchers are just beginning to suspect the full impact of sex hormones—and we're not just talking PMS. Chronic diseases like asthma and lupus—and even minor ailments like laryngitis—may intensify the week or so before menstruation begins. The hormones estrogen and progesterone may contribute to a problem that many women know all too well—the pain and unsightliness of varicose veins. And after menopause, research has shown, lower estrogen levels rob calcium from our bones.

Even the medications we take may need to be stronger, or weaker, at different points in the menstrual cycle.

Until the medical profession has answers, Dr. Werbinski says, it's up to women to read as much as they can, ask questions, demand answers from their doctors—and take part in decision-making about their own care.

The Female Difference

If you're going to be an active participant in your health care, it helps to know something about women's health. Here are some facts that may surprise you:

- The number-one killer of American women is heart disease, not breast cancer. A woman's lifetime risk of heart disease is one in two; for breast cancer, it's one in eight.
- Nine out of ten people with eating disorders are women. Among the many reasons are low self-esteem and intense social pressure to be thin.
- Women are twice as likely as men to become depressed. (But they're also twice as likely to recover, because they are willing to seek treatment.)
- Women are infected more readily than men with certain sexually transmitted diseases. In fact, the soaring death rate has made AIDS the fourth-leading killer of women ages 25 to 44 in the United States.
- Alcohol hits us harder, and it can contribute to osteoporosis, breast cancer and diminished fertility. Yet doctors are less likely to diagnose alcoholism in women than in men.
- Smoking also hits us hard, increasing the risk of developing some kinds of cervical cancer and bringing on early menopause in some women.
- Ninety percent of women in their childbearing years do not get enough folic acid, a deficiency that can lead to neural tube defects in a fetus. Birth control pills, cigarettes and dieting can rob our bodies of folic acid.

Taking Care of Yourself

Our bodies are different. So are our lives.

More of us may be working outside the home, but we're still carrying most of the burdens inside it as well. In one survey, women in dual-income families said they did 81 percent of the shopping and cooking and 71 percent of the child care.

Many women are so busy they haven't found time to take care of themselves. Consider this: 40 percent of women have not had a Pap smear, which is the first line of defense against cervical cancer, in the past three years. And while HIV infections are spreading fastest among women, 70 percent of women surveyed were not concerned about contracting this fatal disease.

Did you know your annual gynecological exam does not include screening for STDs, which can cause infertility, among other problems? Or that if your doctor doesn't know the difference between "good" cholesterol levels in women and men, she may be interpreting your cholesterol test incorrectly?

A doctor/patient checklist developed by the National Women's Health Network starts off with this advice: "Your doctor provides medical knowledge, but it's your body. You're responsible for getting and staying healthy."

As the editors of *Total Health for Women*, we have taken that responsibility seriously to bring you an informed, commonsense guide to women's health. This book is designed to help you understand how your body works, to guard it from disease and to help you make decisions about your own care.

THE EDITORS

Acne

Outmaneuvering Outbreaks

Outbreaks of acne can undermine self-esteem in even the most self-assured of women, from those who thought they'd broken up with breakouts in adolescence to those who reveled in peaches-and-cream complexions.

Acne is more of a problem for women than men, experts agree. An estimated 20 percent of women in their twenties through forties experience acne.

The problem begins under the skin's surface in the sebaceous glands. Sebum, a waxy, oily material that keeps the skin supple and moist, is excreted through the hair follicles. But there are certain times in a woman's life when sebum production increases—most notably during puberty, pregnancy, part of the menstrual cycle and during menopause.

As sebum production lays the groundwork for eruptions, the affected follicles eventually become plugged up. A combination of sebum, bacteria, pigment and dead keratin cells (the top layer of the skin) creates clogged pores—the genesis of breakouts.

Different kinds of blemishes come under the category of acne. Whiteheads are small, closed white bumps that emerge when a follicle clogs and swells. Blackheads are the tiny, dark, raised bumps that appear

GETTING RID OF THE SCARS

Some acne can leave scars—and there are a number of treatments and procedures to smooth them out. Here are some of the options.

Dermabrasion. A refrigerant is sprayed on the area, numbing the skin and creating a firm surface. The area is then sanded with a spinning stainless steel wheel studded with minuscule industrial-grade diamonds. The sharp edges of the scar are planed down, and the base of the scar is also abraded, which may stimulate some growth in the center and overall smoothing of the surface. "Dermabrasion can change the scar from a deep box shape to a smooth dell in the skin," according to Allison Vidimos, M.D., a dermatologic surgeon at the Cleveland Clinic in Ohio.

If scarring is severe and deep, the process can be repeated in six months to a year. One caveat: Beware of the sun. After a dermabrasion, sun exposure can cause problems with darkening of the skin.

Collagen injections. Collagen is a protein that gives skin its form. For injections, physicians use highly purified bovine (cow) collagen, mixed with lidocaine, a numbing agent to anesthetize the treated area.

To find out whether a collagen injection might help clear up scars, place a finger on either side of the scar and stretch the skin. "If the scar disappears," explains Dr. Vidimos, "you're probably a good candidate for this treatment."

The procedure is simple: Your doctor will inject collagen into the scars at the level of the dermis, the second layer of skin, where collagen is normally produced. Since the body "melts away" collagen over time, you'll probably need another round of treatments in three to nine months, depending on where it's injected, says Dr. Vidimos.

when the pore of a clogged follicle remains open. Papules are red, swollen pimples that pop up when a clogged follicle releases its contents into the surrounding tissue and produces inflammation. Pustules are pus-filled inflammations caused by an attack of white cells on the follicle's contents.

Since a small percentage of people have experienced allergic reactions to collagen, your doctor should test a small area for an allergic reaction before you begin full treatments. Also, the safety of collagen injections has not been established for pregnant or nursing women.

Fat injections. Deep scars caused by loss of fat may be corrected with fat injections, sometimes known as lipo injections. For this procedure, fat is surgically removed from another part of the body, rinsed and then injected into the scar, where some of it may grow. This procedure provides correction that usually lasts from 6 to 12 months.

Chemical peels. Mild or superficial peels—which gently remove a top layer of skin cells—are done with trichloroacetic acid or alpha hydroxy acid. For severe acne conditions, doctors use phenol peels, which are usually administered under general anesthesia by cosmetic surgeons.

For average scarring, you might get a trichloroacetic acid peel, administered by a doctor. "These peels work beautifully on shallow crater scars," says Letantia Bussell, M.D., director of Beverly Hills Dermatology Consultants in California.

Punch excision. This procedure can be effective for women who have narrow, deep "icepick" scars. A round, cookie-cutter-type punch is used to physically "lift" the scar out, and the sides of the scar are then stitched together.

Laser dermabrasion. For this treatment, a carbon dioxide laser is used to abrade the skin. "Unlike dermabrasion, laser is a relatively bloodless way of sanding the skin," says Dr. Vidimos. But as with dermabrasion, the laser treatment also has its drawbacks—if performed inappropriately, it can cause new scarring or uneven pigmentation.

Family Ties—And Other Factors

Experts say that heredity plays an important role in determining whether you're acne-prone. "If both parents endured severe acne, their children have a good chance of getting it," says Allison Vidimos, M.D., a dermatologic surgeon at the Cleveland Clinic in Ohio.

Then there are hormones. One group of culprits is comprised of the male hormones, androgens, that even float around in a woman's system. When the balance between female and male hormones in your system is upset and more male hormones start churning through the body, more sebum is produced. As a result, acne develops.

But there's another key player in the system. The female hormone estrogen helps to decrease acne by keeping oil production at a reasonable level. That's why adult acne often occurs during menopause—when estrogen production decreases—and frequently quiets down in postmenopausal women.

Another acne factor is what you spread on top of your skin. "Makeup can clog pores, especially if it's not completely washed off before sleep," says Letantia Bussell, M.D., director of Beverly Hills Dermatology Consultants in California. "Although many cosmetics contain antibacterial agents," Dr. Bussell says, "those agents have a limited life span and wear out." For this reason, she advises women not to use old makeup that's been around more than six months.

And then there's stress. Experts speculate that stress also triggers a temporary increase in sebum production, and they are investigating the link. "We don't know how the connection to sebum works," comments Dr. Vidimos, "but women do break out before weddings, exams or a date. You want to look good, and boom! There's a prominent zit on your forehead."

If your acne has really begun to bother you, or if you just can't put up with unwanted outbreaks, a doctor or dermatologist can prescribe a wide range of treatments. Among the oral antibiotics available are tetracycline (Monodox), erythromycin (Ilosone) and minocycline (Dynacin). To influence hormonal factors, a doctor might recommend oral contraceptives with high doses of estrogen or a drug that regulates androgen (called an androgen antagonist).

Another alternative is isotretinoin (Accutane), a powerful prescription vitamin A derivative. Doctors sometimes recommend it for cystic acne—the most severe kind that can lead to scarring. Accutane must be used with extreme caution, however, since it can cause birth defects.

Complexion Lexicon

For occasional acne, you probably won't need prescription medication. In fact, you may be able to clear up the problem with a few strategic moves. Some items from the pharmacy and a change in your skin-care routine may do the trick. Here's what doctors suggest.

CONSIDER RETIN-A

To rein in your acne and control flare-ups, talk with your dermatologist about using Retin-A. "It's the most effective topical medication," says Sheryl Clark, M.D., a dermatologist at the New York Hospital–Cornell Medical Center in New York City. "It really works at all levels of acne."

Unlike most topical medications that treat surface blemishes, Retin-A contains an active ingredient called tretinoin that penetrates affected hair follicles beneath the skin. By speeding up the elimination of sebum from follicles, the medication loosens existing plugs and pushes them out onto the skin's surface, where they can be shed. Equally important, Retin-A inhibits future outbreaks by preventing the formation of new plugs.

If you already have dry skin, you'll probably benefit from Retin-A in the cream form, which contains nonclogging moisturizers. But it's also available in a more drying gel form for oilier skin. The medication is applied at night after washing your face and allowing 15 to 20 minutes to ensure that your skin is dry. Optimal results take at least 12 weeks.

You can expect to experience some flaking at first from the top layers, according to Dr. Clark. "That means the treatment is doing its job." Although the flaking can be a nuisance, it lasts only four to six weeks—and it shouldn't prompt you to stop treatment prematurely. If you tough it out, the skin usually builds up a tolerance and the shedding ends.

With Retin-A your skin becomes more sensitive to sun exposure, and it's extremely important to take precautions. If you vacation where the hazard of sun exposure is great, Dr. Clark advises you stop treatment for the duration of the vacation and use a sunscreen with a sun protection factor (SPF) of 15.

GO TOPICAL. If you'd like to try a do-it-yourself method for clearing up a case of mild acne, try an over-the-counter medication. A benzoyl peroxide wash, Clearasil product or other drying medication might do the trick.

DISCOVER PEEL APPEAL. Some products have a peeling effect that removes excess skin cells, which helps prevent clogged pores.

"Products containing salicylic acid—a relative of aspirin—act as mild peels and can loosen clogged pores," says Dr. Vidimos. Other products contain sulfur and resorcinol, and these offer a "double whammy," she says. These agents are antibacterial and also act as peeling agents.

Other products that have a superficial peeling effect contain lactic acid, glycolic acid or other alpha hydroxy acids. Many of these preparations can be purchased over the counter, according to Dr. Vidimos. "They can be very effective."

DON'T SCRUB. Frequent scrubbing of your face won't help, even though you might think it will unclog the pores. "Don't wash more than twice a day—it stimulates the follicles," warns Ida M. Tiongco, M.D., clinical assistant professor of dermatology at the New York Hospital–Cornell Medical Center in New York City.

Many women believe grainy cleansers will help to further purge their pores, but it's not so, according to Sheryl Clark, M.D., a dermatologist at the New York Hospital–Cornell Medical Center. "Scrubbing with abrasives can actually make acne worse," she says. "Use a mild cleanser without fragrance, additives or potentially harsh preservatives." Washing gently twice a day with a mild soap like Dove should do the trick.

CAMOUFLAGE CORRECTLY. To avoid provoking flare-ups, lay off oil-based makeups. These foundations stick to the walls of follicles, clogging them with oils, says Dr. Vidimos. Many makeups that do a swell job of covering blemishes are hellish on pores. If you must use regular makeup, try a water-based foundation to cover. Before buying, look for the word "noncomedogenic" on the label.

DON'T GIVE YOUR SKIN A NIGHTCAP. Give a wide berth to thick night creams and products containing petroleum jelly, lanolin, tars, coconut oil or cocoa butter. Covering your skin at night, they clog pores and help promote acne.

JETTISON THOSE GERMS. Without knowing it, you may be infecting your own makeup. "If you're using a powder puff or sponge on blemished areas, germs from the surface of the skin stick to the applicator," explains Dr. Bussell. "When you return the puff to your compact, the germs begin to grow in the makeup."

Instead, use a tissue or disposable cotton pad to apply pressed powder or bleach, Dr. Bussell suggests. For liquid foundation, she recommends application with fresh cotton swabs. Also, avoid washing brushes and reusing them, because the bristles could pick up fungi and bacteria from the water.

SQUELCH THE SQUEEZE. To avoid additional scarring, do not pick or squeeze! "When you try to force the contents of an acne lesion up and out, inadvertently you may force the contents down and in, causing further inflammation and potentially a scar," says Dr. Vidimos.

MONITOR YOUR MEALS. There's no evidence that the traditional "bad" foods—like chocolate, cola, peanuts and potato chips—actually cause acne. But researchers say foods and mineral supplements high in iodine will aggravate the condition. "Foods to watch out for are shellfish, iodized salt, kelp and seaweed," says Dr. Vidimos.

SHUN TOO MUCH SUN. Although most of us are aware that too much sun can be damaging to the skin, many people with acne believe heavy doses of sun will heal lesions. According to Dr. Clark, "While small doses of sun can promote exfoliation of the top layers of skin, too much sun or heat could produce more sebum, which could worsen the acne."

Be extra wary of sun if you're using topical or oral medications, which can make the skin more sensitive to the sun's rays. And after workouts and brisk walks, give yourself a gentle facial wash to remove sweat from the surface of the skin. Be sure to use a sunscreen if you're going to laze on the beach.

GIVE TREATMENTS TIME. If you do get a dermatologist's prescription for acne treatment, be sure to follow the doctor's directions, says Dr. Vidimos. And don't expect instant results. It may take a month or more before you'll know if treatments will work at all. Have patience.

Also, If one treatment fails to give you favorable results, the doctor may recommend other options. Dosages can be increased or decreased, and preparations can be recombined. "I've never, ever seen a patient whose acne couldn't be cleared," says Dr. Clark.

Alcoholism

AGING IS THE CHASER

It's been a hard day. You clear off your desk, grab your keys and head for the car. You're going to meet a few friends, forget all about corporate life and, best of all, have a few beers.

Does that make you an alcoholic?

It might. If you look forward to even a single drink as something that you *need*—to reduce stress, to relax with friends, to achieve orgasm, to cope—chances are good that you're on the way to problem drinking, says Sheila B. Blume, M.D., clinical professor of psychiatry at the State University of New York at Stony Brook and medical director of alcoholism, chemical dependency and compulsive gambling programs at South Oaks Hospital in Amityville, New York.

"Normal drinkers never *need* a drink," says Dr. Blume. That's because the need to drink, the need to make sure booze is plentiful wherever you go and to want a drink when there's no alcohol around are the classic signs of a problem drinker.

Women: Targeted for Destruction?

For too many American women, alcoholism is more than a favorite theme on talk shows and the daytime soaps. It knocks 15 years off a woman's life span and is the third leading cause of death among women between the ages of 35 and 55.

Alcoholism is involved in one-third of suicides, one-fourth of accidental deaths and one-half of traffic deaths. It also contributes to thousands of birth defects and divorces. And it is something that most women are likely to wrestle with alone.

ARE YOU A PROBLEM DRINKER?

Drinking problems in women tend to be more subtle than in men. For the most part, women don't usually go to a bar, get roaring drunk and then let everyone within the tri-county area know about it.

But if you have any question about how serious *your* drinking is, ask yourself the following questions, suggests Sheila B. Blume, M.D., clinical professor of psychiatry at the State University of New York at Stony Brook and medical director of alcoholism, chemical dependency and compulsive gambling programs at South Oaks Hospital in Amityville, New York.

- Am I drinking more now than I was a year ago?
- Do I ever feel I really need a drink in order to function?
- Do I ever feel I must have a drink before I go somewhere?
- Are there times I don't remember things I said or did while drinking?
- Is drinking replacing other activities I used to enjoy?
- Have I tried to cut down on my drinking but only found myself back where I started from?
- Do I feel guilty about my drinking?
- Have other people worried about my drinking?

If the answer to one or more of these questions is yes, or if you have doubts about your drinking, see your doctor or arrange for a confidential visit to your local affiliate of the National Council on Alcoholism and Drug Dependence for an evaluation. You can find your local affiliate by calling 1-800-NCA-CALL.

"Our society is a little more tolerant of alcoholism in men than in women," says Judith Gore Gearhart, M.D., associate professor of family medicine at the University of Mississippi Medical Center in Jackson. "Women are more likely to drink alone and to hide it." Their problem is less likely to be recognized by a physician, and it's more likely to reach advanced stages before it's discovered.

"Unfortunately, many women are single parents, and the only people who can observe their drinking are too young to understand or intervene," says Dr. Blume.

Nonetheless, it's estimated that more than three million women—about half as many as men—suffer from alcoholism.

The beverage industry has targeted women as a growth market, explains Dr. Blume. "Women as a whole drink only about half as much as men. So if the industry can get women to drink like men, there will be a huge increase in sales."

That's one of the reasons problem drinking is increasing among young women, reports the National Institute on Alcohol Abuse and Alcoholism in Rockville, Maryland. Among women 18 through 29, the number of problem drinkers is beginning to equal the number among men, the institute has found.

The Ravages of Drink

Researchers are concerned about the increasing use of alcohol because of the way it affects a woman's health. Women react far more intensely to alcohol than do men. Within moments of drinking exactly the same amount of booze, women will have higher blood alcohol levels than men, and the toxic effects of alcohol will more quickly attack sensitive organs like the liver and brain.

Chronic drinking is known to cause early menopause and may also shrink the ovaries and reduce their production of hormones, interfere with orgasm by depressing the central nervous system, contribute to osteoporosis and breast cancer, and cause infertility, miscarriage, stillbirth, premature birth and birth defects.

What's more, "women tend to become more chemically dependent more easily than men—even when they drink the same amount," says Dr. Gearhart.

Why? "The explanation for that is not entirely clear," she says. But scientists suspect that it's caused by the differing amounts of water and fat in the body. Since women have a higher percentage of body fat and a smaller percentage of water compared with men, says Dr. Gearhart, alcohol is not as diluted with water before it's passed to sensitive organs.

A Woman's Risk Factors

Although men start to drink in their late teens and early twenties, studies indicate that women generally start in their late twenties, thirties and forties.

What sets them off? A ten-year study of women and alcohol at the University of North Dakota at Grand Forks indicates that a low sex drive, the inability to achieve orgasm, a heavy-drinking spouse or significant other, premarital cohabitation, infertility, depression, childhood sexual abuse and unemployment are all risk factors for problem drinking.

Women between the ages of 21 and 34 may develop drinking problems that ebb and flow in response to the shifts in friends, lovers, jobs and roles, says Sharon C. Wilsnack, Ph.D., professor of neuroscience at the University of North Dakota School of Medicine, who conducted the study.

But one-third of these women manage to get themselves on the straight and narrow in a relatively short time. "Leaving the collegiate student scene—where there's a lot of episodic, binge-type drinking—and moving into employment, marital or child-rearing roles causes most women to drastically curtail their drinking," explains Dr. Wilsnack.

For those who do go on to develop a chronic drinking problem, the underlying cause of their drinking is often sexual dysfunction or being unmarried or jobless, the study says.

Preventing Problem Drinking

No woman is destined to be an alcoholic. Studies show that even those who are raised in homes with alcoholic parents are not doomed to become alcoholics themselves.

How can problem drinking be prevented? Here are some suggestions.

DON'T TURN TO ALCOHOL. If you find yourself in an unusually stressful situation—such as going through a divorce, being laid off or having a baby—find ways other than drinking to calm your fears and relieve your tension. Start exercising, talk to friends or, if necessary, get professional counseling, says Dr. Blume.

LEARN THE RISKS. Take a class, talk to your doctor or educate yourself about the genetics of alcoholism. Learning about alcoholism will help you make the right decisions about drinking, based on your family history, according to Dr. Blume.

LOOK AT YOURSELF HONESTLY. Take a personal inventory of your drinking at least once every year, says Dr. Blume. Ask yourself, "How would I feel if my daughter were drinking the way I do?"

TURN BACK AT THE FIRST SIGN. "Alcoholism moves faster in women than in men," says Dr. Blume. And once a woman actually becomes an alcoholic, the disease is very difficult to halt.

That's why you need to understand its natural progression. Know the signs that indicate you're headed for trouble, then stop your drinking.

"The first sign is that a woman starts to drink to make herself feel better, to make herself feel more confident, to make herself feel like she fits in or to counteract anxiety, depression or stress," says Dr. Blume.

"The second sign is that she begins to make sure there's alcohol around. If she's going somewhere, she wants to make sure she can have a drink if she needs it. A later sign is tolerance, which means that for what one drink used to do, it now takes two. For what two drinks used to do, it now takes three." And a fourth sign is saying things or acting in ways while drinking that are not like you at all.

"Any woman who's trying to evaluate herself should ask people frankly if she says or does uncharacteristic things while drinking," says Dr. Blume. She shouldn't trust her own memory, because the alcohol can cause blackouts, which means memory lapses while drinking, not passing out.

"Unfortunately, some women who have alcohol problems are given Xanax or Valium to control stress," says Dr. Blume. Doctors think they're suffering from anxiety when what they're really suffering from is problem drinking.

If you can, discuss your drinking patterns with your doctor. She may be able to recommend treatment programs to suit your needs.

HAVE A DRINK A DAY—OR LESS. Women should limit their drinking to one drink a day, according to the U.S. Department of Agriculture dietary guidelines.

"I would say that women who come from alcoholic families shouldn't drink at all," says Dr. Blume. "Any woman who is the daughter of an alcoholic parent or who comes from a family with alcoholism should accept that if she drinks the way nature moves her, she is at high risk for trouble."

STAY AWAY FROM HEAVY DRINKERS. "One of the strongest predictors of women's drinking is the drinking behavior of husbands or partners," says Dr. Wilsnack.

How does she define heavy? "Two or more drinks a day. To a lot of people that doesn't sound very heavy. But only about 5 percent of women drink that much—and 'problem' drinkers generally drink quite a bit more."

SEE A THERAPIST. Of several hundred possible predictors in a large study, the single strongest predictor of chronic problem drinking was sexual problems, such as having little interest in sex, experiencing pain during intercourse or having an inability to reach orgasm, says Dr. Wilsnack.

The problem gets started because most women believe that alcohol can make sex more pleasurable, eliminate sexual inhibitions and make them feel closer to their partners.

But it doesn't work. Alcohol actually reduces your physical sex drive and makes it less likely that you'll reach orgasm, says Dr. Wilsnack.

Any woman who deliberately uses alcohol to solve sexual problems should see a therapist pronto, says Dr. Wilsnack. Doctors can provide a referral to a specialist in the community.

MAKE A COMMITMENT. Back in the 1970s, researchers thought women drank as a response to the stress of trying to be "superwoman"—the perfect wife, the perfect mother, the perfect career woman, says Dr. Wilsnack. Now they say that some women drink when they have too *few* roles. Some women simply don't have enough opportunities to fulfill themselves and build their self-esteem.

That's why studies show that women who are unmarried or without a full-time career are at greatest risk of developing a chronic drinking problem, says Dr. Wilsnack.

It's not that women need a man or a job, she adds. It's that they need a central focus toward which they can direct their lives.

Allergies
THERE'S NO NEED TO SUFFER

You wake up one morning feeling a little sluggish and not quite with it. But you figure you're just a little tired—nothing a cup of coffee can't handle.

So you shower, dress and jet off to work, with the windows rolled down to let in some cool air. Upon arrival, you fill up that mug and settle down to write some memos.

About an hour later, it hits you.

It's that heavy feeling in your head. Not a headache, really—more like a huge piece of cotton has been stuffed through your nose and back into the deep recesses of your brain. It feels as if the cotton cloud is just sitting there, weighing down your thoughts, blocking your creativity, sapping your mental energy.

You take a brief break. You try switching to a different project.

But no matter what, you just can't seem to shake that foggy, bogged-down feeling.

Then you realize it's that time of year again. Allergy season.

Allergies come in many varieties, affecting about 20 percent of women of childbearing age. Seasonal rhinitis, commonly known as hay fever, affects about 10 to 15 percent of the U.S. population, and women and men are believed to be equally affected. But in addition to seasonal allergies caused by pollen, women can be allergic to a host of other substances—dust, air pollution, molds, chemicals, animals, latex and even medicines. Some women (and men) develop allergic reactions when stung by insects such as bees, wasps and hornets. About 1 percent of the U.S. population has such reactions, and while some are mild, others are life-threatening.

With the exception of skin dermatitis and drug allergies, no one allergy appears to be more common in women than in men, allergists say. Women differ from men, however, in that their allergic symptoms and treatment are sometimes influenced by pregnancy. Hormonal changes during the menstrual cycle and menopause may also affect allergies, although how much is not well-understood.

Understanding Allergies

In their milder forms, allergies are uncomfortable, while the more severe types can be life-threatening. The irony is that an allergy is basically your body's way of trying to defend itself, says Daryl R. Altman, M.D., an allergist and immunologist and director of Allergy Information Services, an allergy consulting service in Lynbrook, New York. But in trying to protect you, it makes you feel miserable.

Here's how it works. A central component of your immune system is antibodies, special proteins that serve as lookout soldiers: Their job is to identify foreign invaders, capture them and transport them to cells in the body that can destroy them. In the case of allergies, your body mistakes certain foreign materials that are usually harmless—dust, pollen and mold, to name a few—as a threat. The antibodies, specifically IgE antibodies, carry the so-called intruder substances to special cells, which then release chemicals to destroy them.

One type of cell that often fights to protect the body is called a mast cell; these cells release histamine, the chemical responsible for runny noses, red, itchy eyes and several of the other symptoms familiar to those with allergies. Other cells are also called into action, and they release different chemicals that cause many of the other symptoms of allergy—congestion, skin rashes and hives. In severe allergies, some individuals experience anaphylaxis, a life-threatening condition in which the throat swells shut, blood pressure plummets and the body goes into shock.

Not everyone develops allergies. That's because it takes a special combination—one which researchers don't completely understand—of your genetic makeup and how much you are exposed to certain substances in the environment. Allergies can be inherited, so if your mother, father, grandparents or cousins have them, there's an increased possibility that you will, too. For some people with environmental allergies, one exposure is enough to trigger an allergy, while for others more repeated exposure is necessary.

Women and Allergies

By and large, women are susceptible to the same allergies as men. Two factors, however—the menstrual cycle and pregnancy—may create differences for women.

Some women notice either worsening or improvement of their allergy symptoms at different phases of the menstrual cycle, says Dr. Altman. Women who get hives, either from a food allergy or an allergy to medication, may find that the start of their menstrual cycle exacerbates the problem, adds Rebecca Gruchalla, M.D., assistant professor of internal medicine in the Division of Allergy at the University of Texas Southwestern Medical Center in Dallas. Physicians are unclear which hormones are responsible for the change in symptoms, but they suspect that progesterone may play a key role.

At menopause, some women who go on hormone replacement therapy—taking both estrogen and progesterone—experience an increase in nasal congestion. And if they have allergies, they may be even more stuffy.

Pregnancy can also affect allergy symptoms, doctors say. Approximately one-third of women find their allergies get worse, one-third experience no change, and one-third experience improvement in their symptoms, says Dr. Altman. In women who experience an improvement, the cause is not clear, says Dr. Gruchalla. Sometimes the improvement will continue even after the woman has had her baby, she says.

While it's difficult to predict how your allergies will respond to pregnancy, it is likely that how you respond the first time will be repeated in subsequent pregnancies, Dr. Gruchalla says.

Women may also have an increase in nasal symptoms during pregnancy, says Michael Schatz, M.D., clinical professor of medicine at the
University of California, San Diego, School of Medicine and a staff allergist at Kaiser Permanente Medical Center in San Diego. About 35
percent of women complain of nasal congestion and sinus headaches at
this time, he says. Hormonal changes that affect tissue elsewhere in the
body also affect the tissues of the nasal passages: The blood vessels there
tend to increase in diameter, causing more congestion. Pregnant
women without allergies can experience this, but if a pregnant woman
has allergies to boot, she can end up with a double whammy. These
problems can make sleeping difficult for some women.

Medications and Pregnancy

Allergy treatment is a special concern for women who are pregnant as well as for those who are thinking about starting a family.
Certain allergy medications are not recommended during pregnancy
because they can have an adverse effect on the fetus. Since pregnancy is
not always that easy to plan, women who are contemplating becoming
pregnant should discuss allergy medications with their doctors ahead of
time, says Dr. Altman.

"The good news is that there are a number of allergy drugs that are
well-known and have been used for a very long time during pregnancy
and have not been shown to increase the risk to the mother or the
fetus," says Dr. Altman. "Although you should have a healthy respect for
medications used during pregnancy, there's no reason for a woman to
suffer and be miserable with allergies during pregnancy," she says.

If you're looking for an over-the-counter antihistamine, those containing diphenhydramine (Benadryl) carry no increased risk for pregnant
women and their fetuses, says Dr. Altman. Women do need to keep an
eye out for—and avoid—a medication called brompheniramine, says
Ellen Garibaldi, M.D., assistant professor of internal medicine in the allergy and immunology division at St. Louis University Health Sciences
Center. "It's known to be harmful to the fetus," she says. "And these
things are available over the counter, so it's really buyer beware."

The prescription anti-inflammatory nasal spray cromolyn (Nasal-
crom) is very poorly absorbed and therefore safe for the fetus as well,
says Dr. Altman. But probably the antihistamine of choice for doctors
and patients is a prescription medication called tripelennamine (PBZ

tablets), says Dr. Garibaldi. It's effective and doesn't pose a risk to the mother or her baby.

Pregnant women or those planning a pregnancy need to pay particularly close attention to the over-the-counter decongestants they choose. "There are certain decongestants that can cause limb or organ malformations in the fetus," says Dr. Garibaldi. "They can be very common products. They can be over-the-counter products," she says.

In particular, pregnant women should avoid phenylpropanolamine (which is in Triaminic Expectorant and some other cold medications), says Dr. Garibaldi. A safe option is pseudoephedrine, found in brands like Guaifed, Bromfed and Tussar. "Pseudoephedrine can be given throughout pregnancy with no ill effects," she says.

While over-the-counter nasal sprays are safe in pregnancy when used as recommended, women often stay on them longer than they should—sometimes months at a time instead of the recommended three days. They also often use them more frequently than they should—sometimes every two hours rather than four times a day, says Dr. Garibaldi. This can cause a dependence on the spray to the point where the woman cannot decongest without it. If women use a lot more than recommended, the drug may endanger the fetus by leading to constriction of the umbilical arteries and veins, she says.

Go for Control

The first step in preventing allergies is to take whatever steps you can to change or control your environment so your exposure to whatever offends you is kept to a minimum. There are a number of lifestyle modifications you can make, both at home and away from home, that can help decrease your allergic reactions.

FIRST, FIND OUT WHAT BOTHERS YOU. The only way to effectively avoid or reduce your exposure to an allergen is to find out what it is. If you think you've got allergies, go to an allergist or immunologist and get tested, says Dr. Altman.

There are several tests doctors can do to determine what you are allergic to. One is a skin-prick test, where the doctor pricks your skin, introduces possible offending agents and waits to see if your arm gets puffy and red in the area where you were pricked. Another test, the RAST test, is a blood test that looks for the IgE antibodies in your system. For referral to an allergist, call the American Academy of Allergy and Immunology's Physician Referral and Information Line at 1-800-822-2762.

When the Problem Is Mites

If you are allergic to dust mites, a very common problem, try the following strategies.

GET DOWN TO THE BASICS. Eliminate the clutter in your home, says Dr. Altman. This means anything that can collect dust—stacks of newspapers, piles of books, knick-knacks and fuzzy stuffed animals. Clothes can harbor dust mites, which feed off human skin flakes. So if you're in the habit of letting your laundry build up into a huge pile, move the laundry basket into a room other than the one you sleep in, says Dr. Altman.

GO MINIMALIST. Carpets and drapes are major dust-mite strongholds, so get rid of the wall-to-wall carpet, says Dr. Altman. "A bare floor is better than carpeting," she says. No amount of vacuuming takes care of dust mites, she says. Shades or mini-blinds may be harder to clean than drapes, but they'll collect less dust.

SCALD THOSE SHEETS. Your sheets and pillowcases can also harbor dust mites. Be sure to wash them in scalding water at least every one or two weeks, says Dr. Garibaldi.

DOUBLE CASE IT. Dust mites can also live in your mattress, box spring and pillows. Since you can't wash your mattress and box spring, and it's not convenient to wash pillows that often, cover all of them before you put sheets and pillowcases on, says Dr. Altman. Some bedding encasings are vinyl, while others have vinyl on one side and cotton on the other.

CLEAN YOUR OFFICE. Keep your work space clear of clutter, says Dr. Altman. Clean your desk once a week with a damp sponge, and don't let paper accumulate in dust-collecting piles.

Send Pollen Packing

If you're allergic to pollen and have a problem with hay fever, here are some suggestions.

USE THE DRYER. Try not to hang your sheets, or any laundry for that matter, out on a line to dry. They'll pick up pollen. Zapping them in the dryer may not be as energy-efficient, but it can help cut down on your hay fever symptoms.

TURN ON THE AC. Keep the windows closed and turn on the air conditioner, says Dr. Altman. Do this in your car as well as at home, she says.

CALL FOR THE COUNT. Find out what the pollen count in your area will be by calling the Pollen Forecast Hotline

(1-800-POLLENS). When you call, you'll be asked to key in your ZIP code or the abbreviation for your state. The hotline then tells you whether the pollen level is low, medium or high, and what plants are pollinating.

CHANGE YOUR EXERCISE ROUTINE. Outdoor activity increases your exposure to offending pollens. In general, pollen counts

WHEN THE PROBLEM'S IN THE AIR

Whether you're in your office or out on the sidewalk, getting a breath of fresh air isn't always easy. Pollen and molds can infiltrate the air and trigger allergies. And a host of other substances can cause reactions that are not allergies but are uncomfortable or dangerous—or both.

A number of different substances can cause problems indoors, says Tom Kurt, M.D., clinical professor in the Department of Internal Medicine at the University of Texas Southwestern Medical Center and founder of Parkland Hospital's North Texas Poison Center, both in Dallas.

The first thing to look for is stagnant air, which can lead to excessive levels of carbon dioxide, says Dr. Kurt. Carbon dioxide is an innocent gas that won't kill you, he says, but it can cause people to hyperventilate and develop a feeling of uneasiness. It's also associated with panic attacks. Carbon dioxide buildup can be detected with a portable air meter, says Dr. Kurt, so ask your employer to measure it if you suspect a problem.

Molds and fungi can grow in air-conditioning ducts and anywhere else where moisture builds up, says Dr. Kurt. If you suspect that molds are a problem, ask your employer or a representative of the Occupational Safety and Health Administration to have a certified industrial hygienist come and inspect the area and take samples. Ask them to check the filters in the air-conditioning system and inspect it for mold growth and also check the place where the air enters and exits the building. This can be an area where mold grows or where animal dander, say from pigeons roosting near air vents, can accumulate.

are highest in the early morning and decline throughout the day, says Dr. Gruchalla. So consider planning your outdoor walk, run or bike ride for late afternoon or early evening, she says. You might also consider moving your exercise routine indoors when pollen counts are really high, says Dr. Altman.

WEAR SUNGLASSES. If you have to be outdoors when

If mold is found and the ducts need to be cleaned out, ask the person or company doing the cleaning not to use masking perfumes when they are finished, says Dr. Kurt. Some companies use the perfumes to create a pleasant smell, but they can bring on symptoms in sensitive individuals, he says.

Recent remodeling or expansion of a building can also cause trouble, says Dr. Kurt, when building materials that contain isocyanates (urethanes) or epoxy glues and paints are used.

Other substances that don't necessarily trigger allergies but can be toxic or dangerous include lead in paint in older buildings (built before 1978), pesticide treatments and some chemicals used in the medical profession.

In terms of outdoor air quality, the substances that can cause the most breathing problems are carbon monoxide, sulfur dioxide, nitrogen oxides, ozone and hydrocarbons. The difficulty with outdoor pollution is that you can do little to avoid the surrounding conditions other than avoiding areas with poor air quality or staying indoors, says Carl A. Brodkin, M.D., assistant professor in the Occupational and Environmental Medicine Program at the University of Washington in Seattle.

When you're in your car, you can limit the amount of dirty air that comes in by turning the air-conditioning system on recirculate, says Dr. Kurt.

The Association of Occupational and Environmental Clinics can refer you to a clinic in your area that specializes in indoor and outdoor air quality issues. The address is 1010 Vermont Avenue NW, Suite 513, Washington, DC 20005.

pollen counts are high, wear wrap-around sunglasses, says Dr. Garibaldi. They'll act as a barrier to prevent pollen from getting into your eyes. Or wear regular glasses for your walk or run.

Fighting Other Reactions

If you have allergies, what's routine for most people can be a nuisance for you. Here are a few things that could be making your allergies worse.

RECONSIDER GETTING A PET. If you have allergies

CAN YOU BE ALLERGIC TO SEX?

You know there are lots of things out there that can cause allergies. But can you actually be allergic to sex?

You sure can. While kissing and hugging don't cause a problem, some women can have allergic reactions after sexual intercourse. Women can be allergic to spermicides, to the latex found in condoms and diaphragms or to their partner's semen.

Allergic reactions to spermicidal jellies and foams aren't all that common, says Daryl R. Altman, M.D., an allergist and immunologist and director of Allergy Information Services, an allergy consulting service in Lynbrook, New York. But women who have them may experience intense vaginal itching, hives or wheezing after intercourse. One solution is to try a different spermicide.

Latex, found in condoms, diaphragms, examination gloves and other medical and surgical equipment, can cause severe reactions, experts say. They may be more common in women, says Stephen I. Wasserman, M.D., professor of medicine at the University of California School of Medicine in San Diego, because we are exposed to these materials more than men are. Women have more surgery, are exposed to latex gloves during their annual gynecological exams and work in health professions, like nursing and dental hygiene, where latex is worn every day, he says.

Severity of an allergic reaction can range from mild to life-threatening. If you've experienced irritation after exposure to latex, experts say, talk to your doctor.

and don't own a pet, think twice before you buy one. If you already have one and you can't bear to part with it, try to keep your symptoms to a minimum. "Don't sleep with it," says Dr. Altman. And if you have a cat, bathing it once a week in warm water, while not always an easy thing to do, can be effective in cutting down on dander, she says. The same goes for dogs, which are generally easier to bathe.

WATCH OUT FOR WICKER. Wicker baskets used for houseplants can be a prime breeding ground for mold. Move the

---

Just how many women are allergic to semen is hard to say, says Jonathan Bernstein, M.D., assistant professor of medicine in the Division of Immunology, Department of Medicine, at the University of Cincinnati Medical Sciences Center. "It's not something that people talk about," nor is it something that may be recognized by either the patient or her doctor, he says. Women who have the allergy can experience burning, swelling or pain in the vaginal area. Or they may have a general reaction that shows up as hives, breathing difficulty, diarrhea and sudden drops in blood pressure, says Dr. Bernstein.

Some women are allergic only to their partner's semen; others are allergic to all semen, says Steven S. Wilkin, Ph.D., an immunologist in the Department of Obstetrics and Gynecology at Cornell University Medical College in New York City.

The allergy doesn't have to mean the end of a woman's sex life. Women can use a condom if they're not allergic to latex. Or they can ask their doctor about prescribing a vaginal cream made of cromolyn, says Ronald Simon, M.D., head of the allergy and immunology division at the Scripps Clinic and Research Foundation in La Jolla, California. Cromolyn is an asthma drug that's believed to prevent allergic reactions.

Women who want to get pregnant can do so, says Dr. Wilkin, since the allergy is to semen, not sperm. Sperm can be washed to rid it of seminal fluid and the woman can then be artificially inseminated.

plant into a nonwicker container. Or place it in a plastic or ceramic pot before putting it in the basket. The pot will keep water from soaking into the wicker basket, preventing mold growth.

STEER CLEAR OF SMOKE. "Try to avoid smoke-filled areas," says Dr. Altman. And if you're a smoker, do your best to give it up. "Smoking makes allergy symptoms worse," she says, because it irritates your eyes, nose and lungs.

GO FOR A FILTER. An air filter will help if you've got dust, pollen or animal dander allergies or are exposed to smoke. A HEPA air filter is very effective, says Dr. Altman. It costs between $100 and $200, but in some cases, insurance may cover it, she says. You can buy a freestanding filtering machine at a hardware or variety store. Or you can have a filter installed in a central heating and air-conditioning system that circulates air.

GET A FILTER TO GO. If you work in an office where you are exposed to things that trigger your allergies—smoke or dust, for example—consider buying a freestanding, self-operating air filter for work.

WEAR YOUR BRACELET. If you are allergic to a medication—penicillin, aspirin, morphine or sulfa—wear a bracelet that identifies your allergy. MedicAlert is one company to call (1-800-423-6333).

When Change Is Not Enough

While changing things in the environment may be enough to control allergies for some women, others with allergies require medication. Here are some tips to help you make your choices.

START WITH OTCs. If you've got hay fever, you can start with antihistamines or decongestants. Just be sure to read the packaging carefully. Many of the stronger over-the-counter antihistamines induce drowsiness and should be taken only at night, says Dr. Gruchalla. And while some packaging may warn you not to take the medication if you are pregnant or think you may be, not all labels carry such warnings. If there's nothing on the label about pregnancy, talk to the pharmacist and ask if it's safe, says Dr. Gruchalla.

Finally, if you've got high blood pressure, see your doctor before taking any allergy medications, says Dr. Gruchalla. Some contain decongestants that may cause elevated blood pressure, she says.

TAKE IT AHEAD OF TIME. If you're going to exercise or walk outdoors, take your antihistamine at least an hour before you go out, says Dr. Garibaldi. This gives the medication time to go to work before you're exposed to pollen.

STAY LUBRICATED. Antihistamines reduce watery eyes and runny noses by causing the tissues in those areas to dry up. But just as your nasal passages dry up, so can your vaginal tissues. If you're taking an antihistamine, you may find you don't lubricate as easily when you're sexually excited. Try a water-based lubricant, says Jo Kessler, a licensed nurse-practitioner and certified sex therapist in San Diego.

CONSIDER PRESCRIPTIONS. If over-the-counter medications don't relieve your symptoms, see an allergist about possible prescription medications.

ARM YOURSELF. If over-the-counter and prescription medications don't control your allergies, allergy shots are a possibility. Your doctor may start you off on a low-dose shot that contains the allergen you react to. Your body will build up an immunity, and the shots will eventually prevent your allergy symptoms from kicking in. Doctors won't start allergy shots if you're pregnant, but if you're already taking the shots when you get pregnant, you can stay on a maintenance dose. Doctors don't like to increase the dose of shots during pregnancy because there is a chance they can cause anaphylaxis.

Anemia

A Reason to Iron Out Your Diet

Remember the One-a-Day-Plus-Iron commercials? A 30-something woman steps up to a golf tee, then turns to the camera and whispers, "I don't have to worry, I took my One-a-Day Plus."

A fit-and-trim brunette trims the sail on her 13-foot sailboat and shouts above the wind, "I take One-a-Day Plus!"

Taking a break from her gardening, a young woman wipes the sweat from her brow and says, "Thanks to One-a-Day!"

But did you ever see a commercial with a guy—playing golf, sailing or whatever—talking about his iron supplements? Probably not.

That's because iron-deficiency anemia—the health concern these commercials targeted—occurs more often in women than in men. Men can get it, too, but women—who have lower iron stores and regularly lose iron in blood during menstruation and childbirth—are more susceptible. An estimated 0.2 percent of men are affected, compared to 2 percent of postmenopausal women and 3 percent of premenopausal women.

When You're Bone-Tired

The term *anemia* means an insufficient supply of red blood cells and hemoglobin, the protein in red blood cells that transports oxygen to cells throughout the body. Anemia can develop when red cells and hemoglobin are lost through bleeding, when the body has trouble producing them, or when they are somehow destroyed.

Because their cells aren't getting enough oxygen, people with anemia may feel fatigued, listless, dizzy and confused.

In iron-deficiency anemia, the type of anemia most common in women, low iron levels are the problem. Iron plays a crucial role in the production of red blood cells and hemoglobin, so if it's not available in sufficient amounts, red cell production drops.

There is a difference between iron deficiency and iron-deficiency anemia, says Craig S. Kitchens, M.D., professor of medicine at the University of Florida in Gainesville. It's possible to be iron-deficient without being anemic, he says. A woman who is iron-deficient has just enough iron to get by, while a woman who is anemic doesn't have enough iron to meet her body's needs, he says.

Other, less common forms of the disease include anemia of chronic disease, in which anemia signals a serious condition such as liver disease, rheumatoid arthritis, inflammatory bowel disease or lupus, a chronic inflammatory disease that affects the skin, joints, kidneys, nervous system and mucous membranes; megaloblastic anemia, due to a deficiency of vitamin B_{12} or folic acid; pernicious anemia, in which there's difficulty absorbing vitamin B_{12}; and aplastic anemia, in which the bone marrow has difficulty producing red blood cells. These types of anemia occur with about the same frequency in women and men.

Women and Iron

One reason women are more susceptible to iron-deficiency anemia is that, besides losing the one to two milligrams of iron that's normally expelled from the body every day, women lose an additional one milligram a day during menstruation.

Pregnant women may develop anemia for two reasons. First, while the number of red blood cells increases during pregnancy, the amount of fluid, or plasma, containing the cells goes up even more. The result is that the ratio of red blood cells to plasma changes. Second, if a woman is low in iron before she conceives, having the fetus draw on her low stores will push her into anemia, says Dr. Kitchens. Iron deficiency during pregnancy has been associated with complications such as low birthweight, premature birth, abnormalities of the fetus and even fetal death.

Women also can lose iron during childbirth, when as much as 250 to 300 milligrams of iron may be lost through bleeding.

Eating habits may make any woman prone to iron-deficiency

WHERE TO GET YOUR IRON

Women who menstruate need approximately 18 milligrams of iron a day, while pregnant women need up to 30 milligrams daily. Check the following table for iron-rich foods that will help you get what you need. Keep in mind that your body absorbs about 20 percent of the heme iron in meat and seafood but only 3 to 5 percent of the nonheme iron in fruits, vegetables and seeds.

FOOD	PORTION	IRON (MG.)
MEAT AND MEAT PRODUCTS		
Beef liver, braised	3 oz.	5.8
Braunschweiger	2 oz.	5.6
Duck, roasted	3 oz.	4.3
Bottom round, lean	3 oz.	2.9
Sirloin, broiled, lean	3 oz.	2.9
Ground beef, lean	3 oz.	2.0
Turkey, light and dark meat	3 oz.	1.6
Pork shoulder	3 oz.	1.2
Chicken, boneless, broiled	3 oz.	0.9
SEAFOOD		
Clams, steamed	3 oz.	25.2
Oysters, steamed	3 oz.	5.6
Sardines, Atlantic, canned	3 oz.	2.1

anemia, says Dr. Kitchens. At the top of the list are eating too little and not eating meat. "If you are a woman who has or is bordering on bulimia or anorexia nervosa, you are at much more risk," he says. And "if you are vegetarian, you're at much, much more risk."

Vegetarians are at higher risk because heme iron, the type used most readily by the body, comes from meat. Another type of iron, nonheme iron, is found in certain vegetables and nonmeat products, but it's not absorbed as well by the body.

FOOD	PORTION	IRON (MG.)
VEGETABLES AND NUTS		
Tofu	¼ block	8.5
Soybeans, boiled	½ cup	4.4
Miso	½ cup	3.8
Cashews, dry-roasted	¼ cup	3.4
Lima beans	½ cup	2.3
Pea (navy) beans	½ cup	2.3
Black-eyed peas, boiled	½ cup	2.2
Pinto beans	½ cup	2.2
Refried beans	½ cup	2.2
Almonds	¼ cup	2.0
Great Northern beans	½ cup	1.9
Black beans	½ cup	1.8
Black walnuts, chopped	¼ cup	1.8
Chick-peas, canned	½ cup	1.3
FRUIT		
Prune juice	1 cup	3.0
Peaches, dried	5 halves (about 2 oz.)	2.6
Apricots, dried	10 halves	1.7
Raisins, seedless	½ cup	1.5
Figs, dried	3 (about 2 oz.)	1.3

Pump Up Your Nutrients

Iron plays an important role in your body's ability to function properly. So do what you can to keep your iron level where it should be, and if you're low, take steps to remedy it. Here's what you can do.

BE AN IRON-WOMAN. If you're not pregnant, doctors recommend that you get the Daily Value (DV) of iron, which is 18 milligrams. For pregnant women, doctors suggest the Recommended Dietary Allowance (RDA) of 30 milligrams. To get the DV, eat well-balanced meals. Record what you eat for a couple of days, add up the iron content of all the foods and see how much you are consuming. Remember that dietary iron is poorly absorbed, with only about 20 percent of the iron in heme iron sources being absorbed and only 3 to 5 percent of the iron in nonheme sources being absorbed, says Eleanor Young, R.D., Ph.D., professor of nutrition in the Department of Medicine at the University of Texas Health Sciences Center in San Antonio. Good food sources of nonheme iron include dried figs, dried apricots or peaches, lima beans and tofu.

REACH FOR LEAN MEAT. You don't have to consume large quantities of meat, but try adding a bit to your diet. Roughly half of the iron found in lean beef and chicken is heme iron.

THINK FOLIC ACID AND B_{12}. Good eating will also help you get adequate amounts of vitamin B_{12} and folic acid. The DV for B_{12} is 6 micrograms. The best food sources are beef liver, clams, oysters, tuna, milk, yogurt, eggs and cheese, Dr. Young says. The DV for folic acid is 400 micrograms for nonpregnant women, which is the same as the RDA for pregnant women. So whether or not you're pregnant, you should try to get the recommended amount of 400 micrograms of folic acid in your daily diet. Good food sources include asparagus, black-eyed peas, kidney beans and orange juice.

TRY A SUPPLEMENT. If you find you're iron-deficient or anemic, talk to your doctor about taking an iron supplement or a multivitamin supplement with iron, says Dr. Young, but don't take iron supplements without a doctor's okay. Multivitamin supplements may also fend off vitamin B_{12} and folic acid deficiencies. The cheapest is iron sulfate, says Dr. Kitchens. Unless the supplement contains a stool softener, it can cause constipation. And some women have the opposite problem—diarrhea. Tell your doctor or switch to another brand if you have either problem.

WASH IT DOWN RIGHT. If you're taking a vitamin supplement with iron, certain drinks will help absorption, while others will hinder it. Vitamin C helps the body absorb iron, so drink some orange or tomato juice with your vitamin supplement. Tannins, chemical compounds found in tea and coffee, deter absorption, says Dr. Young.

TAKE CALCIUM SEPARATELY. Calcium and iron interact, and the result is that the body can't absorb the iron, says Dr. Young. So if you are taking supplements of both calcium and iron, take them at least 90 minutes apart, she says. Remember not to take iron pills within 90 minutes of eating a calcium-rich food, like yogurt, milk or canned salmon. If you're taking a multivitamin that contains both iron and calcium, be aware that you will not absorb as much iron as you would if the calcium wasn't there. You may need to take a separate iron supplement to compensate.

KEEP AN EYE ON MEDICATIONS. Some medications can prevent iron from being properly absorbed, says Dr. Young. Tell your doctor what medications you're taking and ask her if they can interfere with your body's ability to absorb iron.

HAVE A PREPREGNANCY EVALUATION. Get your iron level evaluated before you get pregnant, says Theresa Scholl, Ph.D., professor of obstetrics and gynecology at the University of Medicine and Dentistry of New Jersey in Camden. Research shows that "the real risk of iron-deficiency anemia is in the first and second trimesters," she says. Iron-deficiency anemia during these times has been linked to preterm birth, low birthweight and infant mortality more often than iron-deficiency anemia in the third trimester.

GET YOUR IRON LEVEL CHECKED. If you suspect you're anemic, ask your doctor to check your iron level with a blood test.

Angina

THE PAIN YOU CAN'T IGNORE

The pain stabs your arm, lasts about a minute, then disappears. In a man, it's probably a cramp. But in a woman, it might be angina.

Statistics show that more than 1.3 million women of all ages experience the pain of angina. Sometimes it flashes up an arm, other times it radiates toward the neck. Less often it occurs directly under the breastbone, as it typically does in men.

Since angina may show up differently in women than in men, physicians sometimes fail to diagnose it. Nonetheless, studies conducted by the National Institutes of Health in Bethesda, Maryland, show that twice as many women as men between the ages of 25 and 54 actually get it.

"Nobody knows for sure why more women than men in this age group have angina," says C. Noel Bairey Merz, M.D., medical director of the Cedars-Sinai Prevention and Rehabilitation Cardiac Center in Los Angeles. "Women may just be more body-aware. But there's also reason to think that estrogen may cause the heart's blood vessels to be more constrictive."

Healthy Women Can Have Angina

Scientists used to think that angina, which is triggered when the heart doesn't get enough oxygen, was caused by coronary artery disease, a condition in which arteries stiffened and clogged by a lifetime of fatty food and no exercise are so narrow that the flow of oxygen-rich blood is significantly reduced. In the early stages, the narrowed arteries might not be much of a problem. But when a particular activity—running up a flight of stairs, lugging 25 pounds of kitty litter in from the car, shoveling snow, even eating a heavy meal—suddenly increases the heart's workload, the heart doesn't get enough oxygen to do its job. And angina is the result.

But coronary artery disease in women under 40 is rare, doctors say. And new research indicates that angina in younger women may be caused by a wide variety of substances that actually act directly on arterial walls to constrict arteries and shut down the flow of oxygen-rich blood to the heart.

Doctors have known for years that in rare cases angina could be triggered by a spasm of the coronary arteries. What they are only just beginning to understand, however, is that women's arteries may very well be predisposed to it.

What triggers this type of angina in women? "Estrogen, stress and smoking," says Dr. Bairey Merz. And all three can cause angina in perfectly healthy women with perfectly healthy arteries.

Preventing Twitchy Arteries

Having a set of spastic coronary arteries that are likely to twitch shut at any moment may be not only disconcerting but disabling as well. In a 3½-year study of 159 women, this type of angina caused almost half of the women to limit their activities.

Complicating the problem is the growing awareness among scientists that many substances in the body, such as estrogen, can constrict arteries under some circumstances and dilate them under others.

So how can you prevent arterial spasms? Here are some suggestions.

AVOID SMOKE. Once your doctor has proved that it's arterial constriction and not coronary artery disease that's provoking the angina, avoiding cigarettes and smoky rooms is one way to help keep your arteries open, says Dr. Bairey Merz.

Some doctors feel that women's arteries are actually more reactive to cigarette smoke than men's. What's more, smoking actually provokes angina in different ways, says Jo Dalal, M.D., a cardiologist at Johns Hopkins University School of Medicine in Baltimore. It promotes the deposit of cholesterol within your coronary arteries, thereby narrowing the arteries themselves, and it triggers arterial spasms.

Women who do have heart disease are put in real jeopardy by cigarette smoke. "Smoking causes blockages in the arteries of your heart," says Dr. Dalal. With smoking, "new blockages are created and old blockages are made worse," she says.

IDENTIFY THE PRESSURES IN YOUR LIFE. A second way to prevent arterial spasm or reduce the angina caused by coronary artery disease is to identify everyday situations in which you feel pressured. Try to avoid them, recommends the American Heart Association. Cut down on rushing around and trying to do everything yourself. Let other people prove they've got the "right stuff," while you move on to other tasks.

RELAX AND BREATHE. When it's not possible to avoid all of life's pressures, learn to handle them gracefully with meditation and relaxation techniques. Some doctors suggest you breathe deeply and concentrate on a pleasant thought or experience when you're feeling stressed. Other experts suggest you totally concentrate on relaxing all your muscles—head to toe—for 20 minutes twice a day.

CONSIDER MEDICATION. If you still experience angina, your doctor can prescribe calcium channel blockers or nitroglycerin tablets to prevent it, says Dr. Bairey Merz.

Get Your Arteries in Shape

Focus on preventing the coronary artery disease that can cause angina in the decades ahead, says Dr. Bairey Merz, or if you already have angina from blocked arteries, try to keep your arteries from getting worse. In either case, your strategy should be the same.

KEEP YOUR ARTERIES CLEAN. "That means don't smoke, eat a low-fat diet and try to get some exercise every day," says Dr. Bairey Merz.

HIT THE ROAD. Exercise can be of particular help, she adds. Results from over 40 studies show that inactive individuals are almost two times more likely to develop heart disease than are active people. And these findings are independent of other risk factors for heart disease, such as smoking, high blood pressure, obesity, family history or high cholesterol levels. This means that inactivity carries a risk almost as high as the relative risk of smoking a pack of cigarettes a day. Studies show that even light to moderate exercise, such as walking, climbing stairs and gardening, is associated with lower risk for heart disease.

Exercise does two things, explains Dr. Bairey Merz. It conditions the cardiovascular system so that it requires less oxygen as a whole, and it dilates and tones the arteries themselves, giving clogged or spastic arteries an extra margin for error.

How much exercise would it take for a woman to achieve those kinds of results? "Nobody's done the research," says endocrinologist Irma Ullrich, M.D., professor of medicine at West Virginia University in Morgantown. But there is some evidence in men that regular high-intensity exercise such as running can literally restructure the coronary arteries.

A study conducted at Stanford University compared 11 long-distance runners, who ran at least 40 miles a week, to 11 physically inactive men of equal age. The coronary arteries in the runners' hearts could expand to 265 percent of the original size when dilated as much as possible, compared to the inactive men's hearts, which could only expand to 134 percent. That means that the increase in area in the runners' coronary arteries would lead to about twice the increase in the flow of blood.

No one knows whether this occurs in women, says Dr. Ullrich. But we do know that even moderate amounts of exercise—brisk walking three or four times a week, swimming laps or biking—can help women prevent angina.

And we know that, combined with low-fat eating and avoiding smoking, exercise can also reduce your chances of developing high cholesterol, high blood pressure and diabetes—a deadly trio that is known to interfere with your arteries' natural ability to prevent constriction.

Appendicitis

IT CAN BE THE UNKINDEST CUT

On the lower right side of your abdomen, there's a smoldering pain that won't go away. You've thrown up twice in the past hour, your temperature is climbing, and the thought of food is revolting.

Do you have appendicitis?

Maybe. But if you're a woman, chances are that even if you don't, you could still end up losing your appendix.

A study of more than three million men and women conducted over a six-year period by the Centers for Disease Control and Prevention (CDC) in Atlanta found that women have twice as many appendectomies as men, even though they have about half the number of cases of appendicitis.

The same study showed that a mistaken diagnosis is 12 percent more likely to occur in women than in men and that women between the ages of 35 and 44 are 12 times more likely than men to have a healthy appendix removed.

What's more, the study determined that five out of every six appendixes surgically removed from women ages 35 to 39 are likely to be disease-free—meaning they didn't need to be taken out.

Why Us?

Appendicitis is an inflammation of the small appendage situated near where the small and large intestines meet. The appendix itself doesn't serve much purpose—you can live just fine without it—but once it's diseased it has the potential to reach life-threatening status.

Nobody knows what causes appendicitis. Only 110,000 women have appendicitis every year, but nearly 372,000 women have appendectomies.

"I was surprised by the statistics," says medical epidemiologist David Addiss, M.D., the investigator who led the CDC study.

Studies indicate that the most common reason women undergo more appendectomies than men is the biological makeup of the female anatomy: Doctors often have difficulty differentiating between gynecological problems and appendicitis. And sometimes a doctor will simply decide to remove a normal appendix while operating in the abdomen for other reasons.

"Women tend to get more appendectomies than men because of the confusing picture presented by gynecologic disorders," says gastroenterologist Marie Borum, M.D., assistant professor of medicine at George Washington University Medical Center in Washington, D.C.

ARE YOU SURE IT'S APPENDICITIS?

Many conditions can be mistaken for appendicitis in women, doctors say. Here's a list of the most common.

- Pelvic inflammatory disease
- Ovarian cysts
- Endometriosis
- Intestinal virus
- Cervical inflammation
- Pain in passing a hard stool
- Gallstones
- Cancer
- Abnormal menstruation
- Intestinal adhesions
- Abdominal infection
- Abdominal pain of unknown origin

The problem is that the symptoms of appendicitis—predominantly right-lower abdominal pain—are nearly the same as those of a dozen other conditions ranging from ectopic (outside the uterus) pregnancy to inflammatory bowel disease. "Even though I do a thorough physical and perform lab and radiologic studies," says Dr. Borum, "I still may not be certain what's causing the symptoms."

Confusing the diagnosis even further, she adds, is the fact that the appendix may not be where it should be. "Sometimes the appendix can be in an unusual position and refer pain to the right shoulder, above the stomach or even to the rectum," says Dr. Borum.

Taking Caution's Side

Aside from the complexities of diagnosis, one factor that sends doctors reaching for the scalpel is the knowledge of how dangerous appendicitis can be.

"I too have the concern that women are getting more appendectomies than men," says Dr. Borum. "But I think it's because doctors are concerned that they may miss a potentially catastrophic event like a perforated appendix."

Perforation—a hole or break in the appendix wall—can lead to peritonitis, a condition in which the appendix bursts and spreads pus throughout the abdominal cavity, she explains. The result is a massive infection that threatens every part of the body and can be fatal.

"Those appendixes are the ones that doctors are scared to miss," says Dr. Borum, even though perforations themselves are present in less than 5 percent of all appendectomies and occur mostly in children 10 to 14.

The fear of a perforation in the future may also encourage doctors to cut out a healthy appendix during surgery for other conditions.

"Doctors are just doing it because they're in there," says Dr. Borum. They figure that since the appendix has no known purpose, and since no one's really sure what triggers appendicitis to begin with, they'll get it before it causes a problem.

How to Save Your Appendix

According to some doctors, there's a medical school opinion that removing a large number of healthy appendixes is the only way to make sure you get the ones that are likely to perforate. Based on medical textbooks and studies, in fact, it's expected that somewhere between 15 and 23 percent of procedures will remove a *healthy* appendix.

Here's how you can make sure yours is not one of them.

GET AN ABDOMINAL EXAM. You should have an abdominal exam and, if necessary, a pelvic exam, to rule out as many gynecological problems as possible, says Dr. Borum. If these examinations are inconclusive, lab tests, including a complete blood count, should be performed, she says.

TALK. Any time you have an abdominal operation, discuss the procedure with your physician. Since no one's really sure what purpose the appendix serves, you may or may not want to keep it. If tests show that you do have a diseased appendix, you should have it removed, says Dr. Borum.

CONSIDER A LAPAROSCOPIC EXAMINATION. This diagnostic technique, used by gynecologists and adapted in recent years by surgeons, should mean that there is no longer any reason to remove a woman's appendix because of the difficulty in diagnosing appendicitis, says Gustavo G. R. Kuster, M.D., senior surgical consultant at the Scripps Clinic and Research Foundation in La Jolla, California.

"The laparoscope is like a pencil. It is long, with lenses, a light and microcameras. It is introduced through the belly button, so there's no scar. You can use it to look inside the abdomen, and you can visualize the appendix and all the organs around it—the fallopian tubes, the ovaries, the liver, the gallbladder, the stomach and the intestines."

What to Do If You've Got It

If appendicitis is the problem, the surgeon can insert two narrow tubes through quarter-inch incisions on both sides of the abdomen and use long, narrow instruments to remove the appendix.

"It's something like a video game," says Dr. Kuster. "You look into a TV monitor as you work outside the abdomen to manipulate the instruments."

The surgeon can grasp, cut, stitch and cauterize through the tubes, says Dr. Kuster. Compared with the old-fashioned way of opening up the abdomen, "there's less infection, less adhesions that can lead to bowel obstruction, less chance of infertility due to pelvic infection, less pain and scars and quicker recovery," he says. With laparoscopic surgery, you're out of the hospital the next day, if there is no severe infection. The old way, you're flat on your back for three to five days, and you shouldn't lift or exercise for another five or six weeks.

Arthritis

ACTIVITY IS YOUR BEST DEFENSE

For the last couple of months, your 38-year-old walking partner has had trouble with her knee. Some days she has to take the elevator instead of the stairs and drive to the store instead of walking.

It turns out she has arthritis, a joint disease shared by nearly 40 million people. About two-thirds of those—almost 23 million—are women. Although most of us associate arthritis with the elderly, it can strike in childhood, causing inflammation, swelling, pain and joint destruction. There are more than 100 types of the disease, of which osteoarthritis and rheumatoid arthritis are the most widespread.

Osteoarthritis is the most common form. It plagues 16 million adults, 11.7 million of them women. It's not clear what causes osteoarthritis, but experts believe that hormones, body weight, genetics and mechanical problems in the joints may contribute.

Osteoarthritis develops when certain structures that make up a joint—the ligaments, tendons and cartilage—are damaged and the joint shifts out of alignment. Abnormal weight distribution on small areas of cartilage can cause inflammation and eventual joint destruction.

It's Trouble for Women

Researchers aren't sure why osteoarthritis is more common in women, but preliminary research in Taiwan implicates the female hormone estrogen, which has been found in arthritic cartilage.

Body weight is another factor in osteoarthritis, says Cody Wasner, M.D., assistant clinical professor at the Oregon Health Sciences University in Eugene and a spokesperson for the Arthritis Foundation in Atlanta. If you looked at 100 women, he says, the heaviest 25 would be at three to four times greater risk for osteoarthritis than the women who weighed less. Animal studies show that lowering body weight can decrease the severity of arthritis, says Dr. Wasner, partially because joints are better able to stay in place if they're carrying less weight.

Injury is another major cause of osteoarthritis. This is because damage to the joint can cause misalignment and subsequent osteoarthritis, says W. Joseph McCune, M.D., associate professor of internal medicine at the University of Michigan in Ann Arbor.

Osteoarthritis in women ages 30 to 45 usually strikes in the knee, Dr. Wasner says, and arthritic knees are more prevalent in women than in men by a ratio of two to one.

The hands are another osteoarthritis flashpoint for women, with the usual targets being the joints nearest the fingernails. "This kind of arthritis is associated with bumps at those joints," says Dr. Wasner, and women often start developing problems in their thirties and forties. The bumps are known as Heberden's nodes, and women are at ten times greater risk for developing them than men are.

Part of the reason for that, says Dr. Wasner, is genetics. The gene linked to Heberden's is more often passed from mother to daughter. "There's nothing to prevent that from happening," he says. This problem sometimes develops earlier in women who go through early menopause, he notes. While women can't prevent it, early treatment can help them maintain function in their hands.

Another area where osteoarthritis commonly develops is the hip joint, but there the disease strikes men and women at about the same rate.

Osteoarthritis is difficult to diagnose, Dr. Wasner says. That's because early arthritis, say in the hip, may first be noticed as pain in the groin area. Doctors don't realize that the problem is in the hip until the disease becomes serious.

Investing in Joint Preservation

Osteoarthritis is a condition you can try to prevent. Here's how.

AVOID INJURY. Condition yourself properly for whatever activity you're doing, warm up, stretch, cool down and wear the proper equipment, particularly footwear, Dr. McCune says.

WATCH YOUR WEIGHT. Since heavy people are at greater risk for osteoarthritis, says Dr. Wasner, try to achieve your ideal weight. Consult with your physician about how to combine exercise and healthy low-fat eating to accomplish this goal.

STAY IN SHAPE. Muscles work to stabilize your joints, so the stronger they are, the less susceptible to injury and arthritis they will be. Patients with underlying joint problems should consult a physical therapist, exercise physiologist or an individual trained in exercise science about appropriate exercises and techniques.

Fighting the Pain

If you think you've got osteoarthritis, here's what you can do to cope.

SEE A DOCTOR. The longer you wait, the more damage can be done to your joints and the harder it will be to treat. Rheumatologists specialize in the treatment of arthritis and can either care for your disease themselves or refer you to a physical therapist or to an orthopedic surgeon if your disease is severe enough to warrant joint replacement. To find a rheumatologist in your area, contact your local chapter of the Arthritis Foundation.

ICE DOWN THE PAIN. For the pain and swelling of arthritis, apply ice, says Dr. Wasner. Ice reduces inflammation because it causes blood vessels to constrict, reducing blood flow and fluid buildup. Ice for 20 to 30 minutes after you exercise or after any strenuous activity in which you've placed excessive demands on your joints, he says. You can buy an ice pack at your pharmacy or make one yourself by putting ice in a plastic bag and wrapping it in a towel so the ice doesn't harm your skin.

WARM UP. If you've got joint stiffness, heat can help, says Dr. Wasner. Sit in a hot bath for 20 minutes or apply a heat pack or hot towel for 20 minutes to the joint that's bothering you.

EXERCISE CAREFULLY. Not all leg-strengthening exercises are good for the knees, says physical therapist Mark Taranta, director of the Physical Therapy Practice in Philadelphia. Some exercises, such as squats and knee extensions, can accelerate osteoarthritis. The best are straight-leg raises, because they help strengthen your thigh muscles without straining your joints.

Do stairs properly. Stairs place substantial stress on your knees. Practice the following technique when going up and down: Going up, lead with your "good" leg; this makes that leg carry most of the weight and do most of the work. On the way down, lead with your "bad" leg; this again allows your good leg to absorb the most stress, says Taranta.

Replace doorknobs. Rotating handles and doorknobs can be difficult for arthritic hands, so replace the ones in your home with lever- and latch-type devices, says Dr. Wasner.

Help your hands. If you've got arthritis in your hands, says Taranta, ask your doctor about splints that can hold your wrists and hands in a comfortable position.

Pick up a cane. Using a cane can help ease hip pain by lessening stress on the hip. It may also prolong the time before you have to resort to more serious treatment, such as surgery. It's hard for people to even consider using a cane, says Dr. Wasner. Just remember that you might get more mileage out of your hip if you do, he says.

The "Other" Arthritis

Rheumatoid arthritis affects between 2 and 3 million people, or 1 to 2 percent of adults, says Dr. McCune. Nearly 1.5 million are women, experts say.

Rheumatoid arthritis is a mystery. It can develop gradually or suddenly, says Dr. McCune, and what causes it is unclear. For some reason, certain cells in the immune system misbehave, and their activity causes the cells that line joints to proliferate and start destroying the bone and cartilage they're supposed to protect. The lining of the joint becomes inflamed, causing pain and stiffness. The bone and cartilage sometimes become eroded, causing disability.

The joints most commonly affected are those in the hands, wrists, knees, ankles and toes, says Philip Mease, M.D., clinical associate professor of rheumatology at the University of Washington School of Medicine in Seattle. It appears less often in the elbows, hips, shoulders, neck and low back, he says. Rheumatoid arthritis "tends to affect both sides of the body in a symmetrical fashion," he says. "Flares tend to act in concert."

Genetics is considered to be the major risk factor for rheumatoid arthritis, he says.

One of the unusual things about the disease in women is that it often goes into remission during pregnancy. Studies have shown that more than 75 percent of pregnant women who have it experience improvement during the first and second trimesters. Some researchers believe this remission is due to hormone changes.

Other researchers say remission in pregnancy is related to the genetic makeup of the fetus. In a study at the Fred Hutchinson Cancer Center in Seattle, J. Lee Nelson, M.D., and her colleagues found that the greater the difference between the genetic makeup of the fetus and that of the mother, the more likely that arthritis would go into remission during pregnancy. The researchers suspect that a genetically different fetus somehow signals the maternal immune system, with the interesting effect that the arthritis subsides.

Fighting Back

Rheumatoid arthritis typically strikes in a woman's forties and fifties, the most productive time of life, says Ernest Brahn, M.D., associate professor of medicine in the Division of Rheumatology at the University of California, Los Angeles, School of Medicine. "It's a disease of working-age women," he says. "It affects their capacity to work, to take care of their family."

You can't prevent rheumatoid arthritis, researchers say. But if you know you are at risk because it runs in your family, or if you already have it, here's what you can do.

KEEP BONES AND MUSCLES STRONG. The greater your level of physical fitness before you get arthritis, the better you'll be able to fight the disease, says Dr. McCune. Lift weights, do aerobic exercise at least three times a week for 30 minutes a session and take enough calcium to get the Daily Value of 1,000 milligrams.

DON'T OVERDO IT. If a particular task takes a number of hours, do it in segments with rest breaks in between, Dr. Brahn suggests. Doing this will help prevent stress on joints and avoid pain.

KEEP MOVING. While arthritis pain makes you want to do the opposite—that is, sit still—it's important to maintain some level of activity, says Dr. Brahn. Ask your rheumatologist about seeing a physical therapist, who can give you exercises to maintain your joints' mobility. As far as sports are concerned, swimming is good, says Dr.

Brahn, because it enables you to work your joints through their range of motion without having to fight gravity.

BE PERSISTENT. It's important to do your exercises even when you are feeling good, says Dr. Brahn.

EXERCISE YOUR HEALTHY PARTS. "A major strategy in arthritis is to make sure the unaffected part of the body gets as much real exercise as possible," says Dr. McCune. So if your hands are sore, try riding an exercise bike that doesn't require you to use your hands, he says.

BE INFORMED ABOUT MEDICATIONS. Arthritis medications range from nonsteroidal anti-inflammatory drugs like ibuprofen to very strong prescription drugs like methotrexate (Mexate) and cyclophosphanide (Cytoxan). Ask your doctor how the medication works, what its side effects are, whether it will affect your fertility and what impact it will have on your bones and heart.

GET HELP. If you suspect you have rheumatoid arthritis, see a rheumatologist, says Dr. Brahn. The longer you wait, the more destruction the disease can cause and the harder it will be to get pain relief, he says. To find a rheumatologist in your area, contact the Arthritis Foundation. Or you can check the *Directory of Medical Specialists*, which may be available at your local library, for a list of board-certified rheumatologists, suggests Dr. Brahn.

Asthma
BREATHING EASY AGAIN

Many of us can remember the girl in grade school who had asthma. We can still hear her, wheezing along beside us in gym class or panting for breath after a quick run to the bus stop. And we can still see her standing there, the last one to be picked for a game of soccer, softball or capture the flag.

Then there were the days she couldn't come to school at all because her asthma was so bad. And the times she had to use her inhaler, the one she always had to carry with her in a coat pocket or her book bag. Whenever she had an attack, she'd grab it, clutch it tightly and hold it to her mouth to suck in deep, quick breaths. From the look on her face we could tell that whatever asthma felt like, it was scary, and we were glad it wasn't happening to us.

Even if you never had asthma as a child, it's possible to develop it when you're older. "Of the general asthma population, 30 to 40 percent will get it as adults," says Sally E. Wenzel, M.D., assistant professor of medicine at the National Jewish Center for Immunology and Respiratory Medicine in Denver. And while little boys tend to get asthma more often than young girls, after puberty that trend reverses. After age 20, women are more likely than men to have asthma for the first time.

The disease can also be more difficult for women. Between the ages of 20 and 50, women are nearly three times more likely than men to be hospitalized for asthma. Asthma can also make pregnancy more complicated, and pregnancy sometimes makes asthma symptoms worse. Finally, evidence suggests that hormonal changes may cause asthma to flare right around the time a woman starts her period.

The Asthma/Allergy Link

An estimated 10 to 12 million people in the United States have asthma, and the majority of those—about 7 million—are adults. The number of women with asthma is estimated to be just over 3.5 million.

Doctors don't know the exact cause of asthma. They used to think the disease involved a spasm of the airway due to some defect in the nerves and muscles there. But over the past several years, many allergists and immunologists have come to believe that the breathing difficulty is the result of airway inflammation and constriction that's somehow related to allergy. Through some mechanism that experts don't fully understand, substances like dust, mold, pollen and smoke trigger cell inflammation and mucus production. Both reactions cause the airway to narrow, and the symptoms of allergy—coughing, wheezing and chest tightness—result. A higher percentage of allergic people have asthma than nonallergic folks, says Michael Schatz, M.D., clinical professor of medicine at the University of California, San Diego, School of Medicine and a staff allergist at Kaiser Permanente Medical Center in San Diego.

But not all asthma is triggered by allergies. Women can also have asthma attacks after taking aspirin, while working in certain occupations and even while exercising.

In the case of aspirin-sensitive asthma, researchers suspect that aspirin interferes with a special chemical pathway in the body. When the pathway is blocked, chemicals are released that trigger asthma. Individuals can become asthmatic in response to pure aspirin as well as to some over-the-counter nonsteroidal anti-inflammatory products that contain aspirin (such as Excedrin).

With occupational asthma, people have trouble breathing only when they're exposed to certain chemicals and substances at work. In some cases it's because they're allergic, but in other cases the agents may cause cellular damage that triggers asthma. Occupational asthma can occur in many lines of work, including the pharmaceutical, automobile, textile, hair-care, farming and printing industries.

Exercise-induced asthma is another type of nonallergic asthma. Cold or dry air coming into the lungs or a change in the fluid balance of cells stimulates the airway in such a way that the smooth muscles surrounding the airway constrict. Within about five to ten minutes after beginning exercise, individuals experience asthmatic symptoms such as chest tightness, coughing or wheezing.

Getting It as an Adult

Why asthma develops in adulthood is a mystery, says Dr. Schatz. Yet several things tend to trigger its development then. The first is cigarette smoking—if a person smokes or used to smoke, that may predispose them to asthma, he says. The second is a respiratory infection. Often adults will develop asthma soon after they've had one. Finally, in women with allergies, moving to a new location—with its different dust or air quality—or getting a new pet can sometimes trigger asthma.

Asthma can be just as frightening for adult women as it is for young girls. During a mild attack, a woman may feel as if someone is hugging her just a little too tightly. But in a more severe attack, the airway tightens to the point that airflow is restricted and the woman feels like she's suffocating. "Being unable to breathe or feeling like you can't breathe is one of the single most scary things you can go through," says Dr. Wenzel.

Part of what's so frightening is that asthma attacks are so unpredictable. Those who have asthma don't know when one is going to strike. They worry about having an attack when they're alone, without their medication or far from a hospital. But the scariest thing is that asthma can kill. When an attack is severe and not treated sufficiently or in time, oxygen can be cut off from the brain. Although it's rare, asthma can be fatal.

On a daily basis, asthma can leave women feeling exhausted as well as limited in what they can do. Asthma often wakes women during the night, adding to the fatigue they already feel from raising a family, pursuing a career, or both, says Dr. Wenzel. The disease can also limit the amount of physical activity women can do, she says. "One of the biggest complaints is 'Gee, I used to be able to exercise and do everything I wanted to do and I can't any more.'"

Asthma and the Menstrual Cycle

Although they don't know exactly how, researchers suspect that reproductive hormones may play a key role in the experience women have with asthma.

A study conducted at the Medical College of Pennsylvania in Philadelphia of 203 women who came to the emergency room with a severe asthma attack found that more women had the attack around the beginning of their period than at other times in the menstrual cycle.

Emil Skobeloff, M.D., clinical assistant professor of emergency medicine at the William H. Spivey Research Lab at the Medical College of Pennsylvania, who was the lead researcher on the study, suspects that the occurrence of these severe attacks is somehow related to the declining levels of estrogen at that time in a woman's cycle. This would mean that the days surrounding the start of a woman's period—when estrogen levels are dropping—may be the time when women are most susceptible to severe asthma attacks, he says.

Dr. Skobeloff first suspected that reproductive hormones might play a key role when he noticed that women are admitted to hospitals more often than men for serious flare-ups of asthma and, after puberty begins, new cases of asthma are more likely in females than in males the same age. In one study, 75 percent of the hospital admissions for asthma were women and 25 percent were men. This is in stark contrast to hospital admission rates for children with asthma. In the childhood years, 65 percent of admissions are boys and 35 percent are girls.

Pregnancy and Asthma

A particular concern for women is how pregnancy will affect their asthma. Some women find their symptoms get worse, while others find their symptoms stay the same or get better. Doctors can't predict how a woman's asthma will react, but they do know that women with more severe asthma are more likely to have their asthma worsen during pregnancy than women with milder forms. And the way a woman's asthma responds during her first pregnancy is often the way it will react in later pregnancies.

Studies show that women with asthma tend to have an increase in pregnancy complications compared with women without the disease, says Dr. Schatz. Women, particularly those with severe asthma, have been found to give birth to lower-birthweight babies, deliver their babies prematurely and in some cases, lose their babies through stillbirth.

Women may be wary about taking their asthma medication during pregnancy for fear that it may harm the baby in some way. While some drugs can pose potential harm, there are asthma drugs available that appear to be safe to take during pregnancy. Not taking asthma medication can be more dangerous than taking it, experts say. If a woman doesn't take her medication, she's taking the risk of having an asthma attack. If she has one, the baby is endangered, because when the mother can't breathe properly, oxygen is denied to the baby. Uncontrolled asthma over a period of time can limit the amount of oxygen the baby gets, which can limit the baby's growth and result in low birthweight. And if an attack is severe, the baby can be stillborn; in very severe cases, both the mother and baby can die.

Taking Care of Yourself

Adult asthma can range from unpleasant and bothersome to life-threatening. But there are some things you can do to make living with asthma easier. Here are some suggestions.

AVOID YOUR TRIGGERS. If you have allergies, avoiding the triggers that set them off may help reduce your asthma symptoms, says Dr. Schatz. To fend off dust, cover your mattresses and pillows with vinyl cases, keep wall-to-wall carpeting to a minimum and cut down on piles of clutter. For pollen allergies, keep outdoor activities to a minimum when pollen counts are high and use air conditioning both at home and in the car. (For more details on how to control your allergies, see page 14.)

KNOW YOUR BODY. As much as you can, learn to understand the signals your body sends during an asthma attack, says Dr. Schatz. This will help you make the best decisions about when to increase your medication, call the doctor or go to the hospital, he says. Some women find it helps to keep a journal of their symptoms, says Dr. Skobeloff.

BE AWARE OF YOUR CYCLE. Women may be at more risk for an asthma attack in the days surrounding the start of their period, says Dr. Skobeloff. So they need to keep a close eye on their symptoms around that time and be extra vigilant about responding to them promptly. Women also need to educate their doctors about the possible link between menstruation and asthma attacks, he says.

"Many women for decades have been telling doctors they get flare-ups around their periods. And some doctors have been saying, 'Oh, that's all in your mind' or 'That's PMS.' And it's not true," he says. "They need to educate their doctors to the fact that this is real. And their doc-

ASTHMA

tors need to be more aggressive in their therapy of these women," around the start of their periods.

PREPARE FOR PREGNANCY. Ideally, a woman of child-bearing age with allergies or asthma should discuss her condition and her medication with her doctor before she gets pregnant, says Dr. Schatz. That way she can get herself on the medications that are best suited to pregnancy and attempt to get in better physical shape before she gets pregnant, he says.

MONITOR YOURSELF. If you've got asthma, try a peak flow monitor, which measures the amount of oxygen getting to your lungs. The device basically enables you to monitor your asthma and detect whether you are getting into a real danger zone. Peak flow monitors are now made so you can have one at home. Some are even small enough to fit in a purse, says Dr. Wenzel. One particular monitor, called Personal Best, is about the size of a tampon holder, she says. Look for them at a surgical supply store.

DON'T SKIP YOUR MEDICATION. Take your medications, especially inhaled anti-inflammatory medications like beclomethasone dipropionate (Vanceril), on a regular basis, says Dr. Wenzel. "That's been shown to be most effective," she says. Sometimes women get into a cycle where their asthma isn't as bad and they skip medications, she adds. "Continue taking them even when you are feeling good."

TAKE IT WHEN PREGNANT, TOO. Pregnant women also need to continue their asthma medications. "It's extremely important that asthma be controlled in pregnancy," says Daryl Altman, M.D., an allergist and immunologist and director of Allergy Information Services, an allergy consulting service in Lynbrook, New York. "Uncontrolled asthma is much more hazardous to the mother and fetus than the medications used to control it," she says. "A lot of people say, 'I'm afraid to take my asthma medication because I'm pregnant or I'm contemplating pregnancy.' Wrong. Take the asthma medication." Do check with your doctor that the medication you're on is okay during pregnancy.

GO SMOKE-FREE. Smoking appears to increase your chances of developing asthma. It can also exacerbate your symptoms, and it may increase the risk that your children will become asthmatic. So do your best to quit smoking if you haven't already. If you don't smoke, try to stick to smoke-free environments as much as possible. If you are pregnant, be extra vigilant about avoiding passive tobacco smoke. "The content of poisons from cigarette smoke can easily be found in the hair of newborn babies. So insist on a smoke-free environment," says Ellen Garibaldi, M.D., assistant professor of internal medicine in the allergy and immunology division at St. Louis University Health Sciences Center.

EXERCISE RIGHT. If you've got exercise-induced asthma, there are steps you can take to decrease your symptoms, says Stuart Stoloff, M.D., clinical associate professor of family and community medicine at the University of Nevada School of Medicine in Reno. Five to ten minutes before you exercise, try taking a prescription inhaled bronchodilator drug, known as a beta-agonist, like albuterol (Proventil), he says. If this doesn't help, he suggests adding a nedocromil sodium inhaler (Tilade). Also, warm up slowly. This helps change the temperature of the air coming into your lungs and helps decrease bronchospasm, he says. If it's really cold outside, consider exercising indoors. Or wear a mask over your mouth to help humidify the air coming into your lungs.

CALL ON A FRIEND. If you live alone or have to spend periods of time without a loved one around, enlist the help of a friend. Tell your friend about your asthma and ask if you can call when you're having trouble or if she'll keep in touch with you. That way you can have some peace of mind that someone will check on you and that you don't have to suffer through attacks completely alone.

CALL 911. If your symptoms get worse, use a beta-agonist inhaler like albuterol for up to two puffs every 15 minutes for up to four treatments over an hour, says Dr. Skobeloff. If your symptoms worsen between treatments or if they don't get any better after an hour, go right to the emergency room. "Don't drive. Call 911," he says. Many of the people who are dead on arrival at the emergency room, or near death, are people who had someone drive them to the hospital or who waited too long to call for help, he says. When you call 911, the paramedics have equipment and medication to begin helping you right away.

Back Pain

PUTTING AN END TO THE ACHE

It used to be that the last thing on your mind was your back. In those days, it would bend, twist and move as needed, with nary a twinge.

Now you're past 30, and your back is more apt to protest than perform. Like millions of other Americans, you've got back pain, and it's really slowing you down.

The most common discomfort is low back pain: An estimated 80 percent of Americans have it at some point in their lives. Middle and upper back pain occur much less often.

Women and men appear to be equally affected by back pain, yet women tend to develop it later in life, says Malcolm Pope, Ph.D., director of the Iowa Spine Research Center at the University of Iowa in Iowa City. Some men tend to have problems when they're younger because the heavy manual work they do hastens the deterioration of structures in the back, he says. Women, on the other hand, usually don't run into trouble until their thirties and forties, when natural degenerative changes begin.

Why This Aching Back?

Back pain can be due to sprains or strains of the back muscles and ligaments, damage to the bones in the spinal column or injury to the shock-absorbing disks between the bones. In unusual cases, pain also arises from scoliosis and spondylolisthesis, two types of vertebral misalignment, and from illnesses like cancer. The pain can also be what doctors call mechanical low back pain—there is no apparent physical damage, but pain comes and goes.

The good news is that 80 percent of people who suffer from an episode of low back pain will improve within eight weeks. The bad news is that 80 percent of those with low back pain will experience a mild recurrence.

In women, more than 90 percent of problems doctors see are due to pregnancy, mechanical low back pain and disk injury, says Eugene Carragee, M.D., director of the Orthopedic Spine Center at Stanford University. Infections or diseases like cancer account for the other 10 percent, he says.

The Pain of Pregnancy

The number one cause of back pain in women in their child-bearing years is pregnancy, says Dr. Carragee. Seventy-five percent of women who are pregnant have some low back pain, he says. Women who have their babies in their thirties and forties may experience more back pain than younger women if they're not in as good shape, he says.

Women can get back pain throughout their pregnancy, but some women report an increase in the last few weeks. The pain is usually in the low back and can radiate into the buttocks and the backs of the thighs. Walking, sitting, lifting and bending forward can worsen pain. Many women experience more back pain at night.

There are a number of reasons for the pain. For one thing, the weight and size of the fetus cause a woman's center of gravity to shift forward, so there is more curvature in her lower spinal column. This causes some low back muscles to shorten. In addition, the abdominal muscles, which normally stabilize the pelvis and support the back, are stretched and weakened by the growing uterus.

During pregnancy the body releases higher levels of the hormone relaxin. Relaxin's job is to loosen the ligaments so the pelvis can expand as the fetus grows. But relaxin also slackens the ligaments that support the back, and when more stress is placed on the more lax spine, pain develops.

Back pain during pregnancy can also be due to circulatory changes. As the uterus expands, it presses on a major vein that is responsible for collecting blood from the low back. Blood does not circulate properly and pain is the result—especially when a woman has slept or sat or walked for long periods.

Coping with It

There are things you can do to lessen back pain in pregnancy. Here's what experts recommend.

STAY ACTIVE. Remaining as active and fit as you can throughout pregnancy helps, says physical therapist Sheila Reid, coordinator for rehabilitation services at the Spine Institute of New England in Williston, Vermont, because the stronger your muscles are, the better they'll respond to the increasing weight of the baby. Staying fit may also prevent back problems after pregnancy, when new mothers are lifting, reaching, doing extra laundry and manipulating bulky car seats, says Reid. There's no guarantee, however, that being in good shape will make delivery any easier. Ask your doctor about an exercise program or prenatal and postnatal exercise classes, and about classes where you can learn how to perform child-care tasks in ways that won't hurt your back.

DO BACK-HELPING EXERCISES. Doing exercises such as pelvic tilts and side leg lifts will help relieve back pain by strengthening stomach and hip muscles that support the back. If there are exercises you want to do that require lying on your back, clear them with your physician first. If you do perform exercises on your back and notice any unusual symptoms, such as dizziness or shortness of breath, stop the exercise and notify your doctor.

LIE ON YOUR SIDE. An expanding belly may make lying on your back less comfortable. That's because the weight of the fetus can press on the inferior vena cava, the vein that returns blood from the lower body to the heart, and can aggravate backache. Instead, doctors recommend that you lie on your side with your upper knee bent and supported on a pillow. This position allows blood to flow unrestricted to your heart and to the placenta. It also relieves back strain.

CHANGE POSITIONS OFTEN. Prolonged sitting or

standing can worsen the pain. So if you are sitting at a desk or computer all day, take breaks every 15 minutes and walk around for 30 seconds, says Anne McCue Canty, a physical therapist in Yorktown, Virginia. A chair with a tilt adjustment on the seat can help change your positioning slightly, as can the use of a footstool, she says. If you've got to be on your feet for extended periods of time, stand with one foot up on a footstool, alternating periodically between your left and right foot.

LIFT THINGS CAREFULLY. When you are pregnant, never lift anything over 50 pounds, says Dr. Pope. And do your best to lift only objects that are already at waist height, he says. Avoid awkward twisting postures and lift objects straight up. If there's an object on the floor that needs to be moved, try to find someone to help you, he says.

Other Back Pain Bad Guys

Mechanical low back pain is the second most common type of back problem for women, says Dr. Carragee. Women who do heavy labor and those who are very sedentary are at greatest risk, he says. Improper lifting, poor posture and sitting for long periods can lead to this type of pain, but often a specific cause cannot be identified, according to Dr. Carragee.

Disk problems are the third most common cause of back pain. Normally disks are cushiony, but sometimes they dry up and crack, or herniate, which is sometimes incredibly painful. People with herniated disks may have low back pain as well as radiating pain down the leg, known as sciatica. The pain is a result of the herniated disk compressing a spinal nerve root that runs from the back through the buttock and down the leg. With management, pain from herniation can be resolved in six weeks in 75 percent of individuals, says Dr. Carragee. Two percent of herniations require surgery, he says.

There are several habits that can increase a woman's risk for mechanical low back pain and disk herniation.

The first is smoking, which interferes with the supply of nutrients to the disks, says Dr. Pope. Without them, the disks eventually flatten, shrink and dry out, leading to herniation and pain. Also, surgery to alleviate back pain has been less successful in patients who smoke, he says.

The demands of working and raising a family can also contribute, says Reid. Busy women often don't have time to stay in shape and keep their backs strong, and they're under a lot of stress. "When you are under a lot of stress, you experience muscle tension. The muscles are in contraction and are not relaxed and don't respond in the same way to movement," Reid says. That makes them more susceptible to strain.

The workplace is another source of pain, says Reid. "More women work in sedentary jobs than in jobs that require physical activity," she says. "Sedentary workers have the second highest incidence of back pain." As with smoking, sitting in a fixed posture for a prolonged period of time prevents the natural pumping of nutrition in and out of the disks, says Dr. Pope.

High heels are a problem, Reid says, because they throw off a woman's center of gravity. As the heels bring you upright and forward, you get increased curvature, often called swayback, in the lower back. And the higher the heel, the more the body is thrown off-kilter.

Having a family history of back pain places women, as well as men, at increased risk, says Edward Hanley, M.D., chairman of orthopedic surgery at the Carolinas Medical Center in Charlotte, North Carolina. Researchers aren't sure why, but back pain runs in families.

Basic Back Pain Prevention

Just about everyone has back pain at some time. Here are strategies to prevent it.

WATCH YOUR POSTURE. The spine is healthiest when it's in its natural neutral position. Poor posture such as slouching in a chair, sitting hunched over a desk or standing in a slumped position takes the spine out of position and places excess stress on the back muscles. Do your best to maintain good posture while sitting and standing. One quick method that will help you is to place two fingers on your upper lip and gently push your head back, without lifting your chin, until your ears are in alignment with your shoulders, says physical therapist Mark Taranta, director of the Physical Therapy Practice in Philadelphia.

GIVE YOUR BACK SUPPORT. Another way to help maintain good posture is to place a small pillow or rolled towel in the arch of your lower back when sitting. This provides support to the lower back and keeps excess stress off the muscles. When sleeping, try placing a pillow beneath your knees when you are on your back and between your knees when lying on your side, says Taranta.

ADJUST YOUR WORKSTATION. If you sit at a desk or computer all day, use a chair that's the right height, says Reid. Your feet and back should be supported. Your knees may be slightly lower or higher than your hips, whichever is most comfortable for you. Adjust your computer monitor so that you do not have to bend your neck back or hunch forward to read the screen, she says. Close your eyes and then open them; wherever your gaze falls is where the center of your screen should be.

GIVE BOOKS AND PAPERS A LIFT. Create a work surface that's at a 35-degree angle, says Dr. Pope. This will help you sit upright, he says. Stationery supply stores carry desktop podiums.

TAKE BREAKS AND MOVE. Women who are working in an office and sitting for long periods of time need to "get up and move around at least once an hour," Dr. Pope says. If you can't leave your office, try putting your in-box in a location where you'll have to stand up and walk over to check it. Or try standing when you're making or receiving phone calls, says Reid. Take a walk on your lunch break, she says.

EXTEND YOURSELF. Stretching your back can help prevent back pain as well as relieve it, says Taranta. Stretches should be slow and steady.

STRENGTHEN THOSE ABS. Your abdominal muscles are one of the keys to providing support for your back, so the stronger they are, the better. To strengthen them, half sit-ups are better than full sit-ups, says Reid.

LIFT THINGS PROPERLY. Lifting anything, whether it's a box, a bag of groceries or a child, can cause back pain. "Whenever you are lifting any load, keep the load as close to the body as possible," says Dr. Pope. Don't try to pick it up at arm's length, he says. And instead of bending over at the waist to pick up an object, keep your back straight and bend your knees, lowering yourself to the load. Then straighten your knees, keeping your back as straight as possible, recommends Dr. Pope.

CARRY LOADS CAREFULLY. Hauling heavy loads places major stress on muscles and pulls your back into improper posture. If you carry an overloaded briefcase, shoulder bag or gym bag, it's better to distribute the load between two bags and carry one in each hand rather than having the weight all on one side, says Reid. Another option is to use a knapsack or luggage on wheels.

GIVE UP SMOKING. Research shows a strong association between smoking and back pain, says Dr. Pope. So do your best to cut back or quit.

GET FIT AND TRIM. One way to prevent back pain is to maintain your ideal body weight. Ask your doctor what that is, rather than depending on a weight chart. "If you're overweight, muscles are in poor condition," says Dr. Pope. Doctors recommend 20 to 30 minutes of aerobic exercise four times a week. "Do what you enjoy," urges Dr. Carragee. "That way you'll be more likely to keep it up. Try not to let your exercise routine slip away as the years go by." Watch your diet by eating low-fat, nutritious foods, says Dr. Carragee.

WEAR FLAT SHOES. Heels increase the amount of curvature in your lower back, Dr. Pope says, so wear flat shoes. If you must wear heels at work, wear flats or sneakers to and from the office.

GET YOUR CALCIUM. Women are at increased risk for osteoporosis, which can lead to spinal fractures and back pain. Maintain bone strength by consuming enough calcium, says Dr. Carragee. Doctors recommend 1,000 to 1,200 milligrams for premenopausal women and 1,500 milligrams for postmenopausal women.

When Back Pain Strikes

Here's what to do when the pain hits.

DON'T GO TO BED. Take it easy for a day or two, says Dr. Hanley, *but* "don't go to bed for two weeks." While doctors used to recommend bed rest, they now believe it leads to deconditioning of the muscles. Many recommend a wide range of back exercises.

USE HEAT OR ICE. Either can relieve back pain and help you get up and moving, says Reid. She recommends applying them for 20 minutes at a time.

Heat should be in the form of a hot shower or hot bath, since generalized heat relaxes muscles in the entire body, whereas applying localized heat may cause back muscles to swell and worsen the pain, she says. If you use ice, make sure it doesn't come in contact with your skin. Put it in a freezer bag or wrap it in a wet towel, then apply it to your back. Ice can be used several times a day. It's important to use whichever method allows you to move, says Reid.

TRY MEDICATIONS. Taking a nonsteroidal anti-inflammatory such as aspirin or ibuprofen may help provide some pain relief by reducing any swelling and inflammation, says Dr. Hanley. Follow label directions.

MAKE AN APPOINTMENT. If your back pain persists for more than two weeks or if you have shooting pains down your legs, visit a doctor, says Dr. Hanley. Start with your family practitioner. She can refer you to a specialist, such as an orthopedic surgeon or a neurosurgeon, if necessary.

BE SURE ABOUT SURGERY. Surgery should be considered when there is a specific diagnosis, such as fracture, scoliosis or disk herniation, says Dr. Carragee. It's not recommended as an exploratory procedure, he says.

Bladder Infections

Too Familiar
to Too Many Women

It's Tuesday morning and you're zipping through your to-do list with relative ease. Everything is going smoothly.

Until you take a break to visit the ladies room, that is. You start to urinate, but suddenly you feel a burning pain beyond belief. You know that feeling all too well, because you've felt it before. It's a bladder infection, and you'll have to pay a visit to the doctor, start taking antibiotics and get into that cranberry juice routine. You don't have time for this kind of hassle.

Most of us are all too familiar with bladder infections, frequently referred to as urinary tract infections (UTIs). Besides that burning feeling during urination, there can be a frequent need to urinate, pain in the lower back or pelvic area and pain during intercourse.

An estimated 25 to 35 percent of women between the ages of 20 and 40 have had at least one bladder infection. Men can get UTIs too, but they're much more common in women. They're the reason for an estimated seven million visits to the doctor and one million hospital admissions each year. These infections are not only painful and inconvenient, they can progress to more serious infections of the kidney if not stopped in time.

Why Us?

The bacteria that cause bladder infections—there are several kinds, but one common type is *Escherichia coli*—reside in the bowel, where they cause no problems. But if they migrate the short distance from the anus to the opening of a woman's urinary tract, they can lead to infection, says Grant Mulholland, M.D., chairman of the Department of Urology at Jefferson University Medical College in Philadelphia.

The lining of the vagina contains good bacteria called lactobacillus that can protect against the overgrowth of the bad bacteria. But when the bacterial balance in the vagina is disturbed, the bad guys can take over and ascend into the urinary tract. The result? A bladder infection.

What can throw off the balance? Wiping from back to front after a bowel movement, for one thing, because it can help bad bacteria get into position to multiply and wreak havoc.

Using diaphragms, spermicidal jellies or foams can also change the bacterial balance, says Dr. Mulholland. So can sexual intercourse, since bacteria can be forced up into the bladder. And the use of tampons may also play a role by disrupting the normal defense mechanisms within the vagina. "Women who use tampons may have a higher incidence than women who just use a pad," says Dr. Mulholland.

The hormonal changes that take place at menopause can also spur the development of UTIs. When estrogen levels drop, the pH level of the vagina changes and the number of good bacteria declines, says Kimberly Workowski, M.D., assistant professor of medicine in the Department of Infectious Diseases at Emory University in Atlanta. UTIs increase by 1 to 2 percent each decade after menopause.

Some Are Lucky

Not every woman will get a bladder infection, however—even if she's at risk. That's because some women have a natural defense against bacteria's ability to stick to the bladder wall and cause a raging infection. These women have special substances in their blood called antigens that act as shields, preventing the bacteria from latching on, says Dr.

Mulholland. But most women don't know whether they have this substance in their blood, and this defense is not always foolproof, so it pays to practice good habits.

There are several types of bladder infections, although their symptoms are similar. Some women get what doctors call uncomplicated urinary tract infections—occasional bouts that are easily cured. Other women get complicated infections, which have an underlying cause such as an obstruction in the urinary tract, a malformation of the urethra or kidney stones, which are rare in women. And some women get recurring infections.

Most UTIs can be cured with antibiotics. Others—about 10 percent of total cases—progress into more serious infections of the kidney.

Getting to the Problem

You may have had a bladder infection or two, and you might get another. If you're plagued by bladder infections, here's what you need to know—both to prevent and treat this nuisance.

GO TO THE BATHROOM AFTER SEX. "It's been found to be helpful to urinate right after intercourse," says Dr. Mulholland. This washes out any bacteria that may have worked their way into the bladder.

DRINK FLUIDS. One of the folk remedies for bladder infections is to drink fluids when you feel the symptoms coming on, says Dr. Mulholland. "I suppose this helps because it tends to wash out the urinary tract."

STICK WITH CRANBERRY JUICE. Most of us have heard we should drink cranberry juice for a bladder infection. This advice has been around for a long time, but scientific studies have finally lent credence to the claim.

Animal studies indicate that certain compounds found in cranberry and blueberry juices prevent the *E. coli* bacteria from sticking to the bladder wall. And a study of 153 elderly women, conducted by researchers at Harvard Medical School, provides further support for the cranberry argument. Women were asked to drink about ten ounces of cranberry juice or a placebo drink daily for six months. The women who drank cranberry juice had less bacteria in their urine than women who drank the placebo. While the study did not show that cranberry juice drinkers had fewer urinary tract infections, it indicates that cranberry juice may keep harmful bacteria at lower levels.

SKIP SEX JUST BEFORE YOUR PERIOD. Women who find they are most vulnerable to bladder infections during certain phases of their menstrual cycle may want to avoid having sex then, says Dr. Mulholland. For many women, this susceptible time tends to be right before their period, when levels of estrogen, a hormone that maintains vaginal health, are low.

SWITCH CONTRACEPTIVES. If you are using contraceptive jellies and foams and experience recurrent infections, talk to your doctor about other contraceptives. "The jelly actually has a direct effect on the ease with which bacteria can get into the vagina and infect the bladder," says Dr. Mulholland. Contraceptive jelly is probably the reason that women who use diaphragms often have problems, he says. Whether the cervical cap carries the same risks is not known, he adds.

GET TREATED. Sometimes even if you do all the right things, you'll still get an infection. If you think you've got one, call your doctor immediately for an appointment. Some doctors will prescribe an antibiotic over the phone, but it's a good idea to get a urinalysis to confirm that it's a bladder infection. Antibiotics are used to treat UTIs, and there are now seven-day, three-day and one-day regimens available. Ask your doctor about the pros and cons of each.

While the one-day treatments can be effective, a significant number of women experience a recurrence, says Dr. Mulholland. Most doctors agree that the safest way to treat UTIs is with the three-day regimen, he says.

SELF-TREAT. Women who get recurrent UTIs that are uncomplicated may get a supply of fairly low-dose antibacterial medication from their doctors, says Dr. Mulholland. Taking the prescribed dose after intercourse may prevent an infection.

FIND THE RIGHT DOCTOR. If you get a lot of recurrent infections, say six to eight a year, work with your doctor to identify the problem, says Jerry G. Blaivis, M.D., clinical professor of urology at the New York Hospital–Cornell Medical Center in New York City. Find a health professional who will sit with you and outline a plan for diagnosis and treatment, including a review of a diary of your activities and symptoms. Talk about what seems to bring on the infection, how much you are having sex and what contraceptives you are using.

Breast Cancer
FIGHTING A FEARSOME DISEASE

You see the posters on buses. You hear the ads on the radio. Even while shopping in your favorite drugstore, you're likely to hear a piped-in celebrity voice from an overhead speaker: "See your doctor today. You have a one-in-eight chance of getting breast cancer."

But do you?

Probably not. Nearly 80 percent of all breast cancers occur in women over 50. And only women over 85 have a 1-in-8 chance of getting it. For the rest of us, the risk is considerably less. By age 30, it's 1 chance in 2,426. By age 40, it's 1 in 222. And by age 45, it's 1 in 96.

Still, one chance in however-many is one chance too many for a disease that strikes 182,000 American women every year and kills 40 percent of them within a decade. And some scientists believe that breast cancer among premenopausal women is increasing.

"Many experts believe there has been a real increase in the incidence of breast cancer," says Richard Love, M.D., professor of clinical oncology at the University of Wisconsin at Madison. "The causes of much of the real increase are not known." Among the risk factors that scientists have been able to identify so far are a family history of breast cancer and various factors related to a woman's hormones.

The Enemy Within

It's hard to accept the idea that your own body produces a substance that can encourage tiny breast cells to form cancerous clusters. But "there's overwhelming evidence that the female hormone estrogen plays a central role in causing breast cancer," says Ronald Ross, M.D., professor of preventive medicine at the University of Southern California School of Medicine in Los Angeles.

No one has figured out all the hows and whys, but some studies have found that breast cancer risk is reduced 5 to 15 percent for every year that the onset of menstruation is delayed. Other studies have found that women who experience natural menopause before age 45 have only half the breast cancer risk of women who experience menopause ten years later. Still other studies have found that women who have artificial menopause—when their ovaries are surgically removed, for example—have even less breast cancer risk than women who experience natural menopause.

The common denominator among all these studies seems to be that the less exposure a woman has to her own reproductive hormones, estrogen and progesterone, the lower her risk of developing breast cancer, says Dr. Ross.

That's why pregnancy, breastfeeding, physical activity and a low-fat diet with plenty of plant fiber and little alcohol all decrease a woman's risk of breast cancer: They all reduce the amount of estrogen circulating through her body.

"Any strategy that alters estrogen is going to have an effect on breast cancer risk," says Dr. Ross. Here are strategies that doctors suggest to reduce your risk.

ADJUST FAT AND FIBER. "In countries where women eat a low-fat, high-fiber diet, they have lower estrogen levels and lower breast cancer risk," says Sherwood L. Gorbach, M.D., professor of community health and medicine at Tufts University School of Medicine in Boston. A controversy rages over exactly how much fat you should cut to lower your risk, he adds, but a diet that gets between 20 and 25 percent of its calories from fat is a wise choice until the scientific dust settles.

But fiber may have even more of an impact on estrogen than fat. So as you cut back on fat, start increasing fiber as well, says Dr. Gorbach. You need to get 40 grams of fiber a day to lower estrogen levels.

To accomplish both, cut out processed meats and cheeses, eat red meat no more than three times a week, remove the skin from poultry and eat plenty of whole grains, fruits and vegetables every day.

EAT SOY. "We're particularly interested in soy fiber," says Dr. Gorbach. "We think that there are substances in soy (plant estrogens) that are related to natural estrogens." In animal studies, plant estrogens seem to block the estrogen involved in breast cancer and actually prevent the disease, he says.

Although these plant estrogens are found in their highest concentration in soy products such as tofu, other sources include alfalfa, apples, barley, carrots, cherries, green beans, licorice, oats, parsley, peas, potatoes, red beans, rice, sprouts and wheat.

LOAD UP ON FRUITS AND VEGETABLES. In Harvard University's Nurses' Health Study, which included 89,000 women, researchers found that women who generally ate two or more servings of vegetables a day reduced their risk of breast cancer 17 percent.

No one really knows why, says Dr. Love, but "some studies indicate that intake of adequate vitamin A is important." When women in the Nurses' Health Study who normally didn't get much vitamin A from food took supplements containing 10,000 international units every day, they had half the risk of women who didn't take supplements.

AVOID ALCOHOL. "Reducing the consumption of alcoholic beverages appears to reduce breast cancer risk," says Dr. Love. A study of 34 women between the ages of 21 and 40 conducted by researchers at the National Cancer Institute in Bethesda, Maryland, and the Human Nutrition Research Center in Beltsville, Maryland, found that just two drinks a day significantly elevated total estrogen levels.

GET UP AND GO. A joint study that was conducted by the National Cancer Institute and the Shanghai Cancer Institute in China found that women whose jobs involved moving around rather than sitting reduced their risk of breast cancer somewhere between 30 and 45 percent. In fact, the more physical activity women experienced on the job, the less likely they were to get breast cancer. The difference, researchers concluded, may be explained by the effect that physical activity has on estrogen.

BREASTFEED. "Lactation is protective against breast cancer in younger women," Dr. Love says. "Longer periods of lactation of at least six to eight months appear to provide maximal protection. It seems as though the hormones released during lactation cause a permanent, physical change in breast cells that protects them from the potentially cancer-inducing effects of estrogen."

PUT YOUR OVARIES IN HIBERNATION. Researchers at the University of Southern California are at work on a pill to inactivate the ovaries. "I have no doubt that if you shut down the ovaries, the risk of breast cancer will go down," says Dr. Ross. He and his colleagues estimate that giving a woman medication to suppress ovulation for 5 years will reduce her risk of breast cancer by 38 percent. Suppressing ovulation for 15 years will reduce her risk by 80 percent. While this dramatic method would appear to be only for women with a high risk of breast cancer, Dr. Ross says that the option may someday be available to all women.

The Art of Detection

Breast self-examinations and mammograms are the two best methods for detecting breast cancer. In fact, 90 percent of lumps are found by patients examining themselves.

While many women would rather not do self-exams, doctors emphasize that they're quick and simple to perform, and the effort is certainly worthwhile. Here's what to do.

First put your hands high over your head and look in the mirror for any dimpling, nipple changes or obvious lumps. Then put your hands on your hips and check the mirror again.

WHAT ARE YOUR ODDS?

Your age is still the single biggest risk factor for breast cancer. Here's how the National Cancer Institute and the American Cancer Society assess your risk.

By age 25: 1 in 21,441	By age 60: 1 in 24
By age 30: 1 in 2,426	By age 65: 1 in 18
By age 35: 1 in 622	By age 70: 1 in 14
By age 40: 1 in 222	By age 75: 1 in 12
By age 45: 1 in 96	By age 80: 1 in 10
By age 50: 1 in 52	By age 85: 1 in 9
By age 55: 1 in 34	Lifetime: 1 in 8

Then, if nothing shows up, put the hand on the side you want to examine behind your head. Then check the breast using one of three patterns: Gently use your fingertips to trace concentric circles around your breast, examine the breast in vertical strips from above the breast to below it, or pretend the breast is a pie and gently push on one "slice" at a time.

It's not important which method you choose, or even if you use your own particular variation. What is important, doctors agree, is that you check your breast in the same way and at the same time every month—preferably a week or so after your period.

Finally, put your other hand behind your head and check the other breast.

Most women aren't wild about mammograms, and some are so worried about how they'll feel that they're afraid to get them.

But a mammogram is nothing more than a high-tech x-ray of

QUESTIONS TO ASK YOUR DOCTOR

You've found the lump. Your doctor's confirmed its presence. And you've heard the words that nobody ever wants to hear: "It might be cancer. We need to check it out."

So now—shocked and frightened as you may be—you need to make some decisions. And to help you make those decisions, here are some pertinent questions to ask your doctor, from women who've been in exactly the same position.

• Do you think it's malignant?
• Will you do a needle biopsy or a surgical biopsy?
• How accurate is the biopsy you intend to do?
• Will you phone me with the results as soon as you have them? How long until I'll hear from you?
• If the biopsy is positive, do I meet the surgical criteria for a lumpectomy and radiation?

If the answer is yes, you do have breast cancer, here's what else you'll want to ask.

• Is the breast cancer spreading?
• Is the cancer sensitive to hormones and will it respond to hormone treatment?
• What lab tests were run and what are their results?

your breast. Your breast is placed between two clear plastic plates, x-rays are shot through the breast to a photographic plate beneath, and you're free to go. It takes only a minute and is just slightly uncomfortable.

The advantage of a mammogram is that it can sometimes detect cancer a good two years before you can feel a lump—which gives you an opportunity to get earlier treatment.

When should you have a mammogram? "That varies a little depending on whom you ask," says Kathleen Mayzel, M.D., director of the Faulkner Breast Centre and assistant clinical professor of surgery at Tufts University School of Medicine.

Some doctors feel that there's no reason to get a mammogram until after menopause unless it's to investigate a lump. The American Cancer Society recommends that a regular screening program begin by age 40.

"I generally recommend a baseline mammogram between the ages

- How will you use this information to recommend further tests or treatments?
- Which treatment options do you recommend and why?
- Do you recommend any follow-up hormonal therapy?
- What are the survival statistics after these procedures?
- What are the complications associated with each procedure?
- What type of anesthesia is used?
- How long do I have to stay in the hospital?
- Is the surgeon you're recommending a breast surgeon?
- Is she board-certified?
- How many of the procedures that you recommend has she done?
- How will I know if the surgeon got all the cancer?
- What are the chances that some of the cancer cells have escaped the breast and are now somewhere else in my body?
- How will my breast look after the surgery?
- Am I a candidate for any type of breast reconstruction?
- Should I have it done immediately following the surgery?
- How long will it take me to recover my normal energy level and get my life back on track?

of 35 and 40," says Dr. Mayzel. "Most doctors feel it can be closer to 40 unless you have a mother or sister who developed premenopausal breast cancer. Then it should be closer to 35."

There's no reason to do it any earlier because cancerous cells are usually hidden—even from mammography equipment—by the dense breast tissue characteristic of women under 35.

THE MAMMOGRAM MISSED IT

Matuschka is a sculptor and photographer who lives in New York City. She had been sculpting and photographing a series of torso self-portraits for several years when, at the age of 37, she discovered a lump in her right breast. After a mastectomy, she decided to continue her torso studies. Her provocative work has been exhibited in museums and photography shows around the world. This is her story.

The mammograms never showed my tumor.

I had been going to a breast surgeon and having my breasts checked for ten years because my mother died of breast cancer. But in 1991 I started having a very eerie feeling that I was beginning to look like my mother when she had breast cancer. I had just had my breasts checked six months earlier, but I didn't like the way I was looking or feeling. So I decided to go to a lecture at a local hospital.

One of the things they showed me was how to examine my breasts lying down—I had been doing it standing in the shower. So I went home, followed their instructions and—boom!—I felt a small stone.

I called my breast surgeon, but he said he was too busy to see me, so I went to my physician, my regular GP. He said, "I don't know what this is, but it's not a cyst. You should go get a mammogram and get checked out by a specialist."

The next day, I went for the mammogram. A clinician examined me. She said, "This is nothing, it's noncancerous."

I said, "How do you know? Do you have x-ray vision?" She said, "No, but it's soft and it moves, and cancer doesn't move."

I asked to see the expert on call and he said, "I don't think this is anything to worry about, but you should see if it can be aspirated—if any fluid can be drawn out. And if it can't, you should have a biopsy."

"Between the ages of 40 and 50, women should have a mammogram every one to two years, then yearly after the age of 50," Dr. Mayzel says.

Breast Cancer Treatment

There are three basic options in treating breast cancer: Removing just the cancerous lump of cells with a small margin of healthy tissue

---

The next day I went to his office. It didn't aspirate.

I called my breast surgeon, who had been seeing me for ten years, and insisted that he see me now. And when he felt the suspicious lump he said, "This is nothing to worry about, Matuschka. It's definitely not cancer."

All the doctors I had seen implied it was nothing. They based their judgment on the feel of the lump. The surgeon even said I could go do a show of my work in Helsinki and come back three months later.

I said, "No, I'll have this out immediately."

So I had a biopsy. But because the surgeon didn't think I had breast cancer, he chose to be very cosmetic when he went in to do it. He decided, "Why scar the breast for something that's not cancer?"

When he found out it was cancer, he realized he'd made a mistake. And when the pathology report came back, he recommended a mastectomy.

I didn't know more than he did, so I agreed. I assumed that if you took the breast off, you reduced the chance of having cancer spread to other parts of the body—and of dying. By removing the breast I thought you removed all of the cancer.

A discussion of lumpectomy never occurred. The breast surgeon said later that he actually recommended a mastectomy for cosmetic purposes. He said, "I thought you'd get a better cosmetic result."

In other words, he said that based on what his aesthetic requirements of what a breast should look like, I should have a mastectomy.

After I had the operation, I felt a need to share my experience through the visual arts. The impetus was to help other people. I did public service posters that were created out of my disappointment, sadness, irritation, whatever you want to call it—but not anger, because my work is not compelled by anger—to educate women.

It was my way of sharing.

(lumpectomy), having a lumpectomy followed by local radiation treatments, and amputating the breast (mastectomy).

According to data from the National Cancer Institute, when cancer had not spread to the lymph nodes, 74 percent of women who had a lumpectomy alone were still alive ten years after the surgery. Seventy-five percent of those who had undergone a mastectomy made it to that benchmark.

Even when cancer was found to have spread to the lymph nodes, both procedures were equally effective. The National Cancer Institute found that 51 percent of women who had a lumpectomy alone and 50 percent of women who had a mastectomy survived ten years.

Lumpectomy followed by radiation offered an even better success rate: 78 percent if the cancer had not spread to the lymph nodes, and 58 percent if it had.

"The efficacy of lumpectomy plus radiation has been tested more thoroughly than any other cancer treatment," says Allen Lichter, M.D., chairman of radiation oncology at the University of Michigan in Ann Arbor. "There have been at least six major trials. And every one has demonstrated that women who choose to preserve their breast pay no survival penalty."

What's more, women who choose lumpectomy plus radiation over mastectomy may have a psychological advantage. In a study at the University of Pennsylvania in Philadelphia, women who'd had lumpectomies had a more positive attitude toward their recovery: 87 percent of them felt "cured," while only 36 percent of the women who'd had a mastectomy felt that they were free of cancer.

The missing breast was a source of ongoing anxiety, the researchers concluded, because it was a constant reminder that somehow, somewhere, the women still might have cancer. As a result, 50 percent of the women who had undergone a mastectomy said they regretted their decision. Fifty-five percent said that, given a second chance, they'd have a lumpectomy plus radiation instead.

What's Next?

Once breast surgery is over, your doctor is likely to recommend follow-up treatment.

"Most breast cancers are eight to ten years old by the time you can feel a lump," explains Susan Love, M.D., director of the University of California at Los Angeles Breast Center. "Long before that, cancer cells make their way into the bloodstream and lymphatic system, where they're either killed by the body's own immunity or they begin to establish cancer outposts."

That's why follow-up treatment with either chemotherapy or the estrogen-blocking drug tamoxifen (Nolvadex) is usually recommended by cancer experts. Both these treatments can go after renegade cancer cells and shoot them down.

"Chemotherapy is recommended for premenopausal women with cancerous lymph nodes and occasionally for those with noncancerous nodes as well," says Dr. Mayzel. "The use of tamoxifen in premenopausal women is in clinical trials, although early results suggest that it doesn't work as well as chemotherapy in this group of women. Tamoxifen is recommended for postmenopausal women. It seems to work as well as chemotherapy and has fewer side effects."

Breast Implant Complications

KNOWLEDGE CAN
HEAD OFF PROBLEMS

In 1991, five women in their late thirties to midforties walked into a University of South Florida rheumatology clinic.

One woman complained of chronic fatigue, arthritis, hair loss, sweats and chest wall and shoulder pain.

Another complained of a red area on her breast and dry eyes and mouth, as well as muscle pain in her neck, chest, shoulder and upper back.

Another complained of night sweats, chronic fatigue, lung pain and shortness of breath.

Another complained of chest wall pain, nausea, muscle cramps and a slight fever.

And the fifth complained of a fever, fatigue and joint pain in her knees, wrists and ankles.

Five different women. Five sets of symptoms. One common problem: Each woman had a ruptured silicone implant.

The High Price of Implants

More than 41,000 women had breast implants inserted during 1992—a year *after* news surfaced about implant problems—while more than 25,000 women had their implants removed, reports the American Society of Plastic and Reconstructive Surgeons.

Most women had them removed because of physical problems, often caused by the contraction of the capsule around the implant. But 22 percent of the implants were removed simply because women were afraid.

As reported by Food and Drug Administration (FDA) researchers, one woman wrote: "I am a cancer patient and had double mastectomies. I decided to undergo surgery one more time for breast implants as an attempt to feel normal again. Since the date of my first implant, my health started deteriorating and continued to do so, to the point that I lost my job. I have been unable to work and to conduct any kind of normal life. All along I have questioned the relationship of the implants to the way that I've been feeling."

In 1992, 21 percent of all implants were inserted during postmastectomy surgery, while 79 percent were inserted because women felt their breasts were somehow inadequate.

But women have paid a high price for silicone breast implants. Calls from thousands of concerned women have flooded the FDA since the news first surfaced in 1991 about problems with breast implants; there were 40,000 during a five-month period alone, when a hotline was in operation. The comments revealed that women with breast implants are deeply worried about their health.

In a review of some of the letters that were received in 1992, the FDA reports that 40 percent of the women complained of breast pain, 39 percent complained of joint pain, and 35 percent complained of fatigue. What's more, nearly half of the women had been classified by their doctors as having some type of disease in which the immune system began to attack the body.

The Smoking Gun?

Despite the fact that an estimated 1.5 million women have received implants since they were first marketed nearly 30 years ago, no one knows for sure whether breast implants trigger immunological diseases such as arthritis, lupus, a chronic inflammatory disease that affects the skin, joints, kidneys, nervous system and mucous membranes, or scleroderma, which causes hardening of the skin and scarring of internal organs.

No one knows because there is almost no reliable evidence. Studies conducted by the manufacturers may be tainted by self-interest. And while research at universities across the country is ongoing, it hasn't resulted in data from a large number of women studied over a long period of time, which is what's needed to reach reliable conclusions.

One important study was conducted by researchers at the Mayo

WOMAN TO WOMAN HER PROBLEMS LED TO HELPING OTHERS

Sybil Niden Goldrich, a Beverly Hills homemaker who became a member of the Food and Drug Administration's working group on breast implants, developed breast cancer at the age of 43. She had a double mastectomy, followed by three sets of implants. She is now a member of the Claims Advisory Committee for the Breast Implant Litigation Settlement Program. This is her story.

I was reconstructed 117 days after I had my mastectomies. The implants were polyurethane-foam-covered, silicone gel implants.

There was no indication that there was a problem with the product, nor did my doctor talk about anything but the surgical side effects. And when I developed a rash and fever immediately after the implantation of the devices, I was told that I was allergic to Betadine, the antimicrobial solution they used to wash my chest.

I wasn't. Several years later some technician put it on me by mistake, and no reaction showed up. Later on, however, I found out that the polyurethane foam used in my implants could cause an allergic reaction.

I had the implants removed because they made my breasts very hard. My breasts turned blue—I later found out that was from infection underneath—and one of the scars under my breast didn't heal.

It was a nightmare.

Anyway, I got the second set of implants, which were not polyurethane-foam-covered. But the same thing happened—my breasts got hard. And one

Clinic in Rochester, Minnesota. Women in one Minnesota county who had received breast implants between 1964 and the end of 1991—a total of 749 women—were compared with 1,498 women who had not received implants. The researchers found that the women with implants did not have an increased risk of contracting connective tissue diseases, such as rheumatoid arthritis or lupus, or other illnesses studied.

Although the results of this study are not definitive because the number of women who had implants was small and the illnesses studied were uncommon, there are large studies under way on the safety of breast implants.

Meanwhile, smaller reports suggest two things: first, that silicone

---

implant tried to push its way out through a nipple graft on my breast.

I went right to the doctor and had the implant removed. Then I had another one put in its place, and then finally another set. All of them turned out to be the same. One implant traveled down and the other traveled up underneath the skin. I was hunched over for a year and a half.

Finally I said, "I've got to get rid of these. I'm just too sick all the time."

I heard about a doctor who was doing this new operation in which a flap of abdominal tissue is used to make new breasts. So I went in, he took the breast implants out and I had the abdominal flap operation.

I'm very happy that I did. In 1988 I had a hysterectomy because I had an abnormally large tumor in my uterus. The surgeon took out the tumor, my uterus and my ovaries. He also did a liver biopsy at the same time because my liver looked "funny."

In the lab, doctors found silicone in my uterus, my ovaries and my liver. The tumors were my body's attempt to wall off the silicone from the implants. Other tumors have been removed from my wrist and ankle.

Since then another woman and I have started a self-help group called Command Trust in Beverly Hills that arranges for women to call each other and share their experiences. We've spoken to more than 25,000 women around the world. And if we've saved a few from the pain and difficulty that we've had, we've done well.

gel implants are the suspected cause, and second, that a woman's immune system perceives the silicone gel used in breast implants no differently than it does a splinter or any other foreign substance: It attacks. Also, one study of 31 women found that all implants had leaked after ten years.

In a study of three women at the Medical University of South Carolina in Charleston, researcher Richard Silver, M.D., found that immune system warriors called macrophages attacked the silicone breast implants and tried to destroy them, then tracked down and tried to destroy any silicone that had apparently leaked out of the implant and migrated to the joints, skin or lungs.

"We can't prove that the elemental silicon came from the implant," cautions Dr. Silver. "But the fact that we found macrophages in the implant's capsule suggests that that's where they may have originated."

Which implants are safest to use? "Saline, for now," says Loren Eskenazi, M.D., a member of the clinical faculty at Stanford University and co-chair of the women's caucus for the American Society of Plastic and Reconstructive Surgeons. "They're more prone to leaks than silicone, but saline leaking into the body won't hurt you. And if you do have a problem with leaks, your surgeon can replace the implant."

Another potential problem with saline is that it can obstruct the reading of a mammogram, she explains. "But a mammography technician who is experienced with implants can still get an adequate picture if there is no significant hardening around the breast implant," she says. In Europe, new implant filler materials are being produced that interfere minimally with mammography. They are currently awaiting FDA approval.

Preventing Complications

How can women who have breast implants prevent potential complications? Here's what Dr. Eskenazi suggests.

KEEP UP WITH YOUR CHECKUPS. Keep up a regular routine of breast self-examination and mammography as indicated by your doctor. The gentle compression during a mammogram won't rupture an implant. If you have any questions, see your own surgeon or one recommended by the American Society of Plastic and Reconstructive Surgeons.

LEAVE WELL ENOUGH ALONE. "Many women who have had the most severe problems with their immune system have had multiple revisions and replacements of their implants," says Dr. Eskenazi. "We don't know why, but there seems to be some sort of stimulation of the immune system with repeated surgery that makes any problems worse."

That's why she recommends that women who are not experiencing any symptoms such as joint pains or rashes and are pleased with their implants leave them in place.

CONSIDER REMOVAL. "You should have implants removed if you're significantly uncomfortable, if you're unhappy with the aesthetic result, or if you have any symptoms that began after the implants were inserted and you have no other medical explanation," says Dr. Eskanazi.

But before you go for surgery, she adds, make sure your doctor thoroughly checks out any symptoms you may have. If you have muscle and joint pains, for example, make sure your doctor runs tests for arthritis. If you have neurological symptoms—weakness while walking or unexpected falling, for example—make sure she checks for neurological problems.

EXPLORE POSTREMOVAL OPTIONS. You should be aware that after removal of the implant, your breast will look flatter than it did before the implant was originally inserted. If you don't feel perfectly comfortable having your silicone implants removed and having nothing further done, ask for saline replacements, says Dr. Eskenazi.

So-called tram flap surgery—in which fat, muscle and skin are transferred from the belly to the breast—can be used to rebuild a breast. But the surgery is very expensive and may not be covered by insurance. Few if any surgeons are currently using natural tissue to replace implants originally intended to cosmetically enlarge the breasts. However, for women who have had breast cancer, this is an excellent option.

TAKE AN ACTIVE ROLE. If you decide to have your implants replaced, ask your surgeon to give you any information she has on the replacement implant from its manufacturer or from the American Society of Plastic and Reconstructive Surgeons, says Dr. Eskenazi. Read the information carefully, take a friend to the doctor's office, ask your surgeon about anything you don't understand and tape record your doctor's answers. Then replay the tape, think carefully about what you want to do and make your decision.

Breast Lumpiness
COMMON AND USUALLY HARMLESS

Uh-oh. While smoothing body lotion over your breasts after a shower, you feel something odd—actually, some lumps—under the skin of your left breast. You're not sure what they are or even how they feel. Are they soft? Hard? Sometimes it feels like both. Whatever they are, you don't remember noticing them before.

You finish smoothing lotion over your arms and legs while your mind reels. Should you wait and see if the lumps go away after your period? Or should you make an appointment with your doctor to get them checked? Either way, you won't rest easy tonight.

For most women, lumpy breasts don't mean a thing, healthwise.

"Lumpy breasts are very common," says Kathleen Mayzel, M.D., director of the Faulkner Breast Centre and assistant clinical professor of surgery at Tufts University School of Medicine in Boston. "Most premenopausal women have them. They feel like oatmeal looks—smooth areas interrupted by a series of lumps.

"They get more lumpy before your period and less lumpy afterward because of hormonal changes. As hormone levels go up, they get more lumps. As hormone levels go down, they get less."

The condition used to be called fibrocystic breast disease or benign breast disease, until doctors figured out that it wasn't a disease—it is completely normal, says Dr. Mayzel. Now they call it lumpy breasts, and it's a condition that tends to go away as you get older.

"Starting at the age of 35, fat begins to replace breast tissue," says Dr. Mayzel. "That makes the breast less lumpy."

Here's how she suggests you handle breast lumps.

COUNT. "You have to distinguish between a breast full of lumps and a breast with *a* lump," says Dr. Mayzel. "You don't have to do anything about a breast full of lumps. But a single lump in the breast is something that warrants further evaluation in the form of a mammogram, physician's examination and possible biopsy."

BE THOROUGH. Don't skip any part of that prescription, she adds. Premenopausal women have such dense breasts that mammograms frequently do not detect a malignancy. That's why even if you have a lump and your mammogram is negative, make sure you follow through with a physician's exam and biopsy.

STAY CALM. Don't spend time worrying about the lumps, says Dr. Mayzel. "When women feel a lump, they think that they've got cancer. But something like 80 percent of all lumps are not cancer."

Bronchitis

Quieting the "Bark" That Won't Abate

It's the cough you notice first. Not the polite, get-your-attention kind of cough, but a harsh, sometimes hurtful hacking from deep within your chest. This one's loud and raucous, something like a hound grown hoarse while chasing a hare.

If you're coughing up foul-looking phlegm, maybe producing a curious wheeze from your chest, have chills and possibly a low-grade fever or are experiencing a bit of breathlessness, chances are you've got bronchitis. Despite its serious-sounding name, battles with bronchitis are common enough. An estimated 18 million episodes of it are treated each year in the United States alone. While experts don't know how many of these involve women, they do know that women with bronchitis are keeping doctors busy. And why? Because more women are smoking now than ever before, according to Sally Wenzel, M.D., assistant professor of medicine at the National Jewish Center for Immunology and Respiratory Medicine in Denver.

Just what is this "barking" disease? Picture an upside-down tree and imagine the trunk as your trachea, or windpipe, leading to your lungs. The trunk divides into branches (the bronchi or main airways), the branches into twigs (the bronchioles) and the twigs into leaves (air sacs). When viruses or bacteria enter the trunk through your throat, they make their way into the various branches, twigs and leaves. These nasty little bugs invade and injure cells, causing inflammation and narrowing of the membranes that line the passages. But the body is too smart to allow this irritation to go unchecked: It makes secretions to coat and protect these airways from further damage. That's why you're compelled to cough, sputter and produce phlegm.

So now that you know you've got it, what's next? "Everyone can get acute bronchitis from upper respiratory infections a few times in their life," says Anne L. Davis, M.D., associate professor of clinical medicine at New York University and an attending physician at Bellevue Hospital, both in New York City. "But you must find out which kind you're experiencing—acute or chronic." The differences are significant. And you'll need a doctor's diagnosis.

When It's Acute

This type comes on quite suddenly, announcing itself with what's called a "productive" cough—one that brings up clear or discolored, thin or thick sputum, occasionally mixed with blood. You might feel achy, experience some shortness of breath and run a fever ranging around 101° or 102°. Acute bronchitis often follows on the heels of a simple upper respiratory infection.

"If you've got a cold, it can kick into the bronchial tubes," explains Charles Goodrich, M.D., an internist in New York City. "The usual route is first a cold, then sinus problems, followed by pus dripping into the bronchial tubes and ultimately bronchitis. But some women will get bronchitis first, then the cold kicks in." If your cough persists and the fever lasts longer than three to five days, it's important to see a doctor.

How do you pick up acute bronchitis? Most respiratory infections are transmitted person to person, often by hand contact or sharing food with an infected friend rather than from the sneezing, coughing woman standing beside you in the subway or at the mall. So avoiding them is tricky. But don't be too alarmed—experts say if you have no history of respiratory disease and don't smoke, the usual bout lasts about a week, maybe two. "Acute symptoms last about five to seven days," says Dr. Wenzel, "and you may be left with a cough that lingers for as long as four weeks."

One caveat: "If your cough worsens and if you develop a fever and chest pains, you should see a doctor," counsels Dr. Davis. "Acute bronchitis can go into pneumonia—they sometimes overlap. Be on the safe side and check it out."

When It's Chronic

Unlike its fairly benign, time-limited counterpart, chronic bronchitis can lead to serious complications unless you move to stop it. Chronic bronchitis often emerges just when you think your winter cold has been cured. That's when you notice that all your cold symptoms have disappeared—except that cough and that awful mucus. In time, the coughing and mucus production become second nature; without any true awareness, you're coughing before, during and after colds, all year round.

Since those most affected are smokers, and since most smokers dismiss their morning hack as "just a smoker's cough," it's critical to retire that comment and take the symptom seriously. As a rule, if you have experienced a mucus-producing cough most days of the month, three months of the year, for two successive years without any other underlying causes, you may have chronic bronchitis.

Does this mean you're now immune to acute bronchitis? No such luck. "It's not unusual for women with chronic bronchitis to also have episodes of acute bronchitis," explains Dr. Davis. "You might already have some chronic bronchial impairment, and that makes you more vulnerable to acute infections."

What Causes It?

Either a virus or bacteria—or both—can trigger bronchitis. The underlying causes of this uncontrollable cough aren't too complex. Since latent viruses are always lingering within your cells, it follows that when you're under a lot of stress and pressure, the immune system becomes embattled, your resistance to disease takes a dive, and those viruses are free to take over. "We're not dealing with something unknown and terrifying," explains Dr. Goodrich, "we're talking about super stress—a powerful force in the biology of women today."

Bacterial infections are very different from viral ones. These cruel little bugs arrive uninvited from outside the system, light in your throat and work their way down to the lungs. But even if your bronchitis is viral, a secondary bacterial infection may have entered the equation. "If you notice yellow or green pus in the phlegm, bacteria may be feeding on the raw surface of the virally inflamed bronchial tube," explains Dr. Goodrich.

The distinction between a virus and bacteria is significant when it comes to treatment. Again, you'll need a doctor for this. For instance, "treating viral infections with antibiotics won't help," says Dr. Wenzel. But it's crucial that you see a doctor to rule out bacterial infections—they *can* be treated with antibiotics. And treatments vary, depending on what types of medication you can tolerate and have found to be most effective.

What can you do when you're battling bronchitis?

GET TO A DOCTOR. The only way to discern whether you have acute or chronic, viral or bacterial bronchitis is to let your doctor place a stethoscope on your chest. She'll want to find out if fluids have entered your air sacs, and if they have, send you for a chest x-ray. "You want to make certain you've ruled out a bacterial infection or pneumonia," explains Dr. Goodrich, "and if the results prove it's bacterial, your doctor will prescribe the appropriate antibiotic."

SAY GOOD-BYE TO CIGARETTES. Smoke is an irritant to the lungs and airways. "It not only causes hypersecretion of mucus and disruption in the lining of the airways," says Dr. Wenzel, "smoking makes you very susceptible to further irritant exposure leading to a chronic cough." If you're a smoker, the least you can do for now is give your lungs a rest; the best you can do is give up the habit entirely. "By smoking, you're chronically poisoning your inner bronchial tubes," says Dr. Goodrich.

GET THE VAPORIZER GOING. To keep your air passages moist and the secretions loose, turn on a warm steam vaporizer. For a viral infection, steam is the most healing treatment you can provide for those raw, inflamed surfaces inside the bronchial tubes (for a bacterial infection, it's second only to antibiotics), says Dr. Goodrich.

More good advice: Every hour on the hour that you're awake, heat a pot of water, place a towel over your head and breathe in the steam for four or five minutes, he says. But make sure the water is hot, not boiling, and do not put your face too close. Allow the towel to vent, so you protect your face from a burn.

If you're a smoker and are continually assaulting your lungs, steam is a great treatment.

FLOOD YOURSELF WITH FLUIDS. Since bronchitis commonly flares up during the winter months when the air is dry, guzzling plenty of liquids will help to thin out that thick mucus and keep fluids circulating through your system. "Drink eight to ten glasses of any fluids a day," suggests Dr. Goodrich. But stay away from coffee or cola with caffeine and dehydrating libations—wine, beer or any kind of booze—because they can cause further dehydration.

RELIEVE THAT COUGH. To minimize that hateful hack—the handmaiden of bronchitis—you might try an over-the-counter cough medicine straight from the pharmacy. It won't cure you, but it will provide a bit of TLC, especially when you're craving sleep.

"Look for a cough medicine that contains dextromethorphan," advises Dr. Goodrich. "It's the equivalent of nonprescription codeine." If this medication fails to do the job, and you're still sitting up with a vicious hack at 4:00 A.M., you may continue coughing till the cows come home unless you ask your doctor for something stronger—a prescription cough medicine with codeine.

GET YOUR NUTRIENTS. Of course, you'll want to reduce your fever, relieve your aches and simultaneously build up your system. If your stomach can tolerate it, "take two aspirin and 500 milligrams of vitamin C four times a day," suggests Dr. Goodrich. Foods, too, can help the system-strengthening process. "Start with the fluids," Dr. Goodrich advises, "and gradually add simple re-energizing proteins to your meal plans, such as foods like meat, fish, chicken and tofu—but no dairy products. Then add fruits, vegetables and whole grains."

TAKE A SABBATICAL. This is no time to show off your superwoman stamina! Get under the covers and rest for a few days. Inhale steam, drink water and juice and read a page-turner book. When you start feeling better, you can begin building yourself up with a few stretches—and then return to bed. "Once you've regained your strength and your body says 'Go!'—then, and *only* then, return to work," counsels Dr. Goodrich.

REASSESS YOUR STRESS. If stress plays such a large part in your daily life that it's almost your middle name, it's best to take an inventory and find out what can be done to alleviate or manage it. Stress can lower your resistance, making you more vulnerable to respiratory infections, and these days, women are under a lot of diverse pressures. While most of us only laugh when advised to change our lifestyles, you might consider a few "doable" alterations.

Cervical Cancer
Why You Need a Pap Smear

Every year you report to the gynecologist for a Pap smear. And every year she props open your vagina, prods your uterus, pokes your ovaries, scrapes a few cells off your cervix and sends them to a lab for analysis.

If you get the lab bill a few weeks later, you know you don't have a problem.

But if you get a phone call from your gynecologist instead, it's a good guess that the Pap smear has signaled cellular changes that may indicate or lead to cervical cancer.

Deaths due to cervical cancer have dropped a whopping 68 percent over the past 30 years, largely because these changes have been detected at such an early stage that radiation or surgery has been able to prevent any cancer from evolving.

"The Pap smear is doing its job," says Vicki Baker, M.D., director of the gynecologic oncology division at the University of Michigan Medical Center in Ann Arbor.

Solid figures are hard to come by. But in 1992 alone, Pap tests signaled abnormal cellular growth in the cervixes of somewhere between 250,000 and 1,000,000 women, according to the American College of Obstetricians and Gynecologists.

How many of those women actually developed cervical cancer is unknown. But based on trends in recent years, the American Cancer Society estimates that in 1992, only 13,500 women would have actually developed invasive cervical cancer.

A Continuum of Change

Cervical cancer does not just pop up unannounced. The cellular changes that characterize its progress may evolve over a 10- to 15-year period.

At one end of the continuum is dysplasia, a condition in which new cervical cells begin to grow in odd shapes and sizes instead of the more symmetrical shapes of healthy cells. They also begin to appear as though they've been plunked down haphazardly rather than lined up in the highly structured rows that are typical of a healthy cervix.

Not all women with dysplastic cells will develop cervical cancer. But because these cellular changes are clearly the first step in that direction, dysplasia is called cervical intraepithelial neoplasia (CIN), a precancerous condition.

If abnormal cell growth continues, the dysplasia will evolve into cancerous cells that line the cervix—in about four years. It is somewhere around this point that symptoms such as bleeding between periods, after douching or after sex may appear.

If the cancer is still not detected and treated, it will grow and become invasive cervical cancer.

Ninety percent of the women who are treated with surgery or radiation while the cancer is confined to the cervix will be alive five years after diagnosis. Sixty-seven percent of the women who are treated for invasive cancer that has spread beyond the cervix into the supporting tissue will also be alive. But only 15 percent of those in whom cancer has spread to the bladder and rectum will survive.

Putting the Brakes on Cervical Cancer

Perhaps reflecting the long incubation period that most cervical cancer requires, precancerous cell changes are detected in the cervixes of women most often between the ages of 20 and 35, while invasive cancer is detected most often between the ages of 35 and 65.

Exactly how these changes are triggered is still a mystery, but infection with the human papillomavirus, which causes genital warts, or HIV, which causes AIDS, along with such activities as smoking, maintaining a poor diet and having multiple sex partners can put any woman at risk for cervical cancer, says Dr. Baker.

"We have only a sketchy idea of what's happening at the molecular level," she adds. How any of these risk factors actually initiates changes is unknown. Scientists suspect that they either turn on genes that direct the

CAN YOU TRUST A PAP TEST?

As far as testing for cervical cancer is concerned, you really don't have any options: The Pap is the only test around that will reveal the health of your cervix. But that doesn't mean it's without faults. Chief among them is a high false-negative rate.

Various surveys indicate that around 10 percent of Pap smears are incorrectly read—primarily because reading Pap smears is so boring that lab technicians zone out. Unfortunately, approximately 20 percent of these misreadings incorrectly lead a woman to believe she is healthy when in fact she has signs of cervical cancer.

To reduce the error rate as much as possible, the Centers for Disease Control and Prevention in Atlanta require that laboratories rescreen at least 10 percent of all negative cervical smears. And some laboratories mandate that a supervisor rescreen any Pap smear that comes from a woman with any reported gynecological symptoms or abnormalities or even a history of such problems.

The result of such meticulous attention to accuracy is an error rate of approximately 5 percent.

You can make it easier for technicians to read a Pap smear by making sure the cell sample is as clear as possible, says Vicki Baker, M.D., director of the gynecologic oncology division at the University of Michigan Medical Center in Ann Arbor. Avoid douches and contraceptive creams or jellies for three days prior to the test. Avoid intercourse the night before your test. And schedule a Pap smear before or after your period, not during.

cell to multiply or turn off the cell's tumor suppressor genes, which would normally put the brakes on any uncontrolled growth. Or they may do both.

But even if doctors and researchers aren't sure how these risk factors actually put women in jeopardy, they do have suggestions for how to prevent cervical cancer.

GET A PAP SMEAR. "The single most important thing a woman can do is have an annual Pap smear," says Dr. Baker. "I still see young and middle-aged women who have not had periodic Pap smears." She says she sees these same women having advanced cases of the disease.

Forty percent of all American women have not had a Pap smear within the past three years, reports the American College of Obstetricians and Gynecologists.

The college, the American Cancer Society and the College of Surgeons recommend that a woman have her first Pap smear at age 18 or when she becomes sexually active, whichever comes first, says Dr. Baker. "Following three consecutive, annual negative Pap smears, they can be done at the discretion of the physician."

Depending on whether a woman has human papillomavirus infections or any other conditions that require closer monitoring, most gynecologists like to recommend an annual screening, she adds.

DON'T SMOKE. "Cigarette smoking is an important factor," says Dr. Baker. "It's been recognized for decades that women who smoke are at increased risk for cervical cancer. But only recently has it been recognized that the possible mechanism for this is that the carcinogens in cigarette smoke, by some unknown mechanism, are selectively concentrated in cervical mucus. They're roughly 10- to 15-fold higher than levels found in blood that's measured at the same time." So what you're doing when you smoke is bathing your cervix with cancer-causing chemicals.

BE SEXUALLY CAREFUL. "Cultivate a mutually monogamous relationship," says Dr. Baker. Studies indicate that the more sexual partners a woman has, the more likely she is to get cervical cancer.

But studies also indicate that the more sexual partners her significant other has, the more likely she is to get cervical cancer. A study of over 300 women in India, for example, found that women whose husbands had other sexual relationships both before and during marriage had nearly seven times the risk of cervical cancer when compared with women whose husbands did not.

EAT RIGHT. "Diet may play a role in preventing cervical cancer," says Dr. Baker. "Women who are deficient in folic acid and perhaps vitamin A may be at some increased risk."

A study of more than 450 women at the University of Alabama at Birmingham found that women who did not regularly eat a diet rich in folic acid—and who therefore had little of the vitamin stored in their bodies—were more likely to get cervical dysplasia than women who did.

Researchers couldn't say exactly why, but they pointed out that cells deficient in folic acid were known to be more susceptible to the effects of carcinogens than cells with a rich supply.

In other words, some cancer-causing agents may only trigger cervical cancer if you're deficient in folic acid.

The best sources of folic acid? Cowpeas, beans, lentils, spinach, wheat germ and asparagus. You can also get folic acid by taking a daily multivitamin supplement.

Cesarean Section

WHAT EVERY WOMAN
SHOULD KNOW

You've been in labor since 5:00 A.M. and it's now
11:00 P.M. Your cervix is stalled at eight centimeters. Contractions are
zapping your uterus. You're freezing cold, nauseated and about to pass
out from exhaustion.

Your husband wants to rub your back. Your nurse wants to take your
blood pressure. And your obstetrician wants to do a cesarean section.

Your response?

"Fine! Yes! Anything!"

It is not your most rational moment. That's why any discussion
about having a cesarean—such as defining the circumstances, outlining
the possibilities, weighing the alternatives, scoping out your doctor's
attitude—should take place before you ever set foot in a labor room,
says Bruce Flamm, M.D., associate clinical professor of obstetrics and

gynecology at the University of California at Irvine and research chairman at the Kaiser Permanente Medical Center in Riverside, California.

This is especially true since cesarean sections are the most frequently done operation in the United States. Of the more than four million babies born every year, it's estimated that about one million are delivered by cesarean section, according to data gathered by the Centers for Disease Control and Prevention in Atlanta.

Studies show that in a typical year, about 35 percent are done because the woman delivered a previous baby by cesarean. Thirty percent are done because, for one reason or another, labor does not progress. Twelve percent are done because the baby is in a breech—that is, feet- or buttocks-first—position, 9 percent because the baby is in distress and 14 percent for various miscellaneous reasons such as the mother's herpes infection or diabetes.

But according to a report from the Public Citizens Health Research Group in Washington, D.C., many of the cesareans done each year are unnecessary. Based on estimates by Edward Quilligan, M.D., co-editor-in-chief of the *American Journal of Obstetrics and Gynecology*, the public citizen group estimates that cesarean sections should account for 12 to 14 percent of total births. The actual number of cesareans is closer to 23 percent of all live births. In other words, about half of all cesareans are probably unnecessary.

The Effects of Age

A cesarean section is a major abdominal operation in which a pregnant woman is given either a local or general anesthetic and the baby is surgically removed from the uterus. Although rare, maternal death occurs two to four times more frequently than with a vaginal birth, while rates for complications such as hemorrhage and infection are five to ten times higher. The procedure also requires an extra couple of days in the hospital, costs more and takes about three times longer to recover from than a vaginal birth.

Common reasons for a cesarean section are situations in which the baby is in danger, is too big to fit through the mother's pelvis or is in a poor position for delivery; there's bleeding; there are multiple fetuses such as twins or triplets; the placenta has torn or separated from the mother before birth; there are large fibroids in the lower part of the uterus that might obstruct the baby's delivery; or the mother has complications such as uncontrolled high blood pressure, says Helen Kay, M.D., a specialist in maternal/fetal medicine and associate professor of obstetrics and gynecology at Duke University in Durham, North Carolina.

Nowhere on that list is either maternal age or the fact that a woman has had a previous cesarean section. Yet a study of more than 700 women at Brown University School of Medicine in Providence, Rhode Island, and Yale University School of Medicine found that women 30 to 34 were 63 percent more likely to have a cesarean than women in their twenties, while women over age 35 were twice as likely to have a cesarean. On the other side of the country, a study of women who delivered single babies in civilian hospitals in the state of Washington from 1987 through 1990 revealed that women in the 30-to-34 age range had nearly double the cesarean rate of women 15 to 19.

Why are post-30 women more likely to have a cesarean? "It may have a lot to do with nonmedical things like the fact that women who have their babies when they're 38 may be attorneys or Ph.D.'s," says Dr. Flamm. It's what's called the premium baby concept, he explains. Some doctors think that because a woman put off childbearing, her "last chance" baby has to be perfect. "And the only way a doctor feels he can assure that is to perform a cesarean section at the first hint of trouble," he says.

Given the number of things that can go wrong as a baby makes that rough-and-tumble trip down the birth canal—like the umbilical cord becoming looped around the baby's neck, for example—some doctors feel that a cesarean tips the scales in the baby's favor.

"Other doctors feel that women who are 32 or 33 aren't as strong and healthy as a 22-year-old, which is why they're not able to have a vaginal birth. My personal feeling is that that's baloney. I've delivered many babies to women who are 38 and 39 who have had vaginal deliveries without any problems," Dr. Flamm says.

The Second Time Around

Even if you had a cesarean section to deliver one baby, you may not need one with the next, doctors agree.

"My personal feeling is that almost every woman who had a prior cesarean is a candidate for a normal birth," says Dr. Flamm. The exception, he says, is the woman who had a "classical" incision during the first section. This is a vertical cut in the uterus that usually begins above the belly button and extends down to the pubic area.

If a woman has a classical incision, there is a 10 percent chance that the uterus will rupture in subsequent pregnancies. That may not sound like a big risk, but if it happens, the results can be catastrophic:

CESAREAN SECTION

significant blood loss for the mother and death for the fetus.

Only about 1 percent of cesareans are done with a classical incision, says Dr. Flamm. Today, most surgeons use a "bikini" incision, in which the initial cut is made horizontally across the uterus. (This incision follows the line where the top of a bikini would lie against the abdomen.)

Statistics indicate that increasing numbers of women who have had prior cesareans are having subsequent babies vaginally, he adds. "The vaginal birth after cesarean—VBAC—rate has gone up about tenfold in the last 20 years," says Dr. Flamm. "In 1970 the rate was about 2.2 percent; in 1990 it was about 20.4."

That still means that 80 percent of women who have had a previous cesarean section are not delivering vaginally. But the increase is enough to cause cesarean rates in general to level off for the first time in decades—a trend that Dr. Flamm hopes will continue.

What You Can Do

Here's how you can reduce your chances of having a cesarean section.

USE A CERTIFIED NURSE-MIDWIFE. "Certified nurse-midwives have very low cesarean rates," says Dr. Flamm, who is married to one. "They're nurses to begin with. Then they go through a year-long program and an internship where they work with other midwives. They're very well-trained, and in most cases they work as a team with a physician as backup." About the only thing they can't do that a doctor can is perform major surgery.

The only women who probably shouldn't use a midwife are those who have a medical problem such as diabetes or are on blood pressure medication. To find a certified nurse-midwife near you, write to the American College of Nurse Midwives, 818 Connecticut Avenue NW, Suite 900, Washington, DC 20006.

GET A DOULA. "You should have somebody with you who can support your point of view about birth and cesarean sections," says Dr. Flamm. "In the midst of labor, it's not easy to keep a focus on what you want to do.

"That's why I believe in doulas, or trained labor support people who have been at hundreds of births. They'll sit with a woman in labor, and they've been down this road so many times before that they're not going to panic when there's a little dip on the fetal monitor." They'll also act as the woman's advocate should the need arise. If a woman has said she doesn't want drugs and a doctor starts to give them, the doula may remind the doctor of the woman's wishes.

"In some cities doulas are listed in the phone book under 'labor support,' " says Dr. Flamm. Any childbirth educator associated with a hospital or Lamaze group can probably refer you to one.

ASK FOR YOUR DOCTOR'S STATS. "There are doctors in this country with a cesarean rate of 10 percent and there are doctors with a rate of 80 percent," says Dr. Flamm. "And amazingly, some of those doctors with 80 percent rates are taking care of low-risk women.

"But cesarean rates are a sensitive issue with most doctors," he says. So basic human courtesy dictates that you should ask about your doctor's rates in a sensitive, nonconfrontational way. You might say on your first visit, for example, "You know that I'm interested in a natural vaginal birth and I was just curious as to what your cesarean rate is." "Approached that way, I think most doctors aren't going to get too upset about it," says Dr. Flamm.

A typical obstetrician's rates might hover between 15 and 20 percent, Dr. Flamm says. "If the doctor says the rate is 30, 40 or 50 percent, however, I'd be a little concerned." If that rate seems too high to you, it's probably a good idea to find another doctor.

Chronic Fatigue Syndrome

SORTING THROUGH THE SYMPTOMS

You're exhausted. Your head aches, your muscles hurt, your memory's shot, and you can't seem to shake that cough you got when you had the flu last month.

You know you're going to feel better soon. After all, it was just the flu. But imagine waking up and feeling that way every day for the rest of your life. What would you do?

That's exactly the question that women with chronic fatigue syndrome (CFS) ask themselves every morning, says Anthony Komaroff, M.D., professor of medicine at Harvard Medical School and director of the Chronic Fatigue Syndrome Research Center, funded by the National Institutes of Health, in Boston.

"They're perfectly fine and then one day they come down with a bad cold or the flu. They have a fever, aching muscles, sore throat, maybe a cough. And instead of getting over it like they did with every other flu they've ever had, they never do."

They're not contagious or overtly ill, but the fatigue forces them to reduce their normal activities by 50 percent and rest whenever possible. Many women also have difficulty thinking and concentrating, or they may become forgetful, confused and excessively irritable. They may also have aching muscles, a sore throat, mild fever and swollen glands.

One thing they are not, however, is depressed.

Some researchers had initially suspected that CFS was "all in the head" and that the disease was actually a form of depression, says Dr. Komaroff. But "the majority of our patients at the research center, even though in some sense their lives have been ruined, are not depressed.

"It's amazing," he adds. "If from out of the blue I suddenly couldn't work, if I couldn't play ball with my kids, if I didn't have the energy to be a vigorous social partner to my wife—if all of those things happened and I was suddenly disabled—I would be depressed. But the majority of our patients are not."

Looking for Some Answers

Chronic fatigue syndrome is still a mystery, says Ann Schlueder-berg, Sc.D., former chief of the virology branch in the Division of Microbiology and Infectious Diseases at the National Institute for Allergy and Infectious Diseases in Bethesda, Maryland. Since the mid-1980s, scientists have discussed what symptoms are actually caused by CFS, how many people it might affect, whether it affects more women than men and which laboratory investigations might actually lead to the cause.

"Laboratory tests suggest that an overly active immune system might be important in how the disease gets started," says Dr. Schlueberg.

"Although no one knows the cause of CFS, research has been able to make two observations," says Dr. Komaroff. "One is that the immune system looks as though it's chronically turned on, as though it's fighting a war against something. The second observation is that certain immune system cells, perhaps because they're constantly fighting this war, simply aren't functioning at normal levels. They're not knocked out completely as they are in AIDS, but they're clearly not working as well as they should." It's almost as though they're suffering from a case of battle fatigue, he adds.

Sleep Interference

Most people with CFS have difficulty sleeping, says Dr. Komaroff. "Brain wave studies in sleep laboratories show that people with CFS simply don't get the deep, restorative sleep they need in adequate amounts. In fact, almost 90 percent of those with this illness say that even if they've slept well, they never get up in the morning feeling rested.

"All of us have those mornings," adds Dr. Komaroff. "But these people feel that way every morning of their lives."

Fortunately, a class of prescription drugs called tricyclics—such as Elavil, Tofranil and Norpramin—can improve the quality of sleep, says Dr. Komaroff. "Tricyclics have two uses in medicine," he explains. "When used in high doses, they're antidepressant drugs. When used in low doses—about one-tenth of the antidepressant dose—they improve the quality of sleep."

Doctors don't know how they work, but they do know that the benefits to those with CFS are more than just a good night's sleep. Whether it's the sleep or the medicine, people who take tricyclic drugs also seem to have fewer CFS symptoms—particularly the ones that affect thinking, remembering and concentrating.

Does tricyclic-aided sleep somehow rest the battle-fatigued immune system in someone with CFS?

Researchers aren't sure. "Throughout medical research there is now growing evidence that the immune system is different in certain respects during sleep and wakefulness," says Dr. Komaroff. "But although sleep and the immune system may be connected in some ways, we're just beginning to understand what's going on.

"My very sophisticated, scientific, medical belief is like my grandmother's when she said that if you don't get a good night's sleep you're going to catch things. Her perception was that poor sleep leads to some kind of immune problem, which leads to infections. I think that when we understand science better we'll prove that my grandmother was right."

Living with CFS

It's pretty difficult to do anything about a disease when scientists can't figure out what's causing it, doctors say.

But the fact that CFS is so much a mystery is the very reason that it's important for people who suspect they have the disease to see a doctor, says Orvalene Prewitt, president of the National Chronic Fatigue Syndrome and Fibromyalgia Association in Kansas City, Missouri. Many different diseases—such as cancer, anemia, depression and hepatitis—can cause the same type of overwhelming fatigue that occurs in CFS. And without constant medical monitoring, these conditions could go undetected.

What's more, people who have CFS should see their doctors every six months, adds Prewitt—just to make sure that their CFS isn't hiding the symptoms of some other, more treatable disease.

Until there is a treatment for CFS, here are several strategies that have helped those with CFS get through the day. Most work by dealing with particular symptoms of the syndrome, such as fatigue, pain or disrupted sleep.

SLOW DOWN. "As a general rule, maintaining an even, throttled-down pace—to the extent that life allows you to do it—will protect you against the physical, emotional and intellectual stresses that can just consume someone with CFS," says Dr. Komaroff. But if you're forced to go all-out on one particular day or another, make sure you rest the next. Give yourself a break.

BE INVENTIVE. Jill Anderson, R.N., Ph.D., a clinical nurse specialist at the University of Illinois in Chicago who is studying women with CFS, has found that people with CFS are good at figuring out how to save energy.

For instance, a teacher Dr. Anderson interviewed uses a luggage carrier—the kind flight attendants use to haul their bags around airports—to move her briefcase, books and other teacher-type paraphernalia from one classroom to another. She also naps in her car at lunch.

A second woman with CFS has a machine answer all her calls, then returns them as she has the energy. A third woman who finds reading exhausting orders books on tape from her local library.

Other women use paper plates to cut down on kitchen work, order stamps by mail to avoid a trip to the Post Office and buy clothes from a catalog to avoid shopping. Still others have groceries delivered and tape TV programs on a VCR, then replay them when they can concentrate.

GET CONNECTED. Dr. Anderson also found that women with home computers have logged onto the Prodigy on-line computer service to access the Medical Support Bulletin Board. This electronic bulletin board allows subscribers to network with people with various medical concerns, says Dr. Anderson. Once connected to the bulletin board, women can select the CFS option from the menu and read messages organized by subjects like "ask the doctor," "advice needed," and "CFS and insurance."

Without expending any more energy than it takes to sit and type, someone connected to the Medical Support Bulletin Board or on-line services can learn how others feel about having CFS, how they handle family relationships and the tricks they use to cope with life.

LISTEN TO YOUR BODY. Some people with CFS find that various foods—especially those containing caffeine, alcohol or sugar—aggravate the syndrome, says Dr. Komaroff. Others say that foods have no effect.

"I tell people to listen to the wisdom of their own bodies," he says. If it bothers you—if you feel even more fatigued in the hours after eating something than you usually do—then don't put it in your mouth. If it doesn't bother you, have a ball. Interestingly, 97 percent of all Dr. Komaroff's patients have become teetotalers since the onset of their illness.

USE PAINKILLERS. "The headaches, muscle pain and joint pain should be treated with nonsteroidal anti-inflammatory medications like aspirin and ibuprofen," says Dr. Komaroff. Check with your doctor regarding the appropriate dosage.

Colds and Flu
Relief Is Easy to Find

Your voice sounds like Suzanne Pleshette's on a very bad day. Your eyes are watery slits.

You sneeze and sniff, and although you continually reapply makeup, that nasty shade of vermilion on your nose reappears every time you blow it. Your throat is scratchy, your head feels thick and heavy—you'd love to nap, but no way! Not now, at your desk. Maybe later, after you've fixed dinner, walked the dog and washed the dishes.

You've caught a bug all right, the old "something that's going around." Could be a cold. Maybe it's the flu.

If you're sneezing and sniffling but your aches are minimal, chances are you've got a cold. If you've got the mother of all headaches, a cough and sore throat, major aches and pains and you're running a fever, more likely you've been bitten by the flu bug. Right now, however, with that stuffy nose and sore throat, let's consider the cold.

The Cold Front

Sure you feel miserable, but you're not alone. Each year Americans suffer from 68 million colds caused by any of 120 cold viruses. As we all know, there is no effective "cold" vaccine.

While they don't have figures to prove it, experts believe women are more likely to get colds than men, mostly because of the swirl of germs surrounding the kids we care for at home, in school or at day care.

But even if you have no occasion to be around a sick child, you can get a cold just by mingling with people on a bus, in the mall or in the office. "Women are exposed to a lot more outside contact than they were in the past," says pulmonary specialist Anne L. Davis, M.D., associate professor of clinical medicine at New York University and attending physician at Bellevue Hospital, both in New York City. "This means they have more chance of picking up respiratory infections."

A Roving Virus

Colds are transmitted easily by physical contact or through airborne droplets expelled during a cough or sneeze. If a sick person has managed to transfer her cold germs from her nose or mouth to her hands—which is pretty easy—anything she touches can infect you if you touch it and then touch your nose, mouth or eyes. Door handles, phones, toothbrushes and used tissues can carry germs waiting to get you.

Still, even if you do shake hands with someone with a cold or are awash in droplets spewed by a sneeze, you might not develop a cold. Whether you do may depend on the level of stress in your life and how you cope with it. In a study conducted at the Medical Research Council's Common Cold Unit in Great Britain, 154 men and 266 women were exposed to a cold virus, then placed in quarantine. The study concluded that people struggling with heavier loads of psychological stress were more susceptible to cold infections than those who shared the same living conditions but were less stressed.

"Basically, stress lowers the resistance," says Charles Goodrich, M.D., an internist in New York City. "It assaults the barriers of the immune system in many different ways, gradually decreasing its ability to ward off disease."

The flow chart of symptoms this upper respiratory ailment packs is nothing to sneeze at. Colds are not identical, but they usually start with a runny nose, some sneezing and a stuffy feeling in the head. In addition, you might have a headache, watery eyes, listlessness, an inability to concentrate, a sore throat and perhaps a slight fever. "The virus sets off an inflammation of the mucous membrane, which then may begin to pour out mucus or swell and leave you with that stuffy feeling," says Dr. Davis. "You may start by blowing your nose like mad, then the secretions dry up, mucus thickens and your nose feels swollen."

How Long Will It Last?

The average cold hangs on for 7 to 14 days. Experts agree on one thing: When you're in the midst, forget about a cure—consider your comfort.

Today, pharmacies carry scores of cold-relief products. There are more than 300 products for a combination of cold, allergy and cough. That means product selection can be difficult.

It's up to you and your doctor or pharmacist to evaluate your cold and select products that contain specific ingredients to combat your symptoms. If you're seeking relief from one symptom—say a stuffy nose—you should use a single-ingredient nasal decongestant. If you want relief from a series of symptoms, read the list of ingredients carefully and select a medication targeted for those symptoms only.

When the Inevitable Strikes

What can you do when a cold has you in its uncomfortable grip? Here are some suggestions.

SLEEP IT OFF. You'll feel like it, so do it. "Sleep revitalizes your working parts and plays an important role in getting rid of infections," advises Carole Heilman, Ph.D., chief of the Respiratory Viruses Branch of the National Institute of Allergy and Infectious Diseases in Bethesda, Maryland. While no direct studies prove it, "logic suggests a relationship between sleep and your susceptibility to a variety of infections. If you're worn out, you're simply more prone to picking them up," Dr. Heilman adds. And you're less likely to put up a good fight when the bug takes up residence.

One other thing: Stop trying to do all the things you did when you were well—like work 15 hours a day, go to the grocery, do the wash and clean the bathroom. If you need to take time off from work, do it. It's better than spreading those germs, and you'll get well faster if you give yourself a break.

BREATHE DEEPLY. And make it steamy. Doctors say this moisturizes the lungs and mucous membranes, helping them release germs. "Inhaling steam is the most healing of treatments for viral infections," says Dr. Goodrich. Use a hot-water vaporizer or stand in a hot shower or steamy bathroom. If you can't do that, try putting your head over a sink or bowl of steamy hot water. Drape your head with a towel to keep the steam in your face.

GO OVER THE COUNTER. While some people start taking aspirin at the first sign of colds or flu, experts urge caution if you have flulike symptoms. Because of the rare but potential risk of Reye's syndrome, a life-threatening neurological illness that has been known to affect adults as well as children, you should not take aspirin or aspirin compounds if you have any signs of the flu. Take acetaminophen or ibuprofen instead.

Ibuprofen has emerged as an effective weapon against colds. In a study from Australia, volunteers who were infected with the cold virus and then took aspirin or acetaminophen experienced increased nasal congestion. But those who swallowed ibuprofen suffered no additional stuffiness. Aspirin may relieve headache and other aches and pains, says Dr. Heilman, but it could make the cold virus linger.

SAVOR SOME SOUP. Any hot liquid is helpful for cold symptoms, but good old chicken soup seems to have an especially soothing effect. Although there are no studies to show why it works so well, professionals frequently recommend it. "I'm a firm believer in

WHEN TO SEE THE DOCTOR

When cold or flu symptoms take a turn for the worse and friends and family suggest seeing a doctor, many of us are likely to say, "I just don't have the time. I'll be better soon." But be smart and call your doctor if you have the following symptoms.
- A fever higher than 101°, accompanied by chills.
- Wheezing and/or tightening in the chest.
- A cough that won't abate.
- Coughs that yield yellow or green phlegm.
- Coughs that yield blood-streaked or rust-colored mucus.
- Sharp, stabbing chest pain upon deep breathing or coughing.
- Persistent hoarseness.
- Difficulty breathing or shortness of breath.

If you get help soon enough, you may reduce your risk of complications, including pneumonia or bronchitis.

chicken soup," declares Dr. Heilman. "Even with a fever, if hot soup is what you crave, get yourself a bowl and enjoy." Besides the heat, which relieves congestion and soothes the throat, chicken soup is jam-packed with nutrients to aid in the body's fight against cold invaders.

GARGLE WITH SALT WATER. Most mouthwashes act only as "mouth fresheners." Others, like Listerine, may be too harsh for sore throats. "Gargle with warm salt water," advises Dr. Davis. "The salt is soothing, it flushes away some of the debris and impurities, and it's thought to have a healing effect."

CALM YOUR COUGH. For dry, hacking coughs, a single-ingredient cough suppressant, called an antitussive, is your best bet. For productive coughs, the kind that produce mucus, you can choose to take an expectorant, although a Food and Drug Administration advisory panel has found most expectorants to be harmless but basically ineffective against coughs. In fact, doctors say that the best expectorant is water. For maximum effectiveness, drink lots of warm water, which thins the mucus and increases the amount of fluid in the respiratory tract.

CLEAR YOUR NOSE. For a stuffy nose, drops or nasal sprays may give temporary relief. But be careful. A few hours after using these products, the blood vessels in your nasal passages can dilate, causing a stuffy feeling or rebound effect. You'll want to use the spray again, and the rebound cycle will start over. It's not surprising these products can have an addictive effect. If you want to take an oral decongestant, be aware that they aren't recommended for people with an irregular heartbeat, high blood pressure, heart disease or glaucoma.

SOOTHE YOUR THROAT. Lozenges or hard, sour candy will keep your throat moist and can provide temporary pain relief. If you're taking a lozenge, look for these ingredients: hexylresorcinol, sodium ascorbate and menthol.

BE CAREFUL WITH ANTIHISTAMINES. Studies show the effects of antihistamines are twofold: They have a drying effect on mucous membranes, and they may reduce sneezing. But antihistamines are a very large group, and the side effects can range from irregular heartbeat to drowsiness. So consult your doctor or pharmacist about which antihistamine to take and read labels carefully to find out about side effects.

LISTEN TO YOUR BODY. Should you feed a cold and starve a fever, or vice versa? There's no easy answer. All you can do is let your body tell you what it needs, says Dr. Heilman. If you feel better eating full meals during a cold, go for it, she says. If you'd prefer a lighter diet of soup, crackers and club soda, that's fine, too. Experiment.

SPICE UP YOUR LIFE. Hot spices and pepper increase secretions from your mucous membranes, and this can help relieve cold symptoms. That's because the extra mucus can thin out your phlegm and lubricate your sore, itchy throat.

ZING IT WITH ZINC. Tablets of zinc gluconate with glycine can knock a cold flat. According to a study at Dartmouth University in Hanover, New Hampshire, these tablets can cut the life of a cold by a whopping 42 percent. Look for these tablets at your pharmacy or health food store.

ASSESS YOUR STRESS. If your immune system is fighting an uphill battle against pressure and stress, you're putting yourself at risk for colds and flu. "It's probably a good time to look at your life and make an important stress assessment," says Dr. Goodrich. Since stress lowers resistance to disease, consider making some changes, from getting more sleep and rest to eating more nutritiously and placing relaxation high on your list.

CAN THE KISSES. If you've got a bug, you can bestow it upon your partner, your children or anybody else you kiss. Even hugging can be too close for comfort, says Dr. Heilman. By the same token, avoid kissing and hugging a person who appears to be infected.

DO A LADY MACBETH. Wash your hands frequently. And don't touch your eyes, mouth or nose unless your hands have just been scrubbed. "If your husband and/or children have a cold, be extra vigilant about hand washing," advises Dr. Heilman, "especially after picking up and discarding their used tissues."

DON'T SHARE UTENSILS. To avoid spreading germs, "don't eat off the same fork or drink from the same glass, like the communal bathroom cup," says Dr. Heilman. Use Lysol spray to disinfect phones and doorknobs, and dip your toothbrush in hydrogen peroxide solution after each use.

Fighting the Flu

This acute viral infection of the respiratory tract arrives armed with some mean symptoms. They appear suddenly and soon affect your entire body. Among its calling cards are fever, chills, headache, sore throat, cough, muscle pain and gastrointestinal disturbances. What makes this vicious varmint so unwieldy is its ability to mutate into new and different forms. If you've gotten your yearly flu shot to protect against the current strain, it might also be effective against a closely related mutant strain. Flu shots are always recommended for the elderly and for people with medical conditions such as diabetes.

As with colds, women are more likely than men to become infected with the flu. We're not more vulnerable, but more often than not we're the primary caretakers for children, who easily pick up the bug and then pass it along to us. Additionally, more women than men work in hospitals or nursing homes, where the risk of catching the flu is high.

Once this insidious little bug has entered your system, no drug will kill it. Because the flu is not bacterial, antibiotics won't faze it. Doctors sometimes prescribe antibiotics, but only to ward off secondary bacterial complications such as pneumonia or bronchitis.

Here's small comfort: "If you're feeling bad, you're getting better," says Dr. Heilman. "Your body is reacting to the foreign substance and trying to get rid of it. Take what you need to feel better, let it run its course and get on with your life."

What more can you do? Well, all of the preceding tips for colds will help, along with these strategies.

GET THE SHOT. Doctors advise getting the inoculation between September and November, before flu season, says Dr. Heilman. The vaccine usually reaches its maximum strength in four to six weeks. It is strongly advised for those who work in high-risk settings—nursing homes, hospitals and prisons—along with pregnant women, people over 65 and those with diabetes or chronic heart, lung or kidney disease. The shot may cause soreness at the vaccination site, but serious side effects are rare. Contact your local health department: In many cities, flu shots are free. *Warning:* If you're egg-sensitive, forget the flu shot. The vaccine is grown in eggs and may induce allergic reactions.

ASK ABOUT ANTIVIRALS. If you work in a high-risk environment, ask your doctor about two antiviral drugs, amantadine and rimantadine. While they are not substitutes for the flu vaccine, they can prevent certain strains from infecting you and/or shorten the duration of fever and other symptoms. At high doses, amantadine can cause debilitating side effects, including loss of appetite, nausea and nervousness. It should not be taken by pregnant women or nursing mothers.

PROTECT YOURSELF ABROAD. To ensure a healthy trip overseas, get vaccinated. Although the risk of exposure to the flu virus depends on the season, in certain areas, like the tropics, flu can sweep through anytime of year. But you should get the vaccine more than three days prior to travel. Otherwise, complications related to the shot might occur while you're traveling.

Cold Sores

Wiping Out
a Common Nuisance

Why does a cold sore always pop up when you least want one—right before a big party or a major job interview, or right before your period?

It's not a coincidence. Stress can be one of the primary triggers for the wily cold sore, although exposure to sun and wind, fatigue, dental treatments, certain foods and illnesses with fever can also prompt an appearance of the painful blisters that can last as long as three weeks.

Cold sores are caused by the herpes simplex virus, which, once acquired, lies dormant in your spinal cord and certain areas of your brain until your immune system lets down its guard or becomes pre-occupied with important business, such as fending off the flu or a cold. (That's why they're called *cold* sores.) Given the opportunity, the virus scampers out, usually to the original site of infection, to publicly proclaim its surly power.

Cold sores usually show up on the border of your lips, right where your facial skin begins, but they can also erupt on your nose, fingertips and other areas of your skin. Cancer and AIDS patients are often put on full-time suppressive drug therapy to prevent outbreaks of the herpes virus, which has a field day when the immune system is weakened.

About 90 percent of the adult population has been exposed to herpes simplex type 1, the primary culprit in cold sore eruptions, although herpes simplex type 2, the cause of most genital herpes, can also be responsible. It doesn't matter which virus causes your cold sore: As the lesions begin, they all have the same tingling and discomfort and emerge with the same shallow ulcer that develops a yellow crust. Both types are also similarly contagious.

Some women find that their attacks occur premenstrually, says Mark McCune, M.D., a Kansas City, Kansas, dermatologist who was co-author of a study on cold sores. It is not known exactly why menstruation—or anything else, for that matter—seems to spur outbreaks, he says. The answer probably lies in the subtle interplay of the body's immune system and its varying ability to ward off environmental insults and internal stress.

Women have an advantage over men in that they're more familiar with the cosmetics that can help camouflage cold sores. Cold sores are rarely serious, but they can cause women to feel so unattractive that they socially withdraw, even canceling appointments and dates, says Dr. McCune.

You're in Control

Now for the good news: Because cold sores may be prompted by environmental and psychological factors that you can control, you can often reduce the frequency and duration of recurrence. A person with herpes simplex may feel that the ugly yellow ulcer on her lip diminishes her self-confidence and social desirability, but she does best when she has the conviction that she controls the virus, that it doesn't control her. As Dr. McCune explains, the key to keeping the herpes virus at bay "is to identify your trigger factors and control those the best that you can."

It helps to remember that "you're the same person, whether you're having an outbreak or not," says psychologist Geraldine Hirsch, Ph.D., a medical adviser to Herpetics Engaged in Living Productively (H.E.L.P.), a New York City support group for people with herpes. Being distressed or ashamed over an outbreak can actually prolong and worsen your lesions. "What triggers outbreaks in some people is emotional upset," notes Dr. Hirsch. Women who worry or whose self-esteem sags because of something as minor as a cold sore retard their own recuperation by keeping themselves in the same state that brought on the initial lesion.

Objectively, a cold sore is, at its worst, a discomfort and a drag, but because it is highly contagious, you should be extremely careful to avoid infecting someone else or spreading it to other areas of your own body.

"Make awfully sure you wash your hands with soap and water before you go to the bathroom," in case a hand that has recently touched your lip comes into contact with your genitals while wiping yourself, Dr. McCune says. "The other thing is your eyes: Don't mess with your cold sore and then put your contacts in. Getting herpes in your eye can be very serious."

Women who can't prevent their cold sores with dietary and lifestyle changes, or those who have more than three or four outbreaks a year, should see a dermatologist. Chances are she'll give you a prescription for acyclovir, an antiviral drug usually taken three to five times a day. In a study conducted at the National Institutes of Health in Bethesda, Maryland, researchers found that giving 800 milligrams of acyclovir to adults who had six or more outbreaks per year could reduce the frequency of recurrence by 53 percent. Records kept by the acyclovir patients also revealed that the episodes they did have healed more quickly.

But before you get to the acyclovir stage, you may want to see if you can tame your outbreaks by getting enough sleep, exercising and tinkering with your lifestyle and outlook. Some people find biofeedback and hypnotherapy helpful for getting their emotions and, by association, their immune systems, under control. Some like hot baths, meditation or letting up on a hectic schedule to make time for a passion—be it classical music concerts or ice skating.

If It Calms You, Do It

Dr. Hirsch has a patient who swears by her Positive Visualization exercises. Whenever she feels stressed, she closes her eyes and imagines herself relaxing in a beautiful vacation spot while breathing deeply and evenly. Others may close their eyes and imagine a healthy, swashbuckling immune system trouncing and devouring little herpes microbes. "If you feel it's helpful and calming, it doesn't matter what it is. If it helps you feel in control, then by all means—do it!" says Dr. Hirsch.

Folk wisdom about what works to calm cold sores abounds. Some people swear that pressing warm tea bags on a throbbing sore does the trick. Others say a compress of whole milk at room temperature is soothing and useful. (If you try this, be sure to rinse the milk from your skin afterward.) Others swear by placing cool tea bags or wrapped ice cubes on the affected area. If something helps to banish your blisters, do you really care if you're benefiting from a placebo effect? Go for it.

Here are some other suggestions for battling cold sores.

WATCH WHAT YOU EAT. Herpes needs the amino acid arginine in order to replicate itself, and the arginine in foods can provoke outbreaks in some people. So if you're having frequent episodes, you might want to avoid it. Arginine is found in chocolate, cola, peas, nuts, beer, gelatin and cereals. "Very small amounts of these foods can set some people off," says Dr. McCune. It's worth a try to avoid such foods completely for a while to see if doing so reduces the frequency of your cold sores.

TRY LYSINE. The Food and Drug Administration concluded in 1992 that no orally administered active ingredient—including lysine—has been proven effective in the treatment of cold sores. Yet many doctors and people with herpes continue to swear by it. Dr. McCune says many of his herpes patients have success with the inexpensive supplement, available at health food stores and in the vitamin aisle of grocery stores. He recommends 2,000 to 3,000 milligrams a day. "That's what I recommend if you have outbreaks every six to eight weeks," says Dr. McCune. And while he says he has observed virtually no side effects or dangers connected with high lysine doses, pregnant or nursing women should check with their doctors before deciding to self-medicate.

MAKE SOME RESOLUTIONS. Researchers have found that smoking lowers your immunity, as do drinking and all those other things you know are bad for you: Being overweight, overtired, miserable or lonely. Herpes flourishes when your health suffers, so take good care of yourself. Get enough sleep, eat nourishing, low-fat foods and stay connected to friends and family. Try to dump as much stress as you can.

TRY A NEW ATTITUDE. "The immune system can be affected by the power of suggestion," says Dr. McCune, adding that in studies done on people with herpes simplex, researchers found that 30 to 50 percent responded favorably to a placebo—their sores healed faster or they went longer between outbreaks.

If you feel good about yourself and just see your cold sore as a minor annoyance, other folks are more likely to see you in a positive light, and you're more likely to keep the virus at bay, says Dr. Hirsch.

STOCK UP ON ACYCLOVIR. If your doctor recommends acyclovir, make sure you get a generous prescription with multiple refills, because the earlier you take it, the more effective it is. Start taking it at the first sign of the characteristic tingling that signals the earliest stage of a cold sore, says Dr. McCune. You have an even better chance of aborting or reducing the severity of the sore if you take acyclovir prior to exposure to an unavoidable trigger, like the sun or a stressful situation you can't avoid. Women who have constant cold sores may be put on suppressive doses for long stretches of time to try to drive the virus back to its spinal hideout.

Note: While acyclovir is generally well-tolerated, it should not be taken during pregnancy because there have been no studies showing its effects on pregnant women or fetuses, according to Dr. McCune.

ASK ABOUT ACYCLOVIR OINTMENT. Acyclovir is often prescribed in capsule form, but your doctor can also prescribe an ointment. Topical acyclovir can help the cold sore heal faster, notes Dr. McCune, by keeping the lesion moist and inhibiting the growth of the herpes virus.

Doctors recommend that you use rubber gloves or a finger cot (sheath) while applying acyclovir ointment to prevent spreading the virus. Herpetic whitlow—blisters on the fingertips or other areas of the hands—are often caused by touching a mouth sore with the fingers.

COVER UP. Disguising your dermatological ulcers will no doubt help you feel better. While it's best to keep sores clean, using glossy lipsticks or light foundation on affected areas is unlikely to hinder healing, says Dr. McCune. And they'll make you feel better about how you look. Thick, talc-based makeups can be used as long as you carefully clean makeup residues off the sore's surface with hydrogen peroxide.

BE SAFE IN THE SUN. Numerous studies have shown that the incidence of cold sores rises with exposure to sun. Before you tromp out into the great outdoors, slather your lips and other susceptible areas with a powerful sunscreen. Use a micronized, physical sunblock such as Neutrogena Chemical-Free Sunblocker or Johnson & Johnson's Baby Sunblock. These sunblocks contain minute particles of titanium dioxide, says Albert M. Kligman, M.D., Ph.D., professor of dermatology at the University of Pennsylvania School of Medicine in Philadelphia. They work the same way zinc oxide does to block the sun, but without the white opacity. They have a sun protection factor (SPF) of 16 or above.

WATCH THE WIND. If wind exposure seems to preface your outbreaks, "cover up, even if you don't have a cold sore," Dr. Kligman advises. "Wind is very hard on skin." Wear a ski mask in cold weather, and laugh off the bank robber jokes with your beautiful, untarnished smile.

BE COOL. If you have a cold sore, put your love life on hold until it clears up. "You shouldn't be kissing anybody, anywhere" if you have a cold sore or feel one coming on, Dr. Hirsch says. Most people don't know, she says, that direct contact with any part of another person's body can pass on the virus.

If your cold sore comes in contact with your partner's genital area, for example, you can give him genital herpes. A Scottish study showed that herpes simplex type 1—which once claimed the face as its main domain—was increasingly to blame as the cause of genital herpes. The study, which tracked 1,794 people with herpes over 14 years, found that herpes type 1 infections in the genital area had increased from 20 percent to over 40 percent—and women were more susceptible than men. Similarly, be protective of yourself if you see that your partner has a cold sore and is feeling amorous.

Colorectal Cancer

MORE DETECTABLE—
AND CURABLE—THAN EVER

It's no fun. For a fecal occult exam, a gynecologist slides a gloved finger into your rectum, scoops out a stool sample and smears it on a slide to check for hidden blood.

But even though it's not enjoyable, many gynecologists across the country take the time to do this simple test during a pelvic exam. Early detection methods can help save lives. In fact, because of exams like this one, as well as other factors, deaths due to colon and rectal cancer—collectively known as colorectal cancer—are down 30 percent in women over the past 30 years.

Approximately 74,000 women will develop colorectal cancer this year, making it the second most common cancer in women. Twenty-eight thousand will die. But there are a number of things you can do to help reduce your risk.

Diet and Genetics

Although scientists still haven't figured out exactly what causes colorectal cancer, they have figured out what puts us at risk: "Ninety percent of colorectal cancer is diet-related, while 10 percent occurs in people with a clear-cut genetic predisposition," says Elin Sigurdson, M.D., Ph.D., a surgical oncologist at the Fox Chase Cancer Center in suburban Philadelphia and a researcher on the center's cancer prevention team.

Scientists suspect that diet and genetics may—separately or together—damage cells in a way that sets off the growth of small polyps along the intestinal tract.

Although not all polyps evolve into tumors, all tumors evolve from polyps, says Dr. Sigurdson. So anything that encourages their growth puts a person at risk for cancer.

Some people carry a family gene that triggers polyp formation, while others seem to experience their growth after exposure to free radicals—molecular fragments that are generated by everyone during the body's normal metabolism of dietary substances such as fat.

The theory is that in the colon, these molecular fragments damage genes that control cellular growth, says Dr. Sigurdson. Eventually, a cell's genes can receive so much damage that they no longer function normally, and the uncontrolled cellular growth that becomes cancer can begin.

That's why people who eat a lot of fat, a substance that releases free radicals, may also be at increased risk. A study of 375 women and 270 men at the University of North Carolina at Chapel Hill found that women who ate more than 77 grams of fat per day were more than twice as likely to develop precancerous polyps as those who ate less than 58 grams per day. What's more, a study of more than 88,000 women at Harvard Medical School revealed that women who ate beef, pork or lamb—all high in fat—every day were more than twice as likely to develop colon cancer as those who didn't.

Protect Yourself

Blood in a bowel movement is usually what sends most of us skittering to the doctor. And while it doesn't mean you have colorectal cancer, it is one of the earliest symptoms. Once colorectal cancer strikes, however, early detection can mean the difference between life and death, experts agree.

Ninety-two percent of those who have colon cancer surgically removed while it is still located in a single spot will still be alive five years from diagnosis, making this one of the more survivable cancers, reports the American Cancer Society.

Delayed treatment for rectal cancer has the same result. Eighty-five percent of those who have rectal cancer removed while it is still localized will still be alive five years from diagnosis. Only 51 percent of those who wait for treatment until the cancer spreads will be.

The only way to completely assure survival from colorectal cancer is to prevent it, says Dr. Sigurdson. And here are some ways.

CUT YOUR FAT CONSUMPTION IN HALF. Over the years researchers have noticed that there's a distinct correlation between the amount of colorectal cancer in a country and the amount of fat in the diet of its people, says Dr. Sigurdson. The more fat, the more cancer. The less fat, the less cancer.

The difference is so dramatic, she adds, that "you can go to a country where there's almost no fat in the diet and people don't get colon cancer."

That's why she and other researchers recommend that you abandon the normal American diet, which gets 40 percent of its calories from fat, and aim for a diet in which 15 to 20 percent of calories come from fat.

To get started, get yourself a good low-fat cookbook, avoid high-fat dairy products and check food labels for fat content, suggests Dr. Sigurdson. "It can be a real eye-opener when you realize how much fat is in that yogurt you eat every day for lunch."

BAN BOOZE. "Alcohol is bad," says Dr. Sigurdson. "Maybe it's because the martini crowd is also out eating high-fat steaks or maybe it's because alcohol is an oxidizing agent, but people who drink tend to have more colon cancer."

In a study of more than 15,000 women at Harvard Medical School, for example, researchers found that women who drank more than 30 grams of alcohol a day—the equivalent of two mixed drinks—had nearly double the risk of developing precancerous polyps as those who didn't imbibe at all.

GO FOR THE FIBER. "Fiber seems to have a protective effect on people who are predisposed to colorectal cancer," says gastroenterologist Marie Borum, M.D., assistant professor of medicine at Georgetown University School of Medicine in Washington, D.C.

It adds bulk to the stool and it helps absorb water. And that has three very helpful effects: It dilutes the concentration of any cancer-causing agents in the bowel, decreases the amount of time a potential carcinogen is in the bowel by speeding transit time through the bowel and increases the acidity of the colon, making it less hospitable to cancer-friendly bacteria.

"We generally try to say that you should get 25 grams of fiber into your diet every day," says Dr. Sigurdson. "But since the average North American eats between 2 and 5 grams a day, that's hard. It means eating an African-type diet of vegetables, legumes, beans and rice, with just a little bit of meat to add flavor."

SERVE YOURSELF FRUITS AND VEGGIES. Since fiber from fruits and vegetables has actually been more consistently related to a lower risk of colorectal cancer than fiber from grains, many experts feel that you should eat a balanced diet, but emphasize vegetables. The recommended combination is five servings of fruits and vegetables.

CRUNCH ON CRUCIFERS. Cruciferous vegetables—cabbage, broccoli, cauliflower and brussels sprouts, for example—all seem to activate naturally occurring enzymes in your body, says researcher Christine Szarka, M.D., a medical oncologist at Fox Chase Cancer Center. Those enzymes can actually neutralize cancer-causing substances that are activated by free radicals. Whether cooked or raw cruciferous vegetables are more potent isn't known.

Laboratory tests of crucifers have been so encouraging that human trials are now under way, says Dr. Szarka. At the Fox Chase Cancer Center, for example, high-risk individuals—such as those with a genetic predisposition to colorectal cancer—are being given tablets of crushed and dehydrated broccoli. Study participants take two 500-milligram tablets three times a day. When the study is completed, intestinal biopsies and other tests will reveal whether crucifers can in fact prevent the growth of precancerous polyps, as researchers suspect.

CONSIDER CALCIUM. "Calcium is another way to scavenge up free radicals," says Dr. Sigurdson. It binds to potentially cancer-causing agents and escorts them out of the body.

Good sources of calcium include broccoli, spinach and low-fat dairy products. You should get at least 1,000 milligrams a day, but 1,200 milligrams is recommended if you're pregnant and 1,500 if you're menopausal but not on estrogen replacement therapy.

TALK TO YOUR DOCTOR ABOUT ASPIRIN. "People who take aspirin seem to have a lower mortality from colorectal cancer," says Dr. Sigurdson. And in an American Cancer Society study of more than a million men and women, researchers found that the risk of colon cancer itself was reduced 42 percent in those who used aspirin 16 or more times a month for at least one year.

ASK FOR A CANCER SCREENING. Despite the vigilance of some gynecologists, physicians in general are less likely to check for colorectal cancer. And when they do check, says Dr. Borum, for some unknown reason, they're more likely to check men than women.

In a study of 110 women and 90 men, Dr. Borum found that rectal examinations were performed on 36 percent of the women and 57 percent of the men. Stool samples were checked for hidden blood in 11 percent of the women and 14 percent of the men. A sigmoidoscopy—the insertion of a flexible tube into the lower part of the bowel so the physician can check for polyps—was performed on 13 percent of the women and 29 percent of the men. Because 80 percent of colorectal cancer strikes after age 50, the American Cancer Society recommends that a rectal exam be performed annually after age 40 in both men and women. Stools should be checked for hidden blood beginning at age 50, and sigmoidoscopy should also be performed every three to five years from that age.

There are other conditions that raise your risk of colorectal cancer, says Dr. Borum. Women who have irritable bowel syndrome, Crohn's disease or ulcerative colitis should be screened by colonoscopy—an outpatient procedure in which your doctor can view the entire colon—with a barium enema ten years after they develop the disease. Women who have a family history of colorectal cancer should begin their screening five years before the age at which the relative developed cancer.

Some research shows women who have had gynecologic cancer (breast, uterine, cervical or ovarian) may be at increased risk for colorectal cancer. And women who have a family history of polyps may also be at increased risk for cancer.

HAVE PRECANCEROUS POLYPS REMOVED. Removing any polyps detected by sigmoidoscopy or colonoscopy will prevent them from evolving into cancer, says Dr. Sigurdson. The polyps can be removed painlessly during a colonoscopy.

Constipation

SO EASY TO AVOID

It's been days since your last bowel movement. Your head aches and you're feeling gassy. What's worse, you're bloated—as if there's a clogged drainpipe in your abdomen that's growing larger and larger.

Gulping down a quick mug of coffee, you slip on a loose-fitting dress and rush to the office.

On the way, you think about one of those fast-acting laxatives advertised on TV; that might get things moving. But the ladies room at the office is a little too public to deal with this kind of private problem—and besides that, there's just no time today to deal with constipation.

Maybe you should make time.

Giving your body ample time to have a bowel movement is as crucial in the battle against constipation as eating enough high-fiber foods, drinking plenty of fluids and getting exercise, says Susan Stewart, M.D., a gastroenterologist in New York City and associate medical director at Morgan Guaranty Trust.

A lot of us don't have much extra time, but we do have constipation. An estimated 50 million Americans get that all-blocked-up feeling at least once in a while. And 18 million people—12 million women and 6 million men—are bothered by this uncomfortable problem frequently.

In fact, constipation is something of a national obsession. In 1993 alone, Americans spent $740 million on over-the-counter laxatives.

The funny thing is, many laxative users may not need one at all. Doctors say too many of us have fallen for the myth that anything less than one bowel movement a day means we're constipated. It just isn't so.

When It's Really Constipation

"Regularity is different for everyone," says Dr. Stewart. "If a person has a well-formed stool, not too hard and not too watery, and they go just twice a week without pain or discomfort, I'm not going to worry about them.

"Then again, some people go twice a day. The important things are the comfort of the person and the form of the stool."

Bowel-movement frequency varies for many reasons, including age, diet and differences in your body's natural rhythms.

Constipation comes in two uncomfortable varieties: When relieving yourself is difficult or painful, with hard, dry feces, and when the urge to go is so infrequent—every three days or less—that you get that bloated, all-blocked-up feeling.

Doctors aren't sure why more women than men come to them with complaints about constipation. But factors that can leave you straining on the toilet include hormonal changes during the menstrual cycle, pregnancy, crash diets, depression and side effects from medicines such as antidepressants, codeine and iron and calcium supplements.

Any alteration in your daily routine, from not drinking enough fluids to changing the kind of food you eat to getting less exercise, can also cause it.

That's why many people become constipated while on vacation. Eating patterns change, and in exotic locales you may avoid the local water—not to mention those dirty restrooms. Your body may simply balk at using a different or unclean toilet. Even a public—or unfamiliar—restroom can cause your system to go on hold.

"The act of defecation is a conditioned reflex," says Henry D.

Janowitz, M.D., clinical professor emeritus of medicine and a consultant in gastroenterology at Mount Sinai School of Medicine in New York City and author of *Your Gut Feelings*. "Even if you travel and go to a hotel with a nice private bathroom, it might be hard to move the bowels. The long-established reflex that sets off normal bowel movements is being interrupted," he says.

Then there's the fast-forward pace of daily living.

"In some people, the intestinal tract is not a demand performer," says Dr. Stewart. "If you have one ideal time in the day to have a bowel movement and that time arises when you're on the train or walking through the subway station or talking to the boss, you may not get the urge to go again for another 24 hours."

FILLING UP ON FIBER

You can help prevent constipation by making high-fiber food choices at breakfast, lunch and dinner. Five servings of fresh fruits or vegetables a day plus six servings of whole-grain breads, cereals or legumes will give you the 25 grams of fiber recommended by the National Cancer Institute. Here are some great sources of fiber.

FOOD	PORTION	FIBER (G.)
General Mills Fiber One cereal	½ cup	13.0
Barley, pearled	½ cup	12.3
Pears, dried	5 halves	11.5
Health Valley Fruit & Fitness cereal	¾ cup	11.0
Kellogg's All-Bran cereal	⅓ cup	10.0
Nabisco 100% Bran cereal	½ cup	10.0
Blackberries	1 cup	7.2
Chick-peas	½ cup	7.0
Kidney beans	½ cup	6.9
Lima beans	½ cup	6.8
Refried beans, canned	½ cup	6.7
Black beans	½ cup	6.1

Ignore the call of nature long enough and you won't even notice it anymore. The result can be constipation.

When Constipation Is a Symptom

Chronic constipation can also signal something more serious than a changed bowel-movement schedule or unease with a different bathroom. It can be a symptom of irritable bowel syndrome or Hirschprung's disease, a rare condition in which key nerves in the colon that control the movement of feces through the bowels are lacking.

Researchers also see a link between sexual abuse and severe constipation. In some abuse survivors, pelvic muscles tighten during defecation instead of relaxing. "The harder they strain, the harder it is to evacuate,"

Food	Portion	Fiber (g.)
Raspberries	1 cup	6.0
Whole-wheat spaghetti	1 cup	5.4
Figs, dried	3 (about 2 oz.)	5.2
Lentils	½ cup	5.2
Succotash	½ cup	5.2
Post Raisin Bran cereal	¾ cup	5.0
Guava	1	4.9
Navy beans	½ cup	4.9
Artichoke hearts	½ cup	4.4
Pear	1	4.3
Oatmeal	½ cup	3.9
Raisins	½ cup	3.9
Wheat germ, toasted	¼ cup	3.7
Brussels sprouts	½ cup	3.4
Sweet potato	1	3.4
Orange	1	3.1
Apple	1	3.0

says Douglas A. Drossman, M.D., professor of medicine and psychiatry in the Division of Digestive Diseases and Nutrition at the University of North Carolina School of Medicine at Chapel Hill.

Such cases can be tough to treat, Dr. Drossman says. People with this condition may respond to biofeedback sessions that teach them how to relax specific muscles.

But for garden-variety constipation, the big four—fiber, fluids, exercise and time—usually spell relief, according to Steven Peikin, M.D., professor of medicine and director of gastroenterology at the University of Medicine and Dentistry of New Jersey, Robert Wood Johnson Medical School, Cooper Hospital/University Medical Center in Camden.

Fix It with Fiber

Fiber-rich foods such as fresh fruits, vegetables, grains and beans increase the bulk and water content of your stools. Bigger, wetter stools pass more quickly through the intestines, though doctors are not entirely sure why that is. The National Cancer Institute recommends getting 20 to 30 grams of fiber a day. But most of us eat highly refined foods—white bread instead of whole-wheat, for example, or a chocolate brownie instead of an apple—and get only about a third of the fiber we need every day.

"A high-fiber diet helps 90 percent of the people I see with constipation," says Dr. Peikin. "Our great-grandparents used to come back from grocery shopping with baskets full of fresh fruit and raw vegetables. Today it's processed food and fast food. We've lost the fiber. So you have to change the way you eat. And that can also mean changing the way your family eats, if you're cooking for other people."

A study of elderly patients at a Virginia nursing home found that most cut their laxative use by half or more after just four weeks on a high-fiber regimen combined with more fluids, exercise and scheduled time on the toilet. "If it works in older people, it should work even better in younger people," says Dr. Janowitz. That's because most younger people have better muscle tone and higher activity levels and are less laxative dependent.

Some doctors say fiber supplements such as Metamucil, Perdiem or others containing a high-fiber source like psyllium seeds are an acceptable way to boost your daily fiber intake. But the supplements have a downside, says Carol Walsh, R.D., a clinical dietitian at the University of California at San Diego Medical Center.

If your main source of fiber is a supplement, this can be a problem, says Walsh, because the supplement lacks nutrient content. Walsh suggests instead that you eat foods that are sources of nutrients as well as fiber.

As for laxatives, resist the quick fix. Stimulants such as Ex-Lax, Dulcolax and Fletcher's Castoria work by causing rhythmic, muscular contractions of the small or large intestine. Though they promise prompt relief, such laxatives can lead to dependency and can damage your bowels with repeated daily use.

If You Must Have a Laxative . . .

Ah, the temptation of the quick fix. With dozens of over-the-counter laxatives on sale in drugstores and supermarkets, you may be lured by promises of fast results if you're eager to get your bowels moving again. But beware: Strong laxatives can harm your intestines and with regular use even lead to dependency.

Laxatives should be taken cautiously and only as a last resort, says Henry D. Janowitz, M.D., clinical professor emeritus of medicine and a consultant in gastroenterology at Mount Sinai School of Medicine in New York City and author of *Your Gut Feelings*. "If you've been sick and taking a lot of pain medicines that make you constipated, that's an acceptable time for a laxative. But continual daily use on the assumption that you have to empty your bowels every day is not."

Here's a look at the types of over-the-counter laxatives on the drugstore shelf.

Osmotics, such as Phillips' Milk of Magnesia, make water stay in the intestines for easier bowel movements.

Stimulants use chemicals to prompt rhythmic contractions in the intestines. Active ingredients include phenolphthalein, used in Correctol and Ex-Lax; bisacodyl, used in Dulcolax; castor oil, used in Purge; and senna, found in Fletcher's Castoria.

Stool softeners, such as Colace, provide moisture to the stool and prevent excessive dehydration that makes stools dry, hard and painful to pass. These are sometimes prescribed after childbirth or surgery.

"Jump-starting" your bowels with harsh laxatives can eventually damage the colon, says Dr. Peikin. "You can end up with lazy bowel syndrome, where your intestines don't want to work anymore."

Preventing Constipation

Here are ways to put more fiber into your diet, as well as other tips for coping with constipation.

GO FOR FIVE A DAY. Have five servings a day of fresh fruits and vegetables and six servings of whole grains. Starting the day with a half-cup of high-fiber breakfast cereal and an apple can give you up to 16 grams of fiber. "You can also take dried fruit to work, make your sandwich for lunch with whole-grain bread, snack on a carrot and have some kidney beans with your dinner," suggests Walsh.

If all that fiber gives you gas, back off for a while and add fiber-filled foods more slowly.

WASH IT DOWN. Walsh counsels people to drink eight to ten eight-ounce glasses of fluids a day. "I would include water, juice and milk," she says. "But keep coffee or sodas or tea with caffeine to a minimum. Caffeine is a diuretic that can make you urinate more. And you need the water to bulk up all the fiber you're eating." Also, tea contains substances called tannins, which can cause constipation.

SKIP LOW-FIBER NO-NOS. Chocolate bars, cheese and other high-fat, no-fiber foods are notorious cloggers and can make you feel so full you don't reach for high-fiber choices. Eating lots of meat, refined sugar, pastries, candy and anything made with all white flour has the same effect, says Dr. Peikin.

MOVE IT. If you move, so will your bowels. Walk at least 20 minutes a day three times a week. "Any kind of aerobic activity, such as swimming or running or an aerobics class, seems to improve intestinal transit," says Dr. Drossman.

TAKE A TIME-OUT. Take advantage of the "gastrocolic reflex." Your best chance for having a bowel movement comes 20 to 30 minutes after a meal, when this reflex causes your bowels to start moving. Make sure you're sitting on the toilet then—even if you don't feel the call of nature. "Sitting on the toilet, even if you don't have the urge, may give your body the chance to sense that signal," says Dr. Peikin. "It's a way to retrain your bowels. People with constipation should do this no matter what. Unless you're in the most important board meeting of your career, excuse yourself."

BE PREPARED. Carry paper seat covers or a small can

of disinfectant in your purse if the cleanliness of public bathrooms is a concern. And don't be shy about using them.

"A lot of people wait till they're home," says Nancy Norton, founder of the International Foundation for Bowel Dysfunction, a support group based in Milwaukee. "They don't want to use a ladies' room. It's not pri-

DIVERTICULAR DISEASE: HOW TO KEEP IT AWAY

Back in the 1950s, a British surgeon, Denis P. Burkitt, M.D., discovered a startling link between bowel troubles and refined foods. Dr. Burkitt traveled to Africa, where digestive problems such as diverticular disease were practically unknown, and concluded that local diets high in fiber-rich whole grains, seeds and nuts kept such woes at bay.

"Dr. Burkitt actually weighed people's stools," says Steven R. Peikin, M.D., professor of medicine and director of gastroenterology at the University of Medicine and Dentistry of New Jersey, Robert Wood Johnson Medical School, Cooper Hospital/University Medical Center in Camden and author of *Gastrointestinal Health*. "And the stools of the people eating the high-fiber foods were much, much heavier."

They were bigger, too. And bigger stools, Dr. Peikin says, can prevent diverticulosis, the formation of small pouches in the walls of the intestines, and diverticulitis, inflammation of one or more of the pouches. If you have diverticulitis, you may have a fever and severe pain on the lower left side of your abdomen. The infection is treated with antibiotics, but more serious cases require a hospital stay and even surgery.

Diverticulosis is fairly common in people over 65 but gets its start at a younger age, Dr. Peikin says. "It's really only a problem if any of the pockets become inflamed. Eating high-fiber food can help keep that from happening."

What's the link between fiber, big stools and keeping diverticular disease at bay? Bulky stools are softer and take up more room in the colon. That reduces the pressure inside the colon that can force the pouches to form in the first place.

vate. But it's important to pay attention to the urge to defecate."

SWITCH YOUR CALCIUM SUPPLEMENT. "It's a well-known phenomenon that calcium carbonate can cause constipation," says Dr. Stewart. Try brands that use calcium phosphate and calcium citrate instead; they're available in most drugstores. Or drink orange juice that contains calcium. And don't forget calcium-rich foods such as dairy products, canned salmon with bones, oysters and greens such as collards, mustard and dandelion.

CHOOSE ANOTHER FORM OF IRON. If you suspect your iron supplement is to blame, consider the alternatives. Iron comes in three forms: as ferrous sulfate, ferrous fumarate and ferrous gluconate. Dr. Janowitz says none of these is considered less constipating, but different forms work best for different people. Or choose an iron-rich diet that includes lean beef, molasses, beans, raisins and dried apricots.

DRINK PRUNE JUICE. For a quick fix that works for nearly everyone, drink eight ounces of prune juice in the morning. "It's old-fashioned, but it gets results," Dr. Peikin says.

ADD A FIBER SUPPLEMENT. Also known as bulk-forming laxatives, products like Metamucil, FiberCon and Citrucel absorb water in the intestine and make stools softer. Always take them with at least eight ounces of water, says Dr. Peikin.

TRY A NATURAL UNCLOGGER. Ilana Goldman, M.D., a general practitioner specializing in holistic medicine at the Hoffman Center for Holistic Medicine in New York City, advises people who are constipated to take one to three tablets of magnesium citrate twice a day. "There's no toxicity," Dr. Goldman says. "Pregnant women can take it, too."

GIVE YOURSELF AN ENEMA. Using an enema bag or baby syringe that you can buy at the drugstore, squeeze about a quart of warm tap water into your rectum. The water makes the colon contract, starting a bowel movement. Enemas are safe, says Dr. Peikin, provided you stick with tap water or an over-the-counter enema liquid and keep the stream of water gentle.

SEE YOUR DOCTOR. Bleeding, abdominal pain or constipation that lasts more than three weeks are reasons to consult a physician. "When someone's been regular and all of a sudden they're constipated, especially over age 40, there is the potential for serious disease like cancer," says Dr. Peikin. Constipation can also lead to complications like hemorrhoids or anal fissures.

Depression

FIGHTING THROUGH THE DARKNESS

Betsy can't wake up. She smoked and paced until 4:00 in the morning and now, at 11:00 A.M., she's fast asleep.

Her children—Karen, 5, Kevin, 10, and Jennifer, 12—are used to being on their own. They know it's up to them to make breakfast, do dishes, let out the dog, get dressed and get to school. They know that they can't count on Mom a lot of the time. Dad is usually away on business, so there won't be that ride to the mall, that shoulder to cry on, that game of cards. And they know that, as much as she may love them, Mom often doesn't have the energy to show it. It's all because Betsy is too depressed.

Nearly 12 million American men and women like Betsy experience depression in one form or another every year. Women are twice as likely as men to get it, but they're also more likely to get rid of it, says Frederick K. Goodwin, M.D., former director of the National Institute of Mental Health in Bethesda, Maryland, and now director of the Center on Neuroscience Behavior and Society at George Washington University in Washington, D.C. That's because even though hormones and other biological factors, as well as cultural influences, make a woman more vulnerable to depression, her tendency to reach out to others and to seek professional help frequently gives her the resources to fight off the illness before it can become destructive.

"Men often get caught in the 'stiff upper lip' syndrome," says Dr. Goodwin. "Women don't. This is one of the reasons depressed men are

NINE HIDDEN REASONS YOU MAY BE DEPRESSED

As many as 61 percent of all people diagnosed with depression may actually be suffering from other problems in addition to the depression.

Here are nine commonly overlooked causes of depression in women. Consult your doctor if you believe any of them are causing your depression.

Prescription drugs. Side effects can include depression.

Oral contraceptives. Five to 10 percent of women stop using the Pill because of feelings of depression caused by synthetic hormones in the contraceptive, suggests Janice Peterson, M.D., associate clinical professor of psychiatry at the University of Colorado School of Medicine/Health Sciences Center in Denver.

Thyroid problems. About 10 to 15 percent of depressed people have some form of thyroid imbalance, according to Kimberly A. Yonkers, M.D., assistant professor of psychiatry and gynecology at the University of Texas Southwestern Medical Center at Dallas Southwestern Medical School. Symptoms include unexplained weight change, dry skin, hair loss, constipation, diminished sex drive and chronic fatigue.

Sunlight deficiency. Seasonal affective disorder (SAD)— caused by too little sunlight in fall and winter—can cause the

DEPRESSION

three to four times more likely to commit suicide than depressed women."

What's more, women of the so-called Baby Boom generation have an additional advantage when it comes to beating depression, adds Dr. Goodwin: their attitude. While the number of cases of depression in men and women has doubled in recent decades, the change in the roles and attitudes of women in this group is probably why the earlier three-to-one predominance of women in the depression statistics is now down to two women to every man.

"It's no coincidence that the change in women's depression coincides with a time in which women have more power in society, more independence, more autonomy, more control and more self-esteem

---

symptoms of classic depression, says Dr. Yonkers. Ask your doctor if light therapy would help you.

Poor nutrition. Deficiencies of iron, thiamin, selenium and magnesium may not cause clinical depression, but they certainly can cause your mood to take a nosedive, says Dr. Peterson.

Rapid-weight-loss diets. Depression may be a warning sign that you're pushing your diet too far, too fast, warns Dr. Peterson. Instead of crash dieting, eat balanced meals that include at least five servings of fruits, grains and vegetables daily.

Premenstrual syndrome. If you suffer from depression prior to or during your period, try eating at least one meal a day that is very high in complex carbohydrates, such as cornflakes, potatoes or pasta. Complex carbohydrates may boost brain levels of serotonin, a chemical that keeps your moods stable.

Menopause. Estrogen replacement therapy and antidepressant drugs may relieve the symptoms of menopausal depression. A woman's estrogen level drops at menopause, and some researchers theorize that this lack of estrogen might cause changes in other hormones or chemicals in the brain that affect mood, such as serotonin.

Postpartum depression. Women with a history of depression are particularly at risk for this condition, which is triggered by changing levels of reproductive hormones.

anchored in significant, meaningful, recognized achievement," says Dr. Goodwin.

These women have taken charge of their lives, he adds, and as a result, they're less likely to suffer from depression.

An Illness of the Brain

Most of us have experienced gloomy moods that may be lifted by a walk with the dog, an appointment with the hairdresser or a romp in the sheets. But real depression—what doctors refer to as clinical depression—is actually a serious illness caused by a genetic flaw in our brain's chemical "fight or flight" system, along with some heavy-duty stress.

"Clinical depression is no different from an illness of the heart or the pancreas except that the symptoms are mostly behavioral," says Dr. Goodwin.

Women who are depressed act in the grief-stricken way anyone acts when they've lost a job, moved away from a community or experienced the death of a loved one. "With any of these kinds of losses, people initially have intense sadness and little interest in anything," says Dr. Goodwin. "They are totally distracted from living. They feel helpless and hopeless, maybe even a little bit guilty for what they didn't do or could have done in a particular situation.

"They may also have some of the physical signs of depression—trouble sleeping, waking at night, heaviness in their arms and chest, loss of appetite. And they may get obsessive about things. People who are experiencing grief, for example, frequently try to contain their pain by focusing on small details of things, including the rituals of death—planning the funeral procession, arranging for a memorial service, ordering food for a wake.

"But the difference between a grief reaction and depression is that the grief reaction is time-limited in its severity," says Dr. Goodwin. "Even after a few days, a normal person will begin pulling out of her grief. She'll begin to look for distractions. She'll start dealing with the bank, the insurance and Social Security. She'll do what needs to be done."

On the other hand, a woman who is experiencing depression will frequently get worse. She'll become more withdrawn, negative thoughts will fill her mind, and she'll begin to blame herself for everything that goes wrong in her world.

"Trying to think will become like trying to walk through molasses," says Dr. Goodwin. "And her sadness will intensify into really psychic pain that goes on day after day, week after week, month after month."

The Descent into Darkness

Depression can be triggered by an event or a series of events that shakes people to their very core and makes them feel helpless, says Dr. Goodwin.

The death of a young child, learning you're infertile, losing a job—all these are major adult life stresses that can send women hurtling toward the darkness of depression.

But what determines who will actually drop into the abyss and who will not seems to be something of a family matter. No matter how "strong" you are as a person, no matter how take-it-on-the-chin you may be, whether or not you get depressed may depend less on your strength of character than on two things that are beyond your control: your genes and your childhood.

"Genetic vulnerability is the single biggest predictor of who is going to get clinically depressed and who is not," says Dr. Goodwin. "The brain mechanisms that go awry in depression are the ones programmed by the brain to control the so-called fight-or-flight reaction." In someone who's vulnerable to depression, the genetic program is flawed. It has no brakes. So once some stressful event triggers the fight-or-flight reaction, there's nothing to turn it off. The result is a woman who can feel restless, edgy, irritated, depressed and exhausted, all at the same time.

The second biggest predictor of depression is whether a person had a profound childhood experience such as physical or sexual abuse, the death of a parent or perhaps even just a parent who wasn't emotionally able to meet the child's needs. Scientists are still trying to figure out all the different types of loss that might make women more susceptible to depression, says Dr. Goodwin.

But complicating the issue of who does and does not become depressed are a woman's biology and her hormones.

Biologically, we have the capacity for a more powerful fight-or-flight reaction than men do, says Dr. Goodwin. That's because ounce for ounce, we can pour out far more adrenal hormones—the major fight-or-flight chemicals—than any testosterone-loaded male.

As for our hormones, estrogen and progesterone attach themselves to sensitive tissues in the brain, Dr. Goodwin says. But the levels of these hormones are always changing—most dramatically in puberty, at the onset of menstruation, immediately after childbirth and after menopause.

That may be why we hear so much about "adolescent melancholy," "postpartum blues" and "empty nest syndrome." Women's hormones do not cause depression, says Dr. Goodwin, but they do exacerbate any underlying genetic vulnerability.

En Garde

Although a woman's biology and hormones combine to put her at increased risk for depression, mild episodes of depressive illness can actually be prevented before they get out of control and turn her life upside down.

The key is to recognize the fact that you're beginning to feel depressed before the disease actually drags you under, says Gillian Kaplin Adams, M.D., a family physician in Baltimore who has studied depression. And here's how she suggests you do it.

WATCH FOR CLUES. One of the first warnings of depression is a change in how you think and feel about your world. So watch yourself for sweeping generalizations in which everything's fine or everything's awful and nothing's in between, says Dr. Adams.

"I should" and "I should not" statements—as in "I shouldn't have yelled at my son" or "I shouldn't have had that cherry pie"—are also red flags that your thinking is beginning to be affected by depression. Most people would say "I wish I hadn't yelled at Joe" or "I wish I hadn't had that cherry pie." So if you constantly find "I shoulds" popping up in your conversation, it may be a signal that you're becoming depressed.

Other clues: all-or-nothing condemnations ("I'm always wrong"), minimizing your successes ("It wasn't anything"), magnifying other people's successes ("That presentation was so terrific no else will ever match it"), negative labeling ("I'm a loser") or using emotional reasoning in which your feelings become facts and the real facts don't matter ("I feel that you're having an affair, so don't bother telling me you're not.").

LISTEN TO FRIENDS. When friends start to say things like "Gee, you seem down," or "Have you lost weight?" or "Why haven't you called?" or "We haven't seen you for a while," there's a good chance that you're falling into depression, says Dr. Adams.

TUNE IN TO YOUR FEELINGS. Once a day, sit down, tune in to how you feel and write it down in a diary, says Dr. Adams. Then periodically check the diary for the symptoms of depression. When you start to see that you're feeling increasingly restless, tired, hopeless, worthless, guilty, sad and/or irritable, schedule an appointment with your doctor.

Staving It Off

Studies indicate that 80 percent of women who have one bout of depression will have another. So once you suspect you're beginning to get depressed, says Dr. Adams, try to prevent the illness from taking hold with these strategies.

EXERCISE. "A lot of people who are getting depressed feel incredibly tired," says Dr. Adams, so they may not feel like using what they think is their last bit of energy to exercise.

"But I find that if they can just get out and get going, they really end up feeling better." Experts don't know why exercise helps, but they do know that it can boost production of endorphins—chemicals in the brain that make us feel pleasure and fend off pain. It doesn't matter what kind of exercise you do, Dr. Adams says. Walking, biking, swimming or anything else is fine.

SET A REALISTIC GOAL. One way to get up and moving is to set achievable goals, says Dr. Adams. With exercise, for example, you can decide to walk a half-mile a day for the first week, three-quarters of a mile for the second week and a mile for the third. Set a slightly harder goal each week until you're working out for a minimum of 20 to 30 minutes three times a week.

REWARD YOURSELF. "Don't take the little things lightly," says Dr. Adams. Once you reach whatever goal you've set, pat yourself on the back and treat yourself to something special.

BREAK OUT OF ISOLATION. Friends can save your life, says Dr. Adams. Tell your friends that whenever they suspect you're isolating yourself from the world, they should come over and drag you out to dinner, a movie, a park, a play, a walk—anything at all. Afterward they should point out what a good time you had.

STAY AWAY FROM ALCOHOL AND NICOTINE. Alcohol can literally throw you into depression by depressing the central nervous system, while nicotine, which accelerates your heart rate, can aggravate that jittery, edgy feeling some women get right before or during a depressive episode, says Dr. Goodwin.

GET COUNSELING. "Regular psychotherapy in which women come to understand where the depression is coming from and whether it's related to how they deal with life is important," says Dr. Adams. Therapy can uncover both past and present problems that may be contributing to your illness—an abusive parent, a domineering spouse or a destructive work environment. And once you've identified anything that exacerbates your vulnerability to depression, you're on the way to blocking its effects. If you don't know of any therapists, ask your family doctor for a recommendation.

Defeating Depression

Among people who go for help, 80 percent may be successfully treated, says Dr. Goodwin. Mild to moderate depression usually responds to a short, six- to eight-week course of focused therapy and/or medication. Moderate to severe depression generally requires medication, often in combination with brief psychotherapy.

Most drugs used to treat depression fall into one of three groups: monoamine oxidase inhibitors (Nardil), tricyclic antidepressants (Ludiomil) or serotonin uptake inhibitors (Prozac). All manipulate levels of brain chemicals to bring your mood back to its normally balanced state. One of the most popular—and controversial—drugs is Prozac, which makes more serotonin, the calming chemical messenger, available to your brain. The controversy stems from the fact that the drug is such an effective mood elevator that some doctors are at times prescribing it for people who simply want more upbeat personalities.

"In women who have moderate to severe depression, 65 percent will respond to the first drug they're given," says Dr. Goodwin. "That is, over the course of about four to six weeks they will return essentially to normal. But not everybody will respond to the same drug. It's like antibiotics. Some people will respond to one, others to something else. So if you don't respond to one medication, it's important not to give up but to go to a second drug. In this case, the rate of success of the second drug can reach 85 percent.

"The 15 percent who are still depressed may respond partially, so they're not as depressed as they were. But this 15 percent also includes women who have chronic life situations—a lousy marriage, being in a self-defeating situation at work or substance abuse—that's complicating treatment."

Even in this situation, however, the medication will frequently relieve enough symptoms so that the woman can mobilize some energy.

"The drug isn't going to fix a woman's life," says Dr. Goodwin. "But it can restore her capacity to deal with it."

Dermatitis
THE IRRITATION THAT SHOWS

Chances are you've had it.

Maybe you're a full-time mom, a chef or an artist, and you're up to your elbows every day in soapy water. Or maybe you work in a hospital and wear latex gloves when you treat patients. Or maybe you try a new cosmetic every now and then, wear jewelry or take diuretics. Or you exercise, perm your hair or brush your teeth.

If you do any of these things, you may have had dermatitis, a red, rashlike inflammation that occurs when your skin gets irritated or when you're allergic to something.

Dermatitis is so common, in fact, that most people get it at some point or another, says Elizabeth Whitmore, M.D., clinical director of dermatology at Johns Hopkins University in Baltimore. The most common type is irritant dermatitis, she says, which usually appears as a patch of rough, red, cracked skin. Generally more women than men get this type of dermatitis because we tend to do more "wet work," says Dr. Whitmore.

Another type of dermatitis is allergic contact dermatitis, with nickel allergy being a common cause in women. That's primarily because of the nickel posts commonly used in inexpensive pierced earrings. An estimated 10 percent of women have nickel allergy, compared to 1 percent of men. Allergic contact dermatitis generally appears as a patch of tiny red bumps that itch. Both types of dermatitis may range from mild to severe.

It's Tough to Avoid—But You Can

Because our lives are full of situations that can trigger dermatitis, it seems we are constantly playing roulette with our skin.

But there are ways to prevent dermatitis. The first step is to identify what factors cause problems for you. Then do your best to avoid these things and protect your skin. Finally, there are some things you can do to take better care of your skin and make it less susceptible to dermatitis. Here are some suggestions.

WATCH OUT FOR SOAP AND WATER. Hand dermatitis from overexposure to water and detergents is what dermatologists see most in women, says Dr. Whitmore. It appears quite often in 25- to 40-year-old women who've left their careers to be home with their children and constantly have their hands in water, adds Marianne O'Donoghue, M.D., associate professor of dermatology at Rush Presbyterian–St. Luke's Medical Center in Chicago.

So whenever possible, wear gloves when taking the plunge, and put on moisturizer afterward. If your hands are already irritated, wear a cotton liner inside the vinyl gloves, says Dr. Whitmore. *Never* do your dishes without gloves, and make sure you put them on when working with foods in the kitchen, says Dr. O'Donoghue.

BE GENTLE WITH THE SOAP. When it comes to dermatitis, all soaps and dishwashing liquids are not the same, experts say. Choose milder soaps such as Dove, Tone and Oil of Olay Beauty Bar, says Karen K. Deasey, M.D., attending dermatologist at Bryn Mawr Hospital in Pennsylvania. And reconsider your dishwashing liquids, too. Dawn and Joy can be on the harsh side; try Dove instead, she says.

HOLD ON TO THE BAR. If you have a choice between liquid and bar soap, go for the bar, says Dr. O'Donoghue. "The latest rage is these pump soaps. But with the exception of Dove, liquid soaps are more drying," she says.

CONSIDER YOUR COSMETICS. If you develop dermatitis on your face, you may be allergic to your makeup. Usually it's fragrances or preservatives that cause the reaction, says Dr. O'Donoghue. Also, she says, "it's usually not the foundation that is so much of a problem as the moisturizer you use." Consider hypoallergenic products such as Clinique, Neutrogena, Almay and Allercreme, experts say. If you think you have a problem with fragrances, look for labels that read "fragrance-free," says Dr. Whitmore. Products marked "unscented" usually contain a "masking" fragrance to cover up the natural smell of the product.

SAY NO TO NICKEL. If you develop a rash in an area where you've worn jewelry, it may be an allergic reaction to nickel. Ask retailers about the content of the jewelry you buy, and be aware that studs in jeans, belt buckles and clasps on bras may also contain nickel.

BEWARE THE TOOTHPASTE CONNECTION. Do you often have fine red bumps or a blotchy red rash around your mouth? It might be what doctors call peri-oral dermatitis. "We're tending to see this quite a bit in women," says Thomas Helm, M.D., a dermatologist in Williamsville, New York, and assistant professor of dermatology at the State University of New York at Buffalo. The cause? It might be something as simple as tartar-control toothpaste, says Dr. Helm. Try switching to a nontartar toothpaste and give the rash a couple of weeks to clear up, says Dr. Helm. If it doesn't go away by then, your doctor may prescribe antibiotics.

NAIL IT DOWN. Hand dermatitis sometimes occurs when women have allergic reactions to the glue used for fake nails, says Dr. O'Donoghue. To prevent it, try a patch test, applying a small sample of glue on your skin first to see if it reacts.

PRETEST YOUR PERM. Common causes of dermatitis at the hairline are chemicals in permanent solutions and hair dyes. Again, you can head off this type of allergic dermatitis by patch-testing yourself with the solution or by asking your hair stylist to do so. If you're doing the test yourself, home kits usually have instructions on the box.

BE A GOOD SPORT. Some exercise equipment contains materials that trigger allergic contact dermatitis. Things that can be troublesome include the rubber additives in tennis shoes, masks and mouthpieces, swim caps, swim goggles, diving suits, nose clips, earplugs and swim fins. Athletic tape can also be a problem for people allergic to formaldehyde resins. Also, some of the over-the-counter ointments used for sore muscles contain menthol and methyl salicylate, which can cause allergic dermatitis. So if you have a rash in an area that one of these products touches, consider finding an alternative.

LOOK OUT FOR LATEX. Those innocuous rubber gloves—and even condoms—can cause dermatitis if you're allergic. You may want to try gloves or condoms that are not made of latex.

PAY ATTENTION TO CREAMS AND OINTMENTS. Topical anesthetics like benzocaine (found in some sunscreens, insect bite ointments and hemorrhoidal creams) and neomycin can sometimes cause dermatitis, according to Metta Lou Henderson, Ph.D., professor of pharmacy at the Raabe College of Pharmacy at Ohio Northern University in Ada.

WATCH THE SUN AND YOUR CYCLE. Women with premenstrual syndrome who take a diuretic before their periods may develop dermatitis if they get too much sun. Cover up with sunscreen, Dr. Henderson advises.

CONSIDER YOUR PATCH. If you wear an estrogen or nicotine patch and develop dermatitis in that area, the patch may be the cause. Consult your doctor.

What to Do When You Get It

Besides avoiding things that may trigger dermatitis, you may also do the following to prevent it or ease the discomfort of a flare-up.

KEEP SKIN MOIST. Keeping your skin well-lubricated is the key to preventing dermatitis. "It's the one thing most people get lazy about. Women often don't look after their skin enough," says Dr. O'Donoghue. Remember to apply your lotion immediately after a bath or shower to trap the moisture, experts say. For severe dermatitis, many doctors recommend Vaseline Pure Petroleum Jelly, Nivea, Eucerin, Neutrogena Hand Lotion or Aquaphor.

MAKE IT LOTION, LOTION EVERYWHERE. Buy several bottles of your favorite moisturizer and place each one in a different location so you'll remember to use it often. "I tell my patients to put one bottle beside the bed, another by the phone, another in the kitchen, one by the sofa and one by their favorite reading chair," says Dr. O'Donoghue.

TRY OTCs. If you develop a patch or two of dermatitis, try 1 percent hydrocortisone cream, which is available over the counter. "If it's really dry, try the ointment over the cream," says Dr. O'Donoghue. "It's a nice way to start." If OTCs don't do the trick for you, consult your dermatologist.

Diabetes

The Threat You Can Prevent

You sit all day at a desk. You ride home in a car or bus. Then you sit some more. In fact, the only time you get any exercise is on the way to bed—if your bedroom is upstairs.

Guess who's a possible candidate for diabetes?

If you're a woman whose lifestyle is so inactive that cleaning the house is an indoor sport and running for the bus an Olympic event, you could be putting yourself at risk for diabetes, and it could show up between age 30 and 45.

More than seven million American women have diabetes, about the same number as men. Five to 10 percent have Type I, or insulin-dependent, diabetes, an inherited disease in which the immune system attacks the pancreas and destroys its ability to make insulin, the hormone that transports sugar from food to your body's cells. This type of diabetes usually appears sometime in childhood or adolescence, but it also occurs in adults.

The remaining 90 percent have Type II, or non-insulin-dependent, diabetes, a disease in which the body cannot use all the insulin it produces. Type II has genetic roots, but it's often triggered in women by too much testosterone, the male sex hormone, or a sedentary lifestyle.

Testosterone is not a factor in the development of Type II diabetes in men, studies indicate, but high levels of it seem to double or even triple the risk among women. What's more, a study of 165 women at the University of Texas Health Sciences Center in San Antonio revealed that the more testosterone a woman's body produces, the more likely she is to develop diabetes.

At least half of the women with Type II diabetes don't know they have it, experts say. This is because its development can be insidious. Women can have vague Type I symptoms, such as unusual thirst, extreme hunger or frequent urination, before showing Type II symptoms, which can include blurry vision, frequent infections, cuts and bruises that are slow to heal or tingling or numbness in the hands or feet. The warnings are often so subtle that even doctors can overlook them. Also, some blood tests used to identify the disease frequently fail to detect it.

This failure can be dangerous, since a woman with diabetes has 6 times the risk of heart attack as a woman who does not have it. She also has nearly 20 times the risk of kidney failure, nearly 5 times the risk of stroke and 3 times the risk of death.

Metabolic Mayhem

Diabetes is a disease that forces your body to starve when it's full of food.

Normally your body takes last night's dinner or this morning's breakfast and turns it into a sugar called glucose. Then it dumps the glucose into your blood, where it teams up with insulin secreted by your pancreas. The insulin carries glucose into your muscles and organs, where it provides the energy for everything you do.

A drop in available insulin or the body's resistance to using that insulin can cause metabolic mayhem. With diabetes, glucose builds up in the bloodstream because it's unable to gain admission to muscles and organs. It wears on the heart, kidneys and eyes and then it flows into the bladder and passes out of the body—leaving behind damaged organs starved for fuel.

Left too long in this situation, the body powers down: Symptoms you may have attributed to stress or growing older can, if unheeded, escalate into the complications of diabetes—heart disease, stroke, blindness or kidney failure.

How to Cut Your Risk

Both forms of diabetes can be treated with a smorgasbord of custom-tailored diets, exercise, insulin injections and other medications. But these treatment strategies sometimes fail to prevent the degenerative problems that go with diabetes.

That's why prevention is so important, says Maureen Harris, M.D., Ph.D., director of the National Diabetes Data Group at the National Institutes of Health in Washington, D.C. Here's what you can do.

GET AN EARLY WARNING. Type II diabetes doesn't emerge as a full-blown problem overnight, says Wendy Kohrt, Ph.D., research assistant professor of medicine at Washington University in St. Louis. It generally evolves over a period of years and can be detected in its earliest stages by a blood test that reveals whether your body is beginning to have trouble using insulin.

LOSE WEIGHT. "The higher your weight, the higher your risk of diabetes," says Richard Hamman, M.D., Ph.D., professor of preventive medicine at the University of Colorado School of Medicine in Boulder. "If you're 150 percent of your ideal body weight, your risk is probably three to four times higher than normal. If you're 200 percent of your ideal body weight, your risk is probably six to eight times higher than normal."

But you especially need to lose weight if your body is shaped like an apple—thick in the middle—he adds. Why? Because "the fat in that region is different from other fat in two respects. First, it's metabolically more active, which means it's stored and mobilized more readily," says Dr. Kohrt. Second, that fat is in an area drained by a major vein that picks up the fat's metabolic by-products and takes them to the liver. There they give the liver a false message—that fat is being mobilized because the body is starving. But the liver doesn't know the message is false, so it responds by churning out an emergency ration of glucose into the bloodstream.

"That begins a vicious cycle that just keeps going," says Dr. Kohrt. More glucose in the blood makes the pancreas dump in more insulin. More insulin causes the liver to generate more glucose. More glucose makes the pancreas dump more insulin. Eventually the whole system breaks down, says Dr. Kohrt. Your body will either shut down insulin

(continued on page 146)

WHEN PREGNANCY'S THE PROBLEM

Pregnancy is a time of great adjustment for a woman and her body. Raging hormones cause nausea, fatigue, physical change and an abundance of emotions—all part of a healthy, normal pregnancy. But these same hormones can bring on diabetes in a woman who has never before been diabetic. This condition is known as gestational diabetes.

When a woman has gestational diabetes, one of the hormones affected by pregnancy is insulin, according to Helen Kay, M.D., a specialist in maternal/fetal medicine and associate professor of obstetrics and gynecology at Duke University in Durham, North Carolina. Insulin is produced by the pancreas and influences the way your body absorbs blood sugar, or glucose.

Normally, your digestive system converts food into glucose and sends it into the bloodstream, while insulin helps it get into cells to power the body. When a pregnant woman has gestational diabetes, however, the fetus takes the glucose from its mother's bloodstream, leaving high levels of insulin behind.

High levels of insulin trigger a reaction: The mother's body "reads" that high insulin concentration as a sign of too much glucose and then responds by producing even more insulin. With lots of insulin and little glucose, the result is a diabetic state.

The mother's diabetes also affects the newborn, notes Yvonne S. Thornton, M.D., professor of clinical obstetrics and gynecology at Columbia University College of Physicians and Surgeons in New York City and director of perinatal diagnostic testing at Morristown Memorial Hospital in New Jersey. All babies have a drop in blood sugar after birth, but in babies born to diabetic mothers, the drop is far more severe. "When you cut that umbilical cord at birth, then—boom!—you're significantly decreasing the glucose flow to the baby," says Dr. Thornton. "That's when you have babies with dangerously low blood sugar."

Women who develop gestational diabetes have different risks than women with diabetes who become pregnant. Those who develop diabetes *during* pregnancy tend to have chubbier babies and a higher incidence of unexplained stillbirths. They are also at greater risk for developing pregnancy-related high blood pressure, a condition known as preeclampsia.

Women with diabetes who *become* pregnant, on the other hand, tend to have smaller babies. They have greater risk of birth defects and maternal and fetal death.

Here are some ways to minimize the chances of developing gestational diabetes, or reduce its effects.

EAT FOR ONE. "The woman who starts to gain a lot of weight is more inclined to develop gestational diabetes," says Dr. Thornton. "The American College of Obstetrics and Gynecology says you should gain around 35 pounds. But I'll tell you, if you aim for 25, you'll gain 35." Despite the old story about eating for two, you really need only 300 extra calories a day through the second trimester and 500 in the third.

EAT BEANS. Studies indicate that folic acid, a nutrient that all women need, may prevent the neural tube defects that can occur when diabetes is uncontrolled, says Dr. Kay. (Researchers have found that folic acid helps prevent the overall incidence of spinal defects in the fetus, whether or not the woman has diabetes.) Good sources are beans; ½ cup will give you more than half of the Recommended Dietary Allowance for pregnant women, which is 400 micrograms a day.

GET TESTED. Ask your obstetrician to test you for diabetes between the 24th and 28th weeks of pregnancy, says Dr. Kay. Usually you'll be asked to drink a glucose solution that tastes like "a flat cola," then you'll be given a blood test to measure glucose levels an hour later. If that test shows high levels of glucose, you'll be asked to come back for a second test that measures glucose levels over a three-hour period.

EXERCISE TIGHT CONTROL. If your glucose level is high, your doctor or nutritionist will probably prescribe the American Diabetes Association diet in an attempt to control it, says Dr. Thornton. "If the diet fails and your blood sugar remains high, you'll have to get insulin injections three or four times a day and follow the diet."

production or the muscles and organs will refuse to accept it. Either way, you've got diabetes.

CUT DIETARY FAT. As you start to lose weight, pay particular attention to the amount of fat in your diet, says Dr. Hamman. That's because, independent of its effect on weight, dietary fat seems to increase the risk of diabetes.

Doctors and other experts recommend that you limit your daily diet to less than 30 percent of calories from fat. You can aim for this by limiting your intake of meat, always removing skin from poultry, avoiding processed foods and drinking low-fat milk. (For more tips on following a low-fat lifestyle, see page 393.)

WOMAN TO WOMAN A DISEASE THAT LASTS A LIFETIME

Kate Sullivan is a mother and part-time public affairs officer for the National Kidney Foundation in Philadelphia. She has lived with Type I (insulin-dependent) diabetes since she was born. This is her story.

You know, there is absolutely no aspect of my life, no memory, that isn't completely permeated by this disease.

Diabetes was in my consciousness from before I was really able to think. And I suspect it's influenced me in a number of ways because so much of the disease is a minute-to-minute type of management. If you're out of control there's always the chance that you could lapse into a coma—you know, the ten-seconds-from-now-you-could-be-dead kind of thing.

My mother started giving me the responsibility for handling the disease when I was about eight years old. I remember the first time that I tried to give myself an insulin shot. I really had to sit there and kind of psych myself into it. And this was just injecting into the top of my leg, which isn't really a big deal. But it was very difficult.

I know I found the routine of having to test my urine and record it on a little colored chart extremely tedious and I cheated as often as I possibly could get away with it. I think every kid in the world does.

Long before blood-testing and even before they came up with those handy little dipsticks for urine testing, we used a little chemistry set with little glass test tubes and these little tablets that would dissolve in water. They came in little foil packets. You had to put so many drops of urine and

GET PHYSICAL. "Women who are sedentary probably have a 25 to 40 percent increased risk of diabetes compared to women who are more active at the same weight," Dr. Hamman says.

"Active is walking to the corner grocery rather than driving," Dr. Kohrt says. "It's taking the dog for a one- or two-mile walk instead of putting him outside in a fenced-in yard. It's going up three or four flights of steps rather than taking elevators." It's doing these things every day.

The result? "If you have a 180-pound woman who loses weight—I mean down to her ideal weight, which is very hard to do—maintains it, decreases her dietary fat and increases her physical activity, I suspect she would cut her diabetes risk fivefold," says Dr. Hamman.

---

so many drops of water into the test tube, then put the little pill in and watch the whole thing fizz up and watch for what color it turned.

I also had a metal needle that attached to a glass syringe which came apart. Every morning we boiled all three parts inside a strainer which was inside a saucepan on the stove.

What kept me doing it?

We had a neighbor who lived around the corner who had diabetes. He was minus a foot. And through the years gangrene started to claim parts of his leg. So every time I would see him, you know, he would have less of one leg. And my mother kept saying, "Well, that's a diabetic just like you." You want to talk about keeping a little kid in line?

I mean, I want to live. I don't want to forever be the kid with her nose pressed up against the candy store window looking at the kids inside.

It's only as I've become an adult and looked back on this that I realize that my generation is really the first generation to survive—to get not only to adulthood but to start to get into some of the problems that the middle-aged and aging population normally face. Before, doctors never had to worry about diabetes and heart disease because diabetics never got old. So it's our observations and our experiences that are going to form the body of information for the generation that comes behind us. It's scary because there's no blueprint.

On the other hand, thank God I'm in this generation and not the one before it.

Diarrhea
FINDING THE CAUSE IS THE CURE

Yesterday's picnic was perfect—volleyball, close friends and an awesome feast sparkling in the hot summer sun. The potato salad tasted just like Mom's, down to the mayonnaise and celery seed dressing. No wonder you splurged on seconds.

And no wonder you're sidelined today, shuffling wearily between bathroom and bed, your bowels in an uproar. Your normally well-behaved intestines are a raging river. You call in sick at the office, then heed the gurgling down below and stumble back to the toilet, a prisoner of diarrhea.

The National Institutes of Health in Washington, D.C., estimate that Americans endure 99 million bouts of the runs every year, caused by everything from tainted drinking water to improperly handled food—like the potato salad that sat too long in the sun—to forgetting to wash your hands after changing a dirty diaper.

Add a host of other factors—including travel abroad, stress, lactose intolerance, antibiotics, antacids, caffeine and artificial sweeteners such as Sorbitol—and the number of cases soars well beyond the 100 million mark.

Women and men seem equally disposed to getting diarrhea, defined by doctors as three or more loose bowel movements a day. But researchers note that women are exposed more often to one of the most notorious transmitters of the germs and viruses that cause infectious diarrhea: little kids. One study found that parents of young children in day care were 10 to 25 percent more likely to "catch" the runs from their little ones than parents whose children weren't in day care. And doctors say day care workers face higher risks, too.

"Day care nurseries are a real problem for diarrheal disease," says Ralph Giannella, M.D., professor of medicine and director of the Division of Digestive Diseases at the University of Cincinnati College of Medicine. "You have small children who are not yet toilet-trained. They can pass bacteria or viruses to other kids and to day care workers, who are usually women. Then at home, it's usually mothers who take care of the children, changing the diapers."

Nurses and aides in nursing homes are in the same boat. "These people are usually women, and they're dealing with patients who cannot take care of their own bowels," Dr. Giannella says.

The best defense?

"Wash your hands," says Randall Reves, M.D., associate professor of medicine in the Division of Infectious Diseases at the University of Colorado Health Science Center in Denver. "The ability to get your hands thoroughly clean is the most effective way to prevent the spread of infectious diarrhea—to yourself or anybody else."

Coping When You're Out of Commission

A typical run-in with the runs lasts just two to three days and doesn't merit a trip to the doctor's office. Chances are it's a viral or bacterial infection, and the volumes of watery stool you're seeing are the result of toxins given off by the bug invading your bowels. The toxins stick to the walls of the intestine, making cells there secrete massive amounts of fluid.

While you're lying low, doctors suggest the following tips to help your body weather the thunderstorm in your gut.

DRINK UP. Restoring lost fluids is vital for avoiding dehydration, which can lead to weakness and dizziness. Drink plenty of water or juice, but avoid coffee, tea, colas and other caffeinated drinks. Caffeine is a diuretic and will actually pull water out of your system.

"You have to replace the fluid you're losing," says Sidney F. Phillips, M.D., professor of medicine and director of gastroenterology research at the Mayo Clinic's Gastroenterology Unit in Rochester, Minnesota. "If the problem is a prolonged one, say in the two- to three-day range, or if the infectious process produces nausea or vomiting, then fluids that contain some salt and sugar, like Gatorade, are a good idea. They help replace electrolytes."

Or consider a commercial oral rehydration solution (ORS), available as a powder to mix with water or as a ready-to-use drink. These solutions are tailor-made to replace sugar, salts and other nutrients flushed from the system during diarrhea.

BEATING THE *TURISTA* TRAP

If you're traveling abroad, consider this: Four out of every ten Americans who venture outside the United States for business or pleasure get a little something extra—traveler's diarrhea. The usual culprit is a type of bacteria called *Escherichia coli*, a germ that lives in water and on certain foods.

Robert Salata, M.D., clinical director of infectious diseases at Case Western Reserve Hospital and medical director of the Travelers Health Care Center at University Hospitals, both in Cleveland, gives some basic precautions.

STICK WITH SAFE DRINKS. Only bottled water, soda or juice—with unbroken seals around the caps—or steaming hot coffee and tea can be considered free of bacteria that cause diarrhea. Send back any drink that arrives with ice cubes—the ice was most likely made with contaminated water.

TURN OFF THE TAP. Brush your teeth with mouthwash or bottled water instead of tap water, Dr. Salata suggests.

LEAVE THE LETTUCE ALONE. Leafy vegetables were probably washed in contaminated water and should not be eaten. Ask for fruits and vegetables that can be peeled—and make sure you do the peeling.

MAKE IT WELL-DONE. Order meat cooked through—

"An ORS will keep you feeling better and may even help you avoid hospitalization for dehydration," says Dr. Giannella. "If the diarrhea lasts more than a day and you can't eat any regular food, I would definitely use it. Adults resist trying this, because they think only children or old people or those living in poor countries need them. But we can all benefit."

EAT, BUT LIGHTLY. High-fiber foods, grease and five-alarm spices will only make matters worse in your sensitive gut. Stick with easily digestible fare like white rice, dry toast, applesauce and clear soups or broths.

"The intestine will get a little boost in its function if there are some carbohydrates or simple starches," says Dr. Phillips. "Rice starch is usually thought to be one of the most digestible. And the dry toast; it's just like the dry crackers our grandmothers told us to eat when we were sick."

---

don't accept it if it's rare or even pink in the middle.

KEEP OFF THE STREET. Street vendors offer romantic local color, but their wares may harbor local bacteria.

TAKE YOUR MEDICINE IN ADVANCE. Taking two Pepto-Bismol tablets four times a day has been shown to reduce the risk of getting diarrhea by 70 percent, Dr. Salata says. Side effects can include ringing in the ears and a black tongue, but Dr. Salata says he recommends it for trips of up to two weeks.

BE PREPARED FOR TROUBLE. Ask your doctor for an antibiotic prescription—ciprofloxacin (Cipro) and norfloxacin (Noroxin) are commonly used—that you can fill in advance. Take along an over-the-counter anti-diarrheal drug such as Imodium or the prescription drug Lomotil (available over the counter in some states) to take with the antibiotic. Once diarrhea starts, these drugs work faster than Pepto-Bismol does, Dr. Salata says. And pack some powdered oral rehydration solution to mix with bottled water.

MONITOR YOUR HEALTH. High fever, blood or mucus in the stool and very, very frequent diarrhea, like two to three stools or more an hour, can be cholera. Blood in the stool can signal dysentery. "You must see a doctor immediately," Dr. Salata says.

SKIP DAIRY PRODUCTS. Your diarrhea might be the result of the sudden onset of lactose intolerance—when your stomach lacks the enzyme that digests milk sugar. If that's the case, unabsorbed liquid will back up in your intestines. Avoiding most dairy products—milk, ice cream and most cheeses—could turn the tide, says Dr. Giannella. But follow this advice even if you know you don't have this condition, because your body becomes somewhat lactose-intolerant when you've got diarrhea.

GO EASY ON MEDICINES. If you must haul yourself out of bed for an important business meeting or a social event, or if your diarrhea is intolerable, try an over-the-counter drug like Imodium or Pepto-Bismol. In a milder attack, though, try to avoid taking medicine.

"The purist's point of view is, don't take any anti-diarrheal drugs. Let everything be flushed out of your intestines. Don't slow it down," says Dr. Phillips. "But the more practical approach is, we should try to give people some relief of symptoms. One of the simple anti-diarrheals like Imodium is effective. It probably even helps the intestine reabsorb into the bloodstream some of the excess fluid in the gut."

WATCH THOSE ANTIBIOTICS. Antibiotics can upset the natural balance of bacteria in your intestines and give you the runs. If you suspect that's the cause, call your doctor immediately. "The earlier you can stop the antibiotics, the better, because the diarrhea will be less severe," says Dr. Giannella. He cautions patients not to stop any antibiotic treatment without their doctor's approval, however. "If you cannot stop the antibiotics, though, there's a specific treatment that will be prescribed using another antibiotic and an antimicrobial drug that's very effective. But catching it early is important. Some people end up with recurring bouts of this kind of diarrhea otherwise."

DINE ON YOGURT. Yogurt that contains live cultures of lactobacillus bacteria could recolonize your intestines with "good" bacteria, says Dr. Giannella. "There's some small data that suggest it might be beneficial," he says. "At the very least, yogurt is an excellent foodstuff that's nutritious and well-tolerated by people with diarrheal disease. And the lactose in it has already been broken down, so it won't be a problem."

SEE THE DOCTOR. Diarrhea that lasts three days or more needs a doctor's evaluation, says Nicholas Banatvala, M.D., a medical epidemiologist in the Foodborne and Diarrheal Disease Division of the Centers for Disease Control and Prevention (CDC) in Atlanta.

"Children, the elderly and anyone with a compromised immune system should also see a doctor as soon as diarrhea begins. Infectious diarrhea is often much more serious for them," he says. "Also, diarrhea which lasts more than three days, a high fever, bloody diarrhea or severe abdominal pain are all reasons to consult your physician immediately." All are signs, he says, that your diarrhea may be a more serious infection.

Reaching for Safe Foods

Do you like rare meat? Caesar salad? Chocolate mousse? You could be a candidate for food poisoning—and with it comes diarrhea.

Bacterial infections in food, most often caused by undercooked or mishandled products, account for between 6 and 81 million cases of food poisoning every year in the United States, as well as 9,000 deaths, according to the CDC. In most cases, diarrhea is one of the first symptoms to appear, as it was in the summer of 1993, when hundreds of people in the Pacific Northwest got sick after eating fast-food hamburgers tainted with bacteria. Eventually, four died.

"Food poisoning is widespread, and the sad thing is, it's so preventable," says Morris Potter, D.V.M., assistant director for foodborne diseases in the Division of Bacterial and Mycotic Diseases at the CDC. "For instance, if a hamburger is pink in the middle, or if the juice from it is red or pink, you should take it back and ask for one that's cooked through. It's important."

Eating out? Dr. Potter suggests avoiding dishes made with raw eggs, such as Caesar salad or chocolate mousse (unless they were made with pasteurized eggs), as well as raw foods like sushi, oysters and steak tartare.

Eating in? When you cook, proper food handling can make all the difference. Follow these guidelines.

REFRIGERATE PROMPTLY. Don't leave cooked foods out to cool before refrigerating. It invites bacterial growth. At a picnic or potluck meal, make sure protein foods—including those made with mayonnaise, which contains eggs—are not left unrefrigerated for more than two hours, advises Dr. Potter.

COOK THOROUGHLY. Be careful not to underccok meats, says Dr. Potter. Beef, pork and lamb should be done in the middle. Joints of poultry should not be red. Fish should be flaky.

REHEAT COMPLETELY. "Bring foods to a boil on the stove, leave them in the oven for half an hour at 300° or so, and if you microwave your foods to reheat them, cover the bowl and let them sit afterward for several minutes to heat up any cool spots," Dr. Potter says.

Eating Disorders
YOU CAN STOP THE OBSESSION

Chances are you've known someone with an eating disorder. Maybe she was a high school classmate, the one who became so thin that her clothes just hung on her bones.

Maybe she's the neighbor down the hall, the one who runs five miles every morning no matter what, then appears every night at the gym to ride the exercise bike, swim or work the Stair Master—whatever it takes to get in two workout hours a day.

Maybe she's your housemate, the one who binges quietly in the kitchen late at night—after she's been out to dinner with friends. She tries to hide the pizza boxes, cookie bags and ice cream wrappers, and she vomits in the alley behind the house.

Maybe she's you.

There are three major types of eating disorders—anorexia, bulimia and binge eating disorder—and they can threaten a woman's life.

Ninety to 95 percent of people who have anorexia or bulimia are women. Among those who have binge eating disorder, the majority are also women. Many suffer in silence, so it's hard to determine how many have the problem, but some experts put the figure at seven million women.

Women may be more susceptible to eating disorders than men are because of society's emphasis on thinness, experts say. And other factors—including family history and low self-esteem—may also play a role.

When It Happens after 30

While eating disorders occur most frequently in teenagers, adults suffer as well. Women over 30 who have an eating disorder fall into three categories, says Vivian Meehan, R.N., D.Sc., founder and president of the National Association of Anorexia Nervosa and Associated Disorders (ANAD), based in Highland Park, Illinois. Some develop the problem after 30, some have a recurrence of a disorder they had as teens, and others have battled eating disorders for several years.

Life's upheavals may summon an eating disorder, says Dr. Meehan, especially events that cause a sense of loss, like divorce or the death of a loved one. A woman may try to make up for the loss of control in other areas of her life by controlling her relationship with food, she says.

Sometimes it takes women in the over-30 age group longer to get help, says Dr. Meehan. "We can sometimes intercept the behavior in teenagers because their families are there to support them in the treatment. Their parents decide to put them in a program, to get them into therapy and to participate in family therapy," she observes. But no one can force an adult into treatment, she says.

The Binge Eater's Battle

The most common eating disorder in women over 30 is binge eating disorder, says Susan Yanovski, M.D., who specializes in eating disorders at the National Institute of Diabetes and Digestive and Kidney Diseases in Bethesda, Maryland. People with binge eating disorder overeat but do not vomit, take laxatives or exercise excessively to purge their bodies of food as people with bulimia do.

Binge eating disorder is found in about 2 to 3 percent of adults, and experts say 60 percent of those who have the disorder are women. Binge eating is said by experts to be a problem for 23 to 46 percent of obese women who seek treatment for weight reduction.

Women who binge eat tons of food, and they do it regularly. "If you chow down at Thanksgiving dinner, that's not a binge," says Dr.

Yanovski. "That's not definitely a larger amount than most people would eat under the same circumstances." But if you sit down with the family and eat dinner, then eat a pint of ice cream, a whole bag of cookies and four doughnuts and feel out of control during the episode, that's a binge, she says.

It's important to place a binge in context, says Dr. Yanovski. If you starve yourself through the day, then eat half a cake, that's not necessarily unusual, given that you didn't eat anything all day, she says. "Almost all women have a time when they eat large amounts," she says, but that doesn't mean they have binge eating disorder.

To constitute a true binge eating disorder, such mega-eating must occur at least two days a week for six months, says Dr. Yanovski, and must be accompanied by a feeling of not being able to control what or how much you're eating.

What's going through a woman's mind when she binges? According to Dr. Yanovski, she feels out of control and distressed. Some typical thoughts are "I don't know why I'm eating this," "I really wish I weren't eating this" and "I should really stop now." She feels guilty, depressed or disgusted with herself after the binge.

The binge eater's habits include eating rapidly, chowing down until she feels uncomfortably full and eating alone because of embarrassment over how much she's consuming.

Many women won't go out with friends because they want to stay home and binge. They hide food from their husbands and children, and they eat at night and bury the remains in the trash, says Dr. Yanovski.

Overcome by the Urge to Purge

Bulimia involves bingeing and then trying to get the food out of the body or the calories burned as quickly as possible. Many people with bulimia vomit and take diuretics and laxatives to purge the food. Others exercise excessively or fast for 24 hours or more. Bulimia is the diagnosis when a woman has indulged in this kind of behavior at least two times a week for three months, says Dr. Yanovski.

Bulimia affects from 2 to 3 percent of young women, and women with bulimia outnumber men by ten to one.

While many women with bulimia often appear healthy and are at a normal weight, they have a morbid fear of becoming fat. They often plan their binges, feeling both anxious and excited beforehand and then guilty and disgusted with their behavior afterward, according to Dr. Yanovksi.

Those with bulimia feel shame and often go to great lengths to conceal their habits. Bulimia over a long period of time can severely damage a woman's teeth because of the stomach acids in vomit or cause death from heart arrhythmia or congestive heart failure, which can be triggered by electrolyte imbalances. Women with bulimia may also die from breathing in their own vomit.

When Thinness Is Everything

Like women with bulimia, those with anorexia have an overwhelming fear of gaining weight. Even when they are underweight, they believe they are fat.

Although anorexia nervosa is the least common eating disorder, affecting less than 1 percent of adolescent and young adult women, it has the most serious health consequences. Ninety-five percent of people with anorexia are female.

The woman with anorexia pursues a thinner body by limiting her food intake severely, Dr. Meehan says. She eats so little that her body loses a lot of weight very quickly. Substantial weight loss is often the first sign of the disease.

While many dieters count calories and limit their food intake, women with anorexia carry this behavior to the extreme. They often cut out all carbohydrates and fatty foods. They may be obsessed with calorie counting and become ritualistic about food, allowing themselves to eat only so many pieces of a certain type of food at a certain time.

These women can be very secretive as well, allowing themselves to eat only when they are in a closet or bathroom, where no one will see them.

A diagnosis of anorexia can come when a woman engages in such behavior and is 15 percent below her ideal weight. In extreme cases, people with anorexia have fallen to 60 percent below their ideal weight.

While some women who have anorexia just restrict their eating, others also have episodes of binge eating and purging in addition to food restrictions. The substantial weight loss that occurs can disrupt hormone production, and all women with anorexia develop amenorrhea, or loss of their periods. The lack of estrogen can harm bone health and place women with anorexia at increased risk for osteoporosis. Also, changes in the heart, including decreased heart size, can lead to cardiac complications, a leading cause of death in those with anorexia.

Why Women Are at Risk

Our culture's emphasis on a woman's thinness is a major factor in the development of eating disorders and a big reason why women experience them more than men do, researchers say.

"Women are shown the same TV commercials asking them to eat all the same high-fat foods as men. However, women are then shown magazine covers with impossibly shaped women who are both thin and have breasts. This sends messages to women that 'Yes, you should enjoy yourself, yes, you should be eating all these high-fat foods, but you have to end up looking like these models who are at about 80 percent of their ideal body weight,' " says Dr. Yanovski.

In a study of over 60,000 people conducted by the Centers for Disease Control and Prevention in Atlanta, women were more likely than men to consider themselves overweight: 38 percent of adult women reported that they were trying to lose weight, compared with 24 percent of adult men.

The weight-loss message comes across loud and clear every day. A 1992 study found that ten of the most-read women's magazines contained over ten times more ads and articles promoting weight loss than men's magazines did.

In fact, dieting often precedes a woman's bout with anorexia or bulimia, says Dr. Yanovski. With binge eating disorder, the scenario is a little different. "Over half of women with binge eating disorder report that they began binge eating before they ever started dieting," says Dr. Yanovski.

The Relationship to Emotions

Women with low self-esteem may be at increased risk for anorexia, experts say. These women tend to have a poor body image, place extreme importance on their figure and weight and view thinness as central to self-worth.

Depression has also been associated with eating disorders; an estimated 40 to 80 percent of those with the disorder have a history of depression. Depression's connection to bulimia and binge eating disorder is especially strong, but it's not clear whether depression *causes* those two disorders or vice versa, says Dr. Yanovski. "What we can say very clearly is that bad feelings seem to trigger binge episodes in many people," she says. She cites anger, sadness, boredom and fatigue as feelings that might kick off a binge. In addition to depression, obsessive-compulsive behavior and other psychological disturbances have been observed in individuals with eating disorders.

Having a dysfunctional family is thought to increase a woman's risk for eating disorders, researchers say. People with anorexia, for instance, may come from families that are overprotective, rigid or poor at solving conflicts or have poor boundaries defining the relationships of its members.

A study done at Yale University determined that mothers of girls with eating disorders were less satisfied with family cohesiveness than were mothers whose daughters didn't have such disorders. The study also found that mothers of daughters with eating disorders were more likely to have the disorders themselves than were mothers whose daughters didn't have eating disorders.

Beating the Odds

Women can take steps to protect themselves from falling into the eating disorder trap. Here are some suggestions.

REJECT THE CULTURAL IDEAL. Women are bombarded with images of a body ideal that is unrealistic, experts say. Realize it and don't compare yourself to it or try to achieve it, says Dr. Eckstein. "Begin accepting your body the way it is," Dr. Eckstein says. "Sometimes I give people an exercise to do in the shower: Scrub their bodies and tell every single part of their body, 'I love you, I want to take care of you now,' " she says. And remember this: Most women who feel they need to lose five to ten pounds probably don't need to, says Dr. Eckstein.

AIM FOR A HEALTHY WEIGHT. If you plan to lose weight, talk with your doctor, pick a realistic goal—and stop when you reach it. "If your goal weight keeps getting lower and lower," that may be a sign of trouble, says Dr. Yanovski. Another is when you find yourself telling others that you weigh more than you really do, says Dr. Yanovski.

TALK ABOUT YOUR DIET. If you are going on a diet, be public about it, says Alice Lindeman, R.D., Ph.D., associate professor of applied health science at Indiana University in Bloomington, who studies eating disorders. Tell people how much weight you plan to lose; if you lose more they'll know and point it out, she says. Similarly, if you have a friend who is dieting, speak up if you think she's going too far.

DON'T FEAR A GAIN. If you get very upset if your weight goes up a little and are only content when your weight goes down, that's a clue that you might have an eating disorder. "Anorexics get very upset if their weight goes up. Regardless of what it goes up from, a half-pound is like a catastrophe," says Dr. Simko. So take it easy on yourself and realize that weight fluctuations are normal.

DON'T SKIP MEALS. Skipping a meal will only make

you hungrier and more likely to overeat when you finally are around food, says Dr. Yanovski.

KNOW YOUR TRIGGERS. Alcohol can be a powerful trigger, so if you find you binge every time you drink, avoid alcohol, says Dr. Yanovski. Or if buffets set you off, do your best to steer clear of them, she says. "If you are one who binges every time your husband is out of town because you're bored, plan ahead to spend time with friends," she says.

VARY YOUR ROUTINE. Nip any compulsiveness about eating in the bud, says Dr. Lindeman. For example, thinking things like "I will eat 25 peas" means you might be moving into the danger zone by being ritualistic about food and insisting on the same routine every day. Other examples of this kind of thinking include "I only go down this aisle of the grocery store," "I only buy this cereal," "I eat right at noon."

EAT WITH OTHERS. Make yourself share your eating time with others, so you can eat normally and at a regular pace, says Dr. Lindeman.

TAKE ASSERTIVENESS TRAINING. Anything that strengthens your sense of being an individual, with your own rights and needs, can help, Dr. Eckstein says. Ask your at your local library about assertiveness training classes in your area.

TELL SOMEONE. If you're having a problem with food, tell a friend, family member, doctor or co-worker with whom you can talk openly and easily. Women find telling someone is often a relief and the first step toward healing, says Dr. Eckstein. A support group can also help. Ask your doctor or hospital for help in finding one.

KEEP TRACK OF YOUR PERIODS. If you've been dieting to lose weight and have noticed a change in your menstrual periods, see your doctor. Weight loss severe enough to cause amenorrhea may be a sign of anorexia, and many women with bulimia have irregular periods.

Eczema
MORE THAN JUST AN ITCH

If it's mild, eczema can be just a minor inconvenience—a small, rough, red patch that appears on your elbow and makes you feel self-conscious about wearing a short-sleeved shirt.

But if it's severe, there's a lot more to it. Women with extremely bad cases of eczema say that it affects their social life: Sometimes their skin itches so badly and looks so awful that they're too uncomfortable and embarrassed to be around other people at all.

It affects their relationships in many ways. For example, they might not be able to visit people with pets or be around anyone wearing wool because contact with these things might make their skin break out.

And sometimes they have to stop in the middle of lovemaking and towel down because too much sweat irritates their skin. Even being held in someone's arms can be uncomfortable, because the heat and contact make their skin itch.

It affects their work: Some days they can't go to work because they feel so depressed that all they can do is sleep.

Doctors refer to eczema as "the itch that rashes," says Karen K. Deasey, M.D., attending dermatologist at Bryn Mawr Hospital in Pennsylvania. That's because it generally begins as itching that's so severe that *not* scratching becomes practically impossible. The scratching in turn provokes a rash that can range from red and blistering skin to a thick, discolored patch of skin. It can appear in one spot or cover the entire body.

Most people who develop eczema first get it in childhood: Up to 90 percent of patients have it by the time they are five years old. But it can also appear in adulthood, says Elizabeth Whitmore, M.D., clinical director of dermatology at Johns Hopkins University in Baltimore. With adult onset, the person generally has hay fever or other allergies and then develops eczema, she says. Overall, some 15 million Americans suffer from it.

How do you get eczema? "It runs in families," says Dr. Deasey. So if your parents or someone else in the family has it, it's no surprise that you do, too, she says. If family members have asthma, hay fever or allergies, that can also be related to your susceptibility to eczema. A personal or family history of allergic disease has been noted in 75 to 80 percent of patients with eczema, studies show. And the worse your own hay fever or allergies, the worse your eczema may be, says Dr. Deasey.

The Effect of Hormones and Pregnancy

Many women with eczema notice variations in their skin condition during different phases of the menstrual cycle. And physicians say they often notice changes in eczema during pregnancy.

According to one study from Edinburgh, Scotland, women with premenstrual syndrome experienced worsening of their eczema before menstruation. And while the study also showed that in 52 percent of cases, eczema worsened with pregnancy, 24 percent of women experienced an improvement in their eczema during pregnancy.

One study alone, though, isn't sufficient to represent what's happening for most women, says Sharon Hymes, M.D., clinical associate professor of dermatology at the University of Texas Medical School in Houston. So for the time being, all you can do is take note of the intensity of your eczema at various phases of your cycle and see if you notice any pattern.

There are no definite answers, either, on whether breastfeeding will ultimately prevent a child from developing eczema. "Whether or not nursing the child will delay or prevent the onset of eczema is not clear," says Dr. Hymes. "I recommend that women should nurse if they can, for all the reasons that it's good to nurse."

Eczema and Stress

If you've noticed a relationship between stress and your eczema flare-ups, it's not your imagination. There is a link, Dr. Deasey says.

MEDICAL ALERT: DO A BREAST CHECK

Pay close attention to any eczema on your nipples. Sometimes it will be just eczema, caused either by a bra or shirt that rubs or by nursing a baby for the first couple of weeks. But sometimes it's a sign of a more serious problem called Paget's disease, a form of breast cancer. Don't second-guess it; see a doctor.

Nipple eczema that's caused by irritating clothing can be managed by covering the area with petroleum jelly and applying an adhesive bandage, says Elizabeth Whitmore, M.D., clinical director of dermatology at Johns Hopkins University in Baltimore. Then when it's healed, buy clothing that doesn't chafe, she says.

Nipple eczema from breastfeeding is sometimes seen in the first couple of weeks of nursing, says Sharon Hymes, M.D., clinical associate professor of dermatology at the University of Texas Medical School in Houston. Apply Aquaphor or Eucerin lotion after a session of nursing the baby, she says. Don't use it before feeding time, she says, because it may get in the baby's mouth.

Nipple eczema from Paget's is rare, but it can happen. The eczema will appear on one breast and will be wet and oozing, says Karen K. Deasey, M.D., attending dermatologist at Bryn Mawr Hospital in Pennsylvania. Your doctor will treat it for two weeks as regular eczema. If it doesn't go away, that's the clue that it might be something more serious. Your doctor will then perform a biopsy to test for the possibility of underlying cancer, she says.

"Whether the eczema makes people more stressed or they are just more prone to stress is hard to say," she says.

Stress triggers the nerves to produce substances that, through a series of events, make the inside of the blood vessels sticky, says George Murphy, M.D., professor of dermatology and pathology at the University of Pennsylvania in Philadelphia. These sticky vessels then act like flypaper for white blood cells. When the cells stick, cross through the vessel wall and enter into the tissue, they cause the inflammation of eczema, hives, psoriasis or other skin disorders.

So do your best to keep your stress levels low. It may help keep eczema at bay.

How to Get Control

Managing stress isn't all you can do to cope with eczema. Here are some more strategies.

STAY LUBRICATED. The mainstay of therapy for eczema is keeping the skin hydrated, says Kristin M. Leiferman, M.D., associate professor of dermatology at the Mayo Clinic and the Mayo Clinic Foundation in Rochester, Minnesota. Use mild soaps and bath oils, and apply your moisturizer within minutes of toweling off, she says. "The key is keeping the skin from drying out. Use body lotion day in and day out, whether or not you're itching," Dr. Deasey says. For tough eczema cases, try petroleum jelly and moisturizing lotions such as Nivea, Eucerin, Neutrogena Emulsion or Aquaphor Natural Healing Ointment, experts say.

SURROUND YOURSELF WITH MOISTURE. One trick to remind you to keep laying on the lotion between baths or showers is to place several bottles of moisturizer around the house and in your office or briefcase. This will remind you to use it and make it easy to find, says Marianne O'Donoghue, M.D., associate professor of dermatology at Rush Presbyterian–St. Luke's Medical Center in Chicago.

THINK HUMID. Use a humidifier in your home to keep the air from getting too dry. This will keep your skin from getting too dry as well, says Dr. Deasey.

USE SHOWER SAVVY. Another way to keep your skin from drying out is to keep your showers on the cool side, says Dr. O'Donoghue. And decrease bathing in the winter, when skin is drier, she says.

AVOID SCRATCHY MATERIALS. Rough materials that can irritate the skin can aggravate eczema. "You need to stay away from itchy things like polyester and wool," says Dr. Deasey. "Don't get hot and itchy. And stay with natural fibers like cotton or lightweight, soft-fiber wools like cashmere."

GO TOPICAL. Topical steroid creams are a central part of treatment, says Dr. Leiferman. One percent hydrocortisone cream is a good place to start, experts say, and if that doesn't work, see your doctor about a stronger medication. Doctors generally use low- to midpotency steroids and reserve the ultrahigh-potency medications only for severe cases or severe flare-ups, she says.

SHINE A LIGHT. Natural sunlight or ultraviolet rays can help eczema. Ask your doctor about ultraviolet B light therapy or an

---

WOMAN TO WOMAN LIVING WITH ECZEMA

Shelley Diamond, an editor who lives in San Francisco, has had eczema all her life. She has found several ways to make living with it a little easier. This is her advice.

Sit down when you are feeling good and make a list of all the things that make you feel that way. Then when you are under stress, you can take out the list and look at possible things to do. Treat yourself with those things when you feel bad. I have certain clothes that are comfortable and cozy—I put those on. I love to read, so I buy myself books to feel better. Do whatever it is that makes you feel good. I also refer to my list for reminders to drink lots of water, cut down on caffeine, sugar and salt, and get prescription treatment for bacterial infection of the skin.

The other thing is, be more aware of communication with the people in your life. Tell them beforehand how you want to be treated so that when skin problems flare up they know what to do.

It's important to let yourself feel whatever you are feeling. Sometimes you may just need to sit and sob. Let yourself go through that. If you feel totally hopeless, say "It's okay. Today is just a bad day. I'm going to bed and start over tomorrow." The thing that helps is the freedom to feel what I feel when I feel it. People tell you all these things, all these shoulds. I suffered for years with that. Finally, I said, "I'll listen to myself and my gut reaction." That was when things started to turn around and get better.

You have to figure out what works for you. Everyone is different. You have to find your own way.

ultraviolet light treatment called PUVA. But don't try to do it yourself in the tanning salon, says Dr. Leiferman. The wrong dosage can be painful and permanently damage your skin.

STOP THE ITCH. One way to stop the itching of eczema is to take over-the-counter antihistamines such as Benadryl or Chlor-Trimeton, says Dr. O'Donoghue.

GET SUPPORT. Find someone else who's dealing with eczema, says Shelley Diamond of San Francisco, who has it. "They're the only ones who can really understand what you're going through," she says.

LAUGH IF YOU CAN. Although eczema can be painful and very frustrating, humor is a good way to deal with it, says Corky Stewart, executive director of the Eczema Association for Science and Education in Portland, Oregon. "We call the letters section of our newsletter 'The Scratch Pad.' And we tell our members that if they don't donate each year, they'll get 'scratched' from the list," she says.

KEEP A JOURNAL. "A lot of people with eczema develop a habit of scratching and they are not aware of it," says Stewart. "Some find if they keep a journal, they become more aware. Then they can be more mindful and try not to do it."

Endometrial Cancer
PREVENTION IS NUMBER ONE

Anita, a tall, thin, highly imaginative professional chef from Pennsylvania, was packing for a cross-country tour to promote her latest cookbook when she realized her period was overdue. In fact, now that she took the time to think about it, she might have missed more than one.

She'd had a little spotting here and there as well, she realized. Nothing major, but maybe she'd better stick a box of panty liners in her bag. And maybe she'd better make an appointment with her gynecologist.

It was probably nothing, Anita thought. The skipped periods were probably due to stress. But she'd make an appointment for after the tour and get everything checked out.

Two months and one biopsy later, Anita was sitting in her gynecologist's office wishing she'd gotten there faster. The problem behind the skipped periods and spotting?

Endometrial cancer.

Estrogen: Too Much of a Good Thing

A year after her diagnosis, Anita was declared cancer-free. The cancer was confined to the lining of her uterus—the endometrium—and since her uterus and ovaries were removed, along with some surrounding tissue, at such an early stage, her outlook for survival is excellent.

Not all women are as lucky as Anita. Although the death rate for endometrial cancer has dropped almost 50 percent over the past 30 years, approximately 31,000 women still get the disease every year, and nearly 6,000 women die from it.

"There are two types of endometrial cancer," explains Carolyn Runowicz, M.D., director of gynecologic oncology at Albert Einstein College of Medicine and Montefiore Medical Center in New York City. Type I, which occurs in obese women and is hormone-related, usually occurs after menopause. Type II occurs in underweight women and doesn't seem to be hormone-related at all. It can also occur anytime—either before or after menopause—and is known to produce what doctors respectfully call "a very aggressive tumor."

Doctors don't know what triggers type II, says Dr. Runowicz. But the cause of type I is fairly clear: continuously high levels of the hormone estrogen.

Excessive amounts of estrogen can be found in women who don't ovulate—frequently due to infertility, amenorrhea or polycystic ovaries—and in women who are overweight, says Dr. Runowicz. Women who don't ovulate generally have some type of chemical imbalance. But women who are overweight simply make a lot of estrogen—even after menopause.

"You'd think that at menopause estrogen levels go down," says Dr. Runowicz. "But in an overweight person—a person who is overweight by 20 percent of their body weight—they don't.

"The adrenal glands make androstenedione, a hormone that is converted in the fat cells of every woman to a weak estrogen called estrone," she explains. A weak estrogen in normal amounts is no danger—which is why women of normal weight don't generally get type I endometrial cancer. But if you're overweight, there's so much estrone being released from your fat cells that it acts as a powerful stimulant on the uterus. Cells begin to proliferate, one makes a mistake as it's growing, it mutates, and a tumor is off and running.

Progesterone, a hormone made by your body as it ovulates, can shut down the estrogen-stimulated cell machinery, says Dr. Runowicz.

But once ovulation stops, progesterone's protection stops with it. That's why most endometrial cancer occurs after menopause.

There are ways to prevent endometrial cancer, says Dr. Runowicz.

EAT SENSIBLY AND USE PORTION CONTROL. "The message I would get across to women in their thirties and forties is, don't let yourself get out of shape," says Dr. Runowicz." And if you've picked up some extra weight, get rid of it."

CHANGE YOUR DIET. One of the best ways to trim the fat from your body is to adopt a low-fat, high-fiber diet, doctors agree. A study of 17 women conducted at the U.S. Department of Agriculture Human Nutrition Research Center on Aging at Tufts University in Boston found that reducing dietary fat to 25 percent of calories and increasing fiber to 40 grams a day reduced estrogen levels by an average of 36 percent.

CONSIDER ORAL CONTRACEPTIVES. "There's definitely a decrease in endometrial cancer in women who have taken birth control pills," says Dr. Runowicz. Studies indicate that women who take currently available oral contraceptives that combine estrogen with progesterone throughout the cycle reduce the risk of endometrial cancer by approximately 50 percent. What's more, the protective effects may last for at least 15 years after the pills were taken. In contrast, the old type of oral contraceptives have had the opposite effect.

THINK CAREFULLY ABOUT HORMONE REPLACEMENT THERAPY. Studies show that taking estrogen in the years immediately preceding and following menopause increases your risk of endometrial cancer three to eight times. But there are many ways to take hormones, says Dr. Runowicz. So if you decide to use hormones after menopause, talk to your doctor about taking estrogen cyclically in combination with progesterone, she suggests. If the progesterone dose is adequate, adds Dr. Runowicz, it should prevent endometrial cancer.

SEE A GYNECOLOGIC ONCOLOGIST. If your doctor says you have endometrial cancer, get to a gynecologic oncologist as soon as possible, says Dr. Runowicz. There are only 600 of them in the United States, but cancer specialists say that the extra training and surgical expertise they have is significant.

Generally, gynecologic oncologists are affiliated with teaching hospitals in urban areas. To find the one closest to you, contact the Society of Gynecologic Oncologists at 401 North Michigan Avenue, Chicago, IL 60611; 1-800-444-4441.

Endometriosis

STRATEGIES FOR BEATING THE PAIN

Lynn Repaty's periods were so painful and heavy, she couldn't drive, she couldn't go to work, she was afraid to even leave the house. Sometimes they were so bad that she had a hard time making it to the bathroom to change her tampon. So she'd camp out, literally, on the bathroom floor.

"I couldn't stand. I couldn't walk. For many years—a good 10 to 15 years—I was debilitated three to four days a month," says the director of membership/support services for the Endometriosis Association in Milwaukee.

She remembers exactly when the pain first started—with her first period at the age of 12. She suffered incredibly heavy bleeding and severe menstrual cramps from that day on. At 17 her doctor put her on birth control pills to control the pain, but it wasn't until much later—during an infertility test at the age of 26—that she found out the cause of her discomfort all those years.

Repaty has endometriosis, a virtually incurable, often painful disease in which the endometrium (the lining of the uterus), or tissue resembling the endometrium, grows outside the uterine cavity—where it doesn't belong. Experts estimate that about 7 percent of American women of reproductive age—about five million women—are affected. Some of these women may not have any symptoms, and others may have symptoms that go unrecognized by them or their doctors. Doctors do find endometriosis in teenagers; some 50 percent of teens who undergo surgery for dysmenorrhea, or severe menstrual cramps, have been found to have it.

An Obstacle in a Woman's Life

Endometriosis brings more than just a painful period each month. The disease, especially in severe cases, may control a woman's life. It can interfere with her social plans and influence her career decisions. It can also determine if and when she'll be able to have children. Women with endometriosis plan around their calendar. "They plan around their pain," says Repaty.

For many women, the ability to make and keep social engagements depends on whether the events fall at the right time of the month. And they continually face the possibility of having to cancel activities because their pain arrives at the wrong time. Dinners out, a night at the movies, a friend's surprise party—they may avoid them all because of endometriosis.

Endometriosis costs some women their careers; they may end up choosing a job because it's something they feel they can manage, not because it's what they really want to do. Repaty wanted to be a lawyer. She scored very high on her law school entrance exams and, she says, she showed a real aptitude for the field. Yet she knew she'd have to miss class so many days due to pain, doctor's visits and multiple surgeries that completing law school was out of the question. And the rigorous demands of a lawyer's schedule would also be impossible. Instead she opted for two careers—teaching and running her own business—that would allow her the scheduling flexibility she needed.

Endometriosis can also interfere with a woman's plans to have children. While experts don't know how many women with the disease are infertile, many are unable to conceive because of the damage the disease does to their fallopian tubes and ovaries. Missing out on having children was one of the most painful things for her, says Repaty.

And women who do have the capacity to get pregnant often feel like they're in a pressure-cooker, says Miranda Johnson-Haddad, an English professor at Howard University in Washington, D.C., who has the disease. Women know that the sooner they try to get pregnant, the better, because every day they wait is another day their disease could get worse, she says. They may feel rushed to get married and start a family. Or if they're married but don't feel ready for children yet, they may find themselves in a real dilemma: Should they gamble and wait, or rush when they're not ready? Johnson-Haddad and her husband chose to take a chance and waited three years before having a child.

How Endometriosis Works

A common site for endometriosis is the pelvic cavity. Uterine tissue can also grow on the ovaries, fallopian tubes, bladder and bowel.

The disease causes pain because, just like the lining of the uterus, this out-of-place tissue bleeds when a woman has her period. So she feels cramping wherever it's located. It can also cause pressure on the organs on which it grows. If the tissue is on the floor of the pelvic cavity or on ligaments that support the uterus, the woman may have pain with intercourse. If it has attached itself to the bladder or bowel, she may experience pain during urination or bowel movements.

Some women have no pain, others a little or a lot. And there's often little correlation between the amount of pain and the extent of the disease, says Nancy Petersen, R.N., director of the Endometriosis Treatment Program at St. Charles Medical Center in Bend, Oregon. Some women with advanced disease can have few or no symptoms, and some with milder disease can have excruciating pain, which some describe as knifelike or burning, she says.

While the exact cause of endometriosis is not known, experts have several theories, including that of retrograde menstruation. The hypothesis here is that during menstruation, uterine contractions push blood back through the fallopian tubes into the pelvic cavity. Once there, the endometrial tissue implants itself and grows.

Another theory says that retrograde menstruation couldn't be the answer because endometrial cells are different from uterine tissue. Instead, endometrial cells are laid down in the pelvic cavity during fetal development. Then at adolescence, with the change in estrogen levels, the cells are stimulated and endometriosis develops. Yet another theory says that women may develop endometriosis because their immune system isn't functioning the way it should.

Who's at Risk

If a woman's mother or sister has endometriosis, she's twice as likely to have the disease, says G. David Adamson, M.D., clinical associate professor at Stanford University School of Medicine. And some studies show that when the disease runs in the family, it's usually more severe.

Women who have a cycle that is 27 days or shorter and have menstrual flow that lasts a week or longer are twice as likely to develop endometriosis as women with longer cycles and shorter flows, experts say. Women with dysmenorrhea are also at increased risk. In some studies, it has been found that women with endometriosis began menstruating at a younger age than those without the disease.

Finally, research on monkeys indicates that there may be an association between environmental factors and the development of endometriosis. In one study, monkeys exposed to radiation developed endometriosis. This does not mean that every woman with endometriosis has it because she was exposed to environmental hazards, says Dr. Adamson, but it does indicate that environmental factors may be associated with the development of the disease.

How to Know If You Have It

The symptoms—painful periods, heavy bleeding, pain at midcycle, pain on intercourse, pain while going to the bathroom and infertility—may cause you and your doctor to suspect that you have endometriosis. But the only way to know for sure is through a diagnostic procedure called laparoscopy, says Paula Bernstein, M.D., Ph.D., an attending physician at Cedars-Sinai Medical Center in Los Angeles.

During this procedure, your doctor will take a look through an instrument called a laparoscope, an optical device for viewing the inside of the body, which is inserted into the pelvic cavity through the navel. For years the telltale signs of endometriosis were black lesions called powder burns. Recently, however, red and clear lesions have been identified as endometrial tissue, so now doctors are detecting cases they would not have identified as endometriosis before.

A detection method that doesn't involve surgery is a blood test called CA-125 screening. This test measures the levels of substances that have been found to be high in the presence of endometriosis. It's problematic, though, because a high level doesn't mean you have endometriosis. A study has found that measuring the levels at two different times in the menstrual cycle—once at the beginning of the cycle before ovulation and once during menstruation—gives doctors a better indication of the possibility of disease.

Taking On Endometriosis

There are several options for treating endometriosis, but it's nearly impossible to cure.

Laparoscopy can be used to treat as well as diagnose endometriosis. Through the laparoscope, physicians can use a variety of techniques, including excision and laser vaporization, to get rid of endometrial tissue. Women may need to have the surgery done several times if their disease progresses rapidly.

Women who want to conceive have the best chance of doing so right after they've had laparoscopy, says Dr. Bernstein. "The woman's pelvis is as clean as it's ever going to be right after you've done everything you can surgically. That's her optimum window for pregnancy if she's got moderate to severe disease," she says.

There are also medications available to treat the disease. Oral contraceptives interfere with the normal menstrual cycle, resulting in lighter flow and less cramping. A steroid derivative called danazol (Danocrine), which works by suppressing ovulation and interfering with the normal cycle, has also been used. It also binds to endometriotic tissue and may prevent the cells from proliferating. While women can try danazol, the prescription drug has many possible side effects, including hot flashes, weight gain, acne and irregular vaginal bleeding, and it may cause women to develop male characteristics, such as a deeper voice and hair growth on the face and body.

A newer class of drugs called GnRH agonists, which are drugs similar to the natural brain hormone gonadotropin-releasing hormone (GnRH), affect the key hormones instrumental in the menstrual cycle and interfere with ovulation and menstruation. While women find these prescription drugs—the most commonly used are Lupron and Synarel—somewhat more tolerable in terms of side effects, they can't take them indefinitely. After about six to nine months, women are at increased risk for osteoporosis and heart disease.

Finally, women with endometriosis do have the option of hysterectomy, or removal of the uterus. Advocates say that by removing the uterus, the source of the endometrial tissue is also removed. And if the ovaries are also removed, that eliminates the woman's source of estrogen, which helps endometrial tissue grow.

But other experts argue that the uterus may not be the actual source of the disease in some cases and that because endometrial tissue is located elsewhere, removing the uterus will not cure the disease.

While some women request a hysterectomy because they can no longer tolerate the pain, experts warn that the pain of the disease may return after the procedure. "Having a hysterectomy doesn't always guarantee that someone will necessarily be 100 percent pain-free," says Dr. Bernstein. Surgery usually improves symptoms, but not always, she says.

Coping with Endometriosis

While endometriosis cannot be cured, there are things you can do to alleviate the pain. Here are some suggestions.

TRY TO GET OUT AND ABOUT. Exercise is often helpful for women with milder endometriosis, experts say, and is recommended if a woman can tolerate it. It "increases the natural endorphins . . . the natural painkillers," says Deborah A. Metzger, M.D., Ph.D., director of the Reproductive Medicine Institute of Connecticut in Hartford. Walking for 30 to 45 minutes a day can help, she says.

YOGA-SIZE. Some women have such severe disease that aerobic exercise is out of the question, says Petersen. For these women, yoga is an alternative. "It helps their bodies to be more supple and in some cases it improves muscle tone," she says. "Overall it can decrease stress."

QUESTIONS TO ASK THE DOCTOR

If your doctor thinks you have endometriosis, she may recommend surgery. Here are some questions to ask.

- Why are you recommending laparoscopy?
- How much experience do you have with laparoscopy?
- What's your experience with how patients do?
- What will happen when I go for laparoscopy?
- If you find I have endometriosis, are you going to remove what you can of the disease?
- Do I have any other options for treatment?
- What are my chances of having children?
- How much surgery will I have to have?
- Will it lead to hysterectomy?
- If I have a hysterectomy, will I be pain-free?

EAT REGULARLY. Eating three meals a day will help maintain your blood sugar level, says Dr. Metzger. "When blood sugar gets low, there's a lack of energy, and it can make it harder to deal with pain," she says.

WATCH WHAT YOU EAT. Cut as much caffeine and refined sugar as you can out of your diet, says Dr. Metzger. Cutting back on sugar will keep your energy levels from fluctuating and you'll be better able to deal with your pain, she says. Simple changes like eating a bran muffin made with apples instead of sugar or replacing your morning doughnut with a bagel and light cream cheese can help, she says.

"Caffeine also causes your nerves to be jittery," which can affect your ability to cope, she says. So try decaffeinated coffee and sodas.

Finally, some women find it helpful to eat bananas and drink warm milk at bedtime to help them sleep, says Petersen. Bananas and milk contain tryptophan, which is synthesized by the brain into serotonin, a neurotransmitter that can induce sleep.

MEDITATE AND RELAX. Relaxing through meditation or visual imagery helps many women sleep better, reduces stress and helps women cope with the pain of their disease, says Petersen. Try tapes on visual imagery, pain relief, meditation or deep relaxation and use them to take a break during the day, she says. If you have a private office at work where you can listen to the tape during your lunch break, "think about spending 15 to 20 minutes meditating, allowing the body to sort of reset itself so that you can cope with the rest of the day," she says.

Those who can't take a break at work should find time when they first get home. They should "take 20 minutes, put their feet up, block out the rest of the world, take care of themselves and then move into whatever needs to be taken care of in the evening," says Petersen.

TALK WITH OTHER WOMEN. Networking with other women through support groups is very helpful, says Repaty. "Attending support groups made me feel I wasn't alone, that I wasn't the only woman with my disease," she says. Contact the Endometriosis Association, 8585 North 76th Place, Milwaukee, WI 53223, for information on a group in your area.

CALL FOR HELP. If a support group isn't your style, the Endometriosis Association can connect you with individual women with the disease. If you want to know about endometriosis and drug therapy or hysterectomy, the association can put you in touch with women who have been through it. "The best way is to get firsthand information from women. They can tell you what doctors they've been to, how they were treated, what the doctor's bedside manner was," says Repaty.

INVOLVE YOUR PARTNER. Endometriosis can affect your relationship and your sex life. It's important to talk to your partner and involve him in the process, says Repaty. Take him to the doctor's office with you, and talk to him about your feelings and concerns, she says.

TAKE A NEW VIEW OF SEX. Endometriosis can often cause painful intercourse if the tissue is situated in certain areas. First, realize that there are other ways to be intimate besides having intercourse, says Repaty. Second, if you have more pain at certain times in your menstrual cycle, tell your partner and plan to have sex at times that are better for you, she says. Third, explore different positions, she says. While one may hurt, another may not. If you know one position hurts, try to talk about it before the next time you have sex, she says.

TRY MEDICATION. Over-the-counter and prescription medications may provide relief for women with mild forms of the disease. Look for products that contain ibuprofen, which counters the effects of prostaglandins, the chemicals responsible for menstrual cramping.

CHECK OUT THE PILL. Low-dose oral contraceptives can provide pain relief, says Dr. Bernstein. Being on the Pill often lessens pain because it decreases the amount of menstrual flow; the estrogen in the Pill interferes with the release of the hormones that would normally cause the endometrium to thicken. And the synthetic progesterone in the Pill, called progestin, inhibits the development of the uterine lining. Women can also use the Pill if they've had surgery for endometriosis and their pain returns.

TRY ACUPUNCTURE. Acupuncture, an ancient technique used for pain relief and for the relaxation that comes with it, involves inserting needles into specific points in the skin. "Certain points are associated with relief of pain. Some women I see say it does help them," says Dr. Metzger. "I will not discount any treatment that helps women relax." Ask your doctor to refer you to an acupuncturist.

ASK A LOT OF QUESTIONS. Endometriosis is a complex, difficult disease. Ask as many questions as you have of your doctor. If you ask questions and the answers do not fit with your experience with the disease, consider getting another opinion, says Petersen.

Fatigue

YOU DON'T HAVE TO BE SO TIRED

The alarm goes off at 6:00 A.M. You snuggle with your mate for a moment, then give him a kiss, push the dog off the bed and reach for your moccasins.

You get breakfast for the kids, throw a load in the washer, get dressed, drop the cat at the vet, pick up the dry cleaning and get yourself to work. And it's only 9:00 A.M.

Then you work like a dog trying to meet the deadlines and responsibilities of your job.

It's almost a relief when you stuff a little work into your briefcase at 6:00, grab your keys and head for home.

Once there, of course, life's a breeze. You make dinner, supervise homework, get the kids to bed, fold the laundry and then, with pillows propped behind you and a cup of hot tea at your side, you pull out the work you brought home from the office.

Long, Hard Hours

Women have always worked hard. But today, doctors say, women are exhausted. Married or single, with or without kids, working in an office, a laundry or at home, it seems as true as ever that a woman's work is never done.

The result is that fatigue is one of the top ten complaints in doctors' offices across the country.

That's not to say that the deadening fatigue of which women are complaining can't be caused by physical ailments. It can. Fatigue is a side effect of almost every disease and condition known to woman. It can be caused by pregnancy, menopause, an approaching period, overweight, flu, anemia, mononucleosis, cancer, a low-grade urinary tract infection, a vaginal infection, diabetes, hypoglycemia, depression, fibromyalgia, the common cold, smoking, stress or just having your thyroid out of whack.

It can also be caused by drugs. Antihistamines, tranquilizers, muscle relaxants, sedatives, narcotics, birth control pills, heart medications and pain relievers can all cause fatigue.

Then there is chronic fatigue syndrome, which is something completely different. Some doctors believe it's caused by some kind of malfunction in the immune system.

But when a woman shows up in a doctor's office with fatigue as her chief complaint—rather than fever, itching, sneezing or pain—the problem is not usually illness or medication.

"I think that people feel chronically tired for a very simple reason," says fatigue researcher Anthony Komaroff, M.D., professor of medicine at Harvard Medical School. "They're working long, hard hours."

The work week in the United States has been steadily increasing since the mid-1960s, says Dr. Komaroff, particularly for women. It's one of the most important phenomena of our time, he adds. Yet it's a cultural trend that most Americans haven't yet recognized.

Why? They're too busy working.

The Incomplete Revolution

Why are women working so hard? The problem for most women is that they're caught between social revolutions, experts agree. While one social revolution has expanded women's roles to provide increased career opportunities, a second, hoped-for social revolution—that of increased men's roles in the family—hasn't come to fruition.

In the 1993 National Study of the Changing Workforce, researchers at the Work and Families Institute, a New York City–based think tank, surveyed 3,000 working Americans and found that while men were spending more time working in the home than their fathers, women were still working twice as many hours as men at home. The overwhelming majority of women (81 percent) did most of the shopping and cooking, 78 percent did the bulk of the cleaning, 71 percent assumed primary responsibility for child care, and 63 percent took charge of the check-writing and bill-paying.

Most men (91 percent) did the household repairs, and 35 percent of men did most of the check-writing. Eighteen percent did the shopping, 15 percent did most of the cooking, 7 percent did the cleaning, and 5 percent took responsibility for child care.

"Men think they're doing more, but when you compare what they say they're doing with what their wives say they're doing, there's a 50-point spread," says Dana Friedman, Ed.D., co-president of the Families and Work Institute and one of the researchers who conducted the study.

It's not that the guys are fibbing, she adds. It's that guys look at tasks—specifically the tasks related to the kids—and ignore all the planning that goes into executing various family activities.

"With regard to school, for example, women take all the responsibility for the kids," says Dr. Friedman. "*She* selects the school, *she* visits the school, *she* finds the parents to car pool, *she* sets the car pool schedule. And then, one day, *he* drives.

"You hear what's happening?" asks Dr. Friedman. "*She* did the 42 steps to set something up, he drove, and *he* thinks he's sharing in the child care!"

Fighting Fatigue in the 1990s

Since these circumstances are not about to change overnight, how do you fight fatigue in the 1990s? Here's what experts say.

PRIORITIZE. "Most of us are still assuming the traditional responsibilities that society says a 'real' woman does," says Claire Etaugh, Ph.D., professor of psychology and dean of the College of Liberal Arts and Sciences at Bradley University in Peoria, Illinois.

But just because our moms baked apple pies, had hot chocolate waiting after school and kept the toilet bowl sparkling doesn't mean that we should—especially not in a world where an attorney who works 40 hours a week is considered a part-timer.

"There are too many 'shoulds' in our lives," says Dr. Etaugh. "You have to decide what's most important, set priorities and then—whether it's cleaning, family, friendships or career—let the rest go."

DROP THE GUILT. If not fulfilling your own image of a perfect wife, mom, worker or housekeeper makes you feel guilty, see a therapist, adds Dr. Etaugh. Otherwise, feeling guilty over not baking your son's favorite cherry pie could leave you feeling just as exhausted as if you'd taken the time to make it.

LEARN TO MANAGE YOUR TIME. Most working women—particularly working mothers—are highly efficient at managing their time. They wouldn't survive if they weren't. But it always helps to have someone else look at your workload—both at home and at work—with a critical eye. There's a good chance that somewhere, somehow, there's a more efficient—that is, less fatiguing—way to get things done.

DO TWO THINGS AT ONCE. Become an expert at figuring out how to do more than one thing at a time, says Dr. Etaugh. Hang an extra cleaning brush on the shower caddy and scrub down the walls when you shower. Fold laundry while you listen to a theme your child has written for tomorrow's class.

USE THE PHONE. Bank by phone. Pay by phone. Use direct-mail catalogs and 800 numbers to shop at home. Order gifts by phone—then have them wrapped and sent, says Dr. Etaugh.

TAKE CONTROL OF YOUR WORKLIFE. "Probably the most tiring situation is to have responsibility without authority in the

THE PERFECT PICKUP

Low-fat, high-carbohydrate foods such as cereals and breads, pasta, potatoes, vegetables and fruit are most likely to add energy to your day, nutritionists say. But an excellent choice for a quick pickup during that 4:00 P.M. energy sag would be one of the following foods.

- 1 medium banana
- 1 orange
- ¼ cup raisins
- 5 dates, dried or fresh
- ¼ honeydew melon
- ½ medium cantaloupe
- 3 medium apricots, fresh, canned or dried
- ½ medium apple
- 2 figs, dried or fresh

workplace," says Susan Schenkel, Ph.D., Cambridge psychologist and author of *Giving Away Success: Why Women Get Stuck and What to Do about It:* "It makes things difficult, unpleasant and exhausting. And it's a big workplace issue for a lot of women," she says.

Moving up the corporate ladder—or even sideways—into a different job is one answer, as is looking for another job or quitting and starting your own business. Either way, says Dr. Schenkel, taking control of what you do and when you do it is a big energy booster.

TALK TO YOUR BOSS. If you're finding more and more work on your desk, Dr. Etaugh says, talk to your supervisor and try to work out a more manageable workload.

CHECK THE PARKING LOT. To avoid taking the kind of job in which a 60-hour week is the norm, cruise through the parking lot of any company you're thinking of working for at about 6:00 A.M. or 6:00 P.M. during the week, suggests Dr. Friedman. Count the number of cars. If there are one or two, no problem. But if the lot is a quarter full, there's a good chance that this is a corporation that pushes its people to the wall.

EXERCISE. "Fatigue is a big problem for me," says Dr. Schenkel. "That's why I spend a considerable amount of time working out. I do sit-ups and stretches every morning. And I try to spend about 25 minutes a day on the exercise bike. Then every other day I try to do water walking or walking on the sidewalk for anywhere from 40 minutes to an hour."

Besides keeping your energy levels up on a long-term basis, exercise can also energize you on the spot, doctors agree.

In a study at California State University, for example, researchers compared the energy levels of a group of volunteers who took a ten-minute walk and a group who ate candy instead. The researchers found that the walkers increased their energy more than the munchers, and the effects of walking lasted much longer than those of munching—up to two hours.

WAKE UP TO YOUR DIET. "Another factor that makes a lot of women tired is that they have poor nutrition," says Dr. Schenkel. "Part of the problem is ignorance, some of it is that women are too busy to pay attention, and some of it is that every woman in America thinks she's at least ten pounds overweight."

Whatever the cause, the solution is to keep an eye on your diet, says Dr. Schenkel. Nutrition experts suggest that a high-energy diet is one that's high in complex carbohydrates like those found in grains, beans, pasta and most baked goods, with less than 25 percent of its calories coming from fatty foods. And if you really must lose weight, keep your energy levels up by keeping your calorie intake above 1,000 a day.

GET HELP. One thing that's going to be slow to change is the lack of support women get at home from their men. Social changes take time, says Dr. Etaugh. So instead of draining your emotional energies along with your physical ones by trying to speed up the redefinition of men's roles, hire some outside assistance. If you can afford it, hire someone to clean the house, mow the lawn and babysit the kids, and have the pizza delivered.

The Alternative Route

Since so many illnesses can cause an overwhelming sense of fatigue, check with your family doctor whenever you feel exhausted for more than a few weeks.

But if your doctor gives you a clean bill of health even when you're still exhausted, think about consulting a professional who practices alternative medicine, says Dr. Schenkel.

"If you go to your average doctor and say that you're tired and she doesn't find anything interesting on the tests, she will say, 'You need to reduce your stress, and God be with you, Madam,'" she says. But a physician who practices alternative medicine will take the fact that you're tired as important information. Ask your doctor to refer you to someone who practices this kind of medicine.

For instance, Dr. Schenkel says, "in oriental medicine, doctors organize their whole medical system around energy—around the concept of *chi*. So someone who practices oriental medicine will be curious about where in your body the *chi* is blocked, and they'll help you try to unblock it," possibly with acupuncture, herbs and exercise.

Who knows? says Dr. Schenkel. Maybe an of hour or two of slow, flowing movements of the Chinese exercise tai chi chuan every week is all you need to reenergize.

Fibroids

GROWTHS YOU CAN LIVE WITH— OR WITHOUT

Many of us have fibroids, and unless they're big enough to require removal, most of us don't even know it. Some experts say 50 percent of women of childbearing age have fibroids of one size or another.

Fibroids are benign growths that arise from the muscle tissue of the uterus. They sometimes grow within the uterine wall itself, causing a general enlargement of the uterus. They can also project into the uterine cavity or extend outward into the abdominal cavity. They may hug the wall of the uterus or grow on threadlike stalks. They may show no symptoms at all or cause severe pain, bleeding and permanent damage to other organs. Treatment of fibroids is the number one reason for hysterectomy in the United States today.

As far as medical science knows, absolutely nothing can be done to prevent fibroids, says Francis L. Hutchins, Jr., M.D., director of gynecology and women's services at Graduate Hospital and clinical associate professor of gynecology at Hahnemann University Hospital and Thomas Jefferson University Hospital, all in Philadelphia. Dr. Hutchins says numerous therapies—including diet and vitamin regimens and homeopathic and naturopathic remedies—have been tried, but so far none has been substantiated as a way to prevent fibroids.

The Estrogen Connection

There is no question that estrogen causes fibroids to grow, according to Dr. Hutchins. The estrogen connection means that women are most susceptible to fibroids during their reproductive years, when their systems are pumping estrogen. In addition, some fibroids grow faster and larger during pregnancy or when a woman takes birth control pills. African American women develop fibroids at a rate about three times that of other women—again, nobody knows why.

A few studies have linked fibroids to excess weight, although the exact relationship is unclear. Fatty tissue converts androgen hormones into estrogen, leading to higher-than-normal levels of estrogen in overweight women.

Even the rate of growth of fibroids is unpredictable. "In the women we're talking about—mostly between ages 19 and 50—fibroids appear to grow at varying rates. Nobody has successfully defined the normal rate of growth of fibroids," says Dr. Hutchins. What is certain is that fibroids do grow—little ones become big ones, and the potential for painful, debilitating symptoms increases.

The good news is that fewer than half of all women who have fibroids experience symptoms. When they do, the most common signs are abnormal menstrual flow and pain. Bleeding sometimes is so heavy and prolonged that anemia results. Pain can range from a feeling of pelvic pressure or heaviness to discomfort during intercourse. Sometimes fibroids grow so fast that they outstrip their blood supply and shrivel up, causing severe pain.

Other, less common complications occur when the fibroids put pressure on surrounding organs. "Even though they're benign, fibroids can get big enough to cause real problems, particularly if they compress the ureters, the tubes leading from the kidneys," according to Julia V. Johnson, M.D., assistant professor of obstetrics and gynecology at the University of Vermont in Burlington. The compression can do permanent damage. Dr. Johnson says a uterus enlarged by fibroids may also press on the bladder, causing frequent urination, or on the rectum and colon, resulting in constipation.

When Surgery May Help

When symptoms compromise quality of life or pose a danger to health, surgery is often the only solution. "If a woman is 25 years old and already has very large fibroids, it's unlikely she's going to make it through her reproductive years without having to have surgery," says Dr. Johnson. "On the other hand, if a woman is 49 years old and her uterus is not too large or she has mild symptoms but nothing else, she may want to wait, because the fibroids are going to shrink when she goes through menopause."

Surgical options include hysterectomy or myomectomy, a less drastic procedure in which only the fibroids—not the uterus—are removed. A myomectomy can be performed in a variety of ways, through an abdominal incision or using the newer techniques of hysteroscopy or laparoscopy. With hysteroscopy, the fibroids are removed with small instruments inserted into the uterus through the cervix. With laparoscopy, they are removed with tools inserted through a tiny slit in the abdomen. An even newer technique, laparoscopic myolysis, destroys the fibroid with electricity.

The disadvantage of myomectomy is that it requires more specialized training to perform than a hysterectomy. In addition, fibroids have a recurrence rate of about 15 to 30 percent. But it should be noted that the majority of women with recurrences won't require further surgery.

Key to the decision on which procedure to have is whether you wish to keep your uterus. If so, myomectomy would be the choice to discuss with your doctor.

Hysterectomy used to be the operation of choice for many doctors caring for patients with fibroids. In recent years, however, a growing number of doctors—perhaps spurred by greater health-care activism on the part of their women patients—have jumped off the hysterectomy bandwagon. Hysterectomy and oophorectomy—in which the uterus and ovaries are removed—plunge a woman into instant menopause, with all its symptoms and the need for estrogen replacement therapy. In addition, many women report depression, fatigue and decreased sexual desire after hysterectomy.

Dr. Hutchins believes doctors should not be so quick to advocate hysterectomy. "In every other area of medicine, we practice what is referred to as 'preservation of tissue,' so to sacrifice the organ when you could easily save it with no significant risk to the patient is inappropriate," he says.

Fibroids and Pregnancy

Pregnancy may be complicated by fibroids, says Ruth Schwartz, M.D., clinical professor of obstetrics and gynecology at the University of Rochester School of Medicine and Dentistry in New York. "If fibroids poke into the endometrial cavity, that can cause miscarriage. If they're in the lower portion of the uterus, they can get large and obstruct delivery of the baby; some may cause preterm labor." Occasionally, fibroids grow rapidly during pregnancy and deteriorate, becoming acutely tender and painful. "Some women need pain medication," says Dr. Schwartz, "but we try to wait it out until it quiets down—very few fibroids are operated on during pregnancy because of the potential for excessive bleeding."

Dr. Schwartz cautions that a woman who wants to get pregnant shouldn't necessarily have fibroids removed ahead of time. "Many women with fibroids successfully go through pregnancy, so we don't know if there's going to be a problem until she makes a try. With myomectomy, you often have to cut all the way through the uterus to remove the fibroid; that's a risk in later pregnancy because the uterus can rupture during labor."

Treating Fibroids

Although there are many situations in which surgery is the best answer, a woman has options. Here are the major ones.

WAIT AND WATCH. Less than half of all women with fibroids have symptoms. This means, says Dr. Hutchins, "the majority of fibroids can simply be observed." This is particularly true when symptoms are mild or nonexistent, the rate of growth of the fibroids is slow, or the woman is nearing menopause. Because growth of fibroids is related to levels of estrogen in the body, the fibroids stop growing and usually shrink as natural estrogen tapers off during menopause. And estrogen replacement therapy doesn't stimulate fibroids—the amount of hormone in these preparations is so minute that it rarely causes fibroids to grow.

In fact, if fibroids grow rapidly after menopause, it could be a tip-off to a more serious problem and should be investigated.

TRY PROGESTERONE. Taking doses of this hormone

inhibits the action of estrogen, says Dr. Hutchins. "It's very safe and effective in management of bleeding for fibroids and can be given as long as desired." Unfortunately, many women experience unpleasant side effects at higher doses—the most prominent being fluid retention, weight gain and mood fluctuation—after taking the drug for a while.

ASK ABOUT GnRH AGONISTS. This group of compounds simulates the action of gonadotropin-releasing hormone (GnRH), a substance that occurs naturally in the body. At normal levels, GnRH stimulates production of estrogen, but at therapeutic levels, it desensitizes the pituitary, resulting in a dramatic drop in estrogen. The result is artificial, reversible menopause and a significant reduction in the size and symptoms of fibroids. Although GnRH agonists are still being investigated, Dr. Hutchins characterizes them as "the most exciting form of medicine for fibroids today." A GnRH agonist is given for three months, usually to shrink fibroids prior to surgery. After the treatment is discontinued, fibroids tend to grow to their former size, although symptoms may not be as severe.

The downside is that GnRH agonists are expensive and often not covered by medical insurance, points out Dr. Schwartz, because they haven't yet been approved by the Food and Drug Administration for treatment of fibroids.

DIAGNOSE AND TREAT TOGETHER. If you experience heavy bleeding, it's possible for your doctor to view the inside of your uterus with a hysteroscope inserted vaginally to determine whether fibroids are the cause of the problem. "Diagnosing these problems with a blind D&C is no longer considered optimal," says Dr. Johnson, "but hysteroscopy is new and not all physicians offer it."

Hysteroscopy offers the benefits of both diagnosis and treatment with no more time or anesthetic risk than a standard D&C. "If fibroids are poking into the endometrial cavity," says Dr. Schwartz, "some of them can be removed with the hysteroscopy." No further surgery is necessary.

ASK ABOUT MYOMECTOMY. For a woman who needs surgery, "it's important she get the option of myomectomy, especially if there's any chance she might want a pregnancy in the future," says Dr. Schwartz. "It's certainly not fair to do a hysterectomy otherwise."

Sometimes myomectomy can be performed with a laparoscopic, or "belly-button," incision. This is particularly true for fibroids on the outside of the uterus. Sometimes a fibroid is so close to the ovaries that it's difficult to tell whether it's really a fibroid or a mass on the ovary. "The closer you get to menopause, the more you worry about ovarian cancer," says Dr. Schwartz. "In these cases, I do a laparoscopy just to look at the growth. When I'm assured it's not an ovarian tumor, I just leave it alone."

Laparoscopy is not always a good choice, however, because it's much more difficult to repair the wall of the uterus. "They can't all be removed through the laparoscope," says Dr. Johnson. "A few can be, and a few can be removed through the hysteroscope, but the majority are still going to have to be removed through open abdominal incision."

KNOW ALL ABOUT HYSTERECTOMY. The most dramatic solution to fibroids has a couple of advantages: The fibroids will never regrow, there's less risk of complications of surgery, and you won't have any withdrawal bleeding with hormone therapy during menopause, says Dr. Schwartz. In addition, there's some evidence that women who have a hysterectomy are less likely to develop ovarian cancer later in life.

One of the most common reasons given for hysterectomy for fibroids is that they're growing rapidly and could signal a more serious condition. "If it grows fast, that says it may not be a fibroid," says Dr. Johnson, "so that's clearly a reason for surgery." She wants women to understand that fibroids are not malignant and are not thought to "turn into" cancers. Growths that are thought to be fibroids, however, could be malignant tumors. While the risk of a malignant tumor is less than 1 percent, this is of particular concern for postmenopausal women— the group at greatest risk for uterine cancer.

Fibromyalgia
PAIN, PAIN GO AWAY

You hurt. In your shoulders, your arms, your hips. Even your feet feel as though someone slammed them with the mallet you use to tenderize meat.

Not only that, you're exhausted—as though you haven't slept for a week. Every day it gets harder to drag yourself out of bed—and harder still not to climb back in after breakfast.

Women who have fibromyalgia, a pain-all-over condition characterized by at least 11 tender points in muscles scattered all over their bodies, wake up to pain and fatigue every morning.

They also wake up to a world in which many doctors tell them the disease is "all in their heads." Add to this employers who suspect they're malingering and families who wonder how it could hurt as much as Mom says it does.

Part of the problem with fibromyalgia is that there's no outward sign that anything is wrong—no bruises, no breaks, no swelling.

The Chemical Connection

Fibromyalgia affects somewhere from three to six million Americans, 80 percent of them women. Many are unable to work and are able to leave their beds for only short periods of time.

The reason that fibromyalgia affects women more than men is a mystery, says rheumatologist I. Jon Russell, M.D., Ph.D., director of the University Clinical Research Center at the University of Texas Health Sciences Center in San Antonio and editor of the *Journal of Musculoskeletal Pain*. But until recently, just about everything about fibromyalgia was a mystery.

Now, largely because of the work of Dr. Russell and a handful of colleagues across the country, scientists are beginning to suspect that fibromyalgia is a syndrome in which a series of chemical imbalances in the body trigger cascades of pain and fatigue. They are giving special attention to substance P, the chemical that initiates the process that tells the brain the body is in pain. And they are also looking at the effects of low serotonin, a chemical in the body and brain that blocks the release of substance P and decreases the severity of perceived pain.

Scientists have found that serotonin in the brain also regulates the deepest stage of sleep, says Dr. Russell. Less serotonin would mean less deep sleep. That may be one reason people with fibromyalgia feel so exhausted every morning.

Digging for a Diagnosis

Although the causes of fibromyalgia are just beginning to emerge, doctors have been struggling to identify the disease for nearly 150 years. The difficulty was—and still is—the wide variety of symptoms that can accompany the pain and fatigue that characterize the disease.

"Seventy percent of people with fibromyalgia will tell you that they sleep very poorly," says Dr. Russell. They'll also tell you that their symptoms get worse when the weather changes, that their hands and toes frequently feel cold, numb or tingling, that they have pain in their joints as well as their muscles and that they have chronic, intermittent headaches—particularly in the back of the head or behind the eyes.

"They also report having bowel and bladder trouble," says Dr. Russell. Forty percent will have either constipation or diarrhea along with cramping abdominal pain. About 20 to 30 percent will also have jaw pain, and sometimes fibromyalgia accompanies other diseases such as Lyme disease or rheumatoid arthritis.

"All that's needed for the diagnosis of fibromyalgia is a three-month history of widespread pain and the demonstration of pain to the touch on 11 of 18 specific sites on the body," says Dr. Russell.

Getting Relief

Until fibromyalgia is diagnosed, women with this syndrome are so desperate to be free of pain that they—and their doctors—will try just about any pain reliever. But aspirin, acetaminophen and ibuprofen—and even prescription painkillers—are only marginally helpful.

That's why Dr. Russell and his colleagues are developing medications that directly influence serotonin availability and its effects in those with fibromyalgia. But until such drugs are generally available, here's how doctors suggest you handle the syndrome.

HIT THE ROAD. "Exercise increases the availability of serotonin somewhat," says Dr. Russell. In two studies where researchers evaluated the sleep patterns of healthy young people, exercisers were also less likely to develop muscular pain.

How can you get the same effect? "Develop a regular exercise program. Walk a mile or exercise for about 20 minutes in a pool every other day," suggests Dr. Russell. Start out with whatever amount you can, then build up gradually as your body allows.

TAKE TO A HOT TUB. "Symptoms improve when people with fibromyalgia get into a hot bath or shower," says Dr. Russell. "The improvement is temporary, but it's substantial.

"We don't quite know what it means," he adds, "but it may be that the heat is increasing the availability of serotonin."

GET A MASSAGE. "When someone with fibromyalgia is given a massage, they usually do feel better for a period of time," says Dr. Russell.

CONSIDER ELECTROACUPUNCTURE. A Swiss study of 55 men and women with fibromyalgia found that six sessions of electroacupunture over a three-week period cut fibromyalgia pain in half.

Stainless steel needles connected to a weak electrical current were implanted at four to ten acupuncture points. Study participants reported a significantly higher pain threshold, less pain in general and less need for pain-relief tablets.

GET THE RIGHT PRESCRIPTION. Until a drug specifically developed to treat fibromyalgia is available, there are a number of prescription drugs that scientists have found to help people with fibromyalgia, says Dr. Russell. With some of these medications it's also helpful to take an over-the-counter pain reliever. Ask your doctor whether a prescribed medication is compatible with these OTCs.

A Helping Hand

More than 25,000 people who have fibromyalgia have become part of the Fibromyalgia Network, a self-help organization (P.O. Box 31750, Tucson, AZ 85751-1750). The network assists more than 250 local self-help groups around the country and produces a newsletter that keeps members up to date on research. Members also share tips on how to live with fibromyalgia. Here are some of their favorites.

MAKE SURE YOUR DOCTOR'S UP TO SPEED. Most women with fibromyalgia spend a lot of time going from one doctor to another and being told to think "happy thoughts," says Kristin Thorson, founder of the Fibromyalgia Network. So if your doctor has a tendency to pat you on the head and hasn't any idea where the tender points in fibromyalgia are supposed to be, head for the door. Then check the Yellow Pages in your local telephone directory for a doctor certified in rheumatology or contact the Fibromyalgia Network for a list of self-help groups and physician referrals in your area.

LIVE FOR THE MOMENT. Fibromyalgia pain can be unbearable one moment, better the next. Take advantage of the good moments by doing such things as spur-of-the moment entertaining, suggests one woman with fibromyalgia. Instead of draining your energy reserves with elaborate dinner parties planned weeks ahead, simply call up friends and invite them over for pizza when you're having a good day.

BELT OUT YOUR PAIN. When one woman with fibromyalgia is home alone and in pain, she slips a tape of Carly Simon's "Haven't Got Time for the Pain" into a Karaoke machine, turns down the right channel of the machine to tune Carly out, then belts out the song at the top of her lungs.

PACE YOURSELF. Keep a diary of your activities, then use it to try to spread those activities out. Try to pace your activities so you don't get into situations where you have to do so much at once that you end up utterly exhausted.

USE THE WINDOW. Most women with fibromyalgia seem to feel best between 10:00 A.M. and 3:00 P.M., says Thorson. Use this window to do things like shopping, chores and career tasks.

GET SOME SUPPORT. Minimize muscular strain by using back supports and arm rests where you can. Neck supports, particularly while sleeping, may also help.

INVOLVE YOUR FAMILY. It's hard for your family to understand what's going on. But if you take the time to talk about how you feel—about your pain, your exhaustion, your inability to be the

---

WOMAN TO WOMAN MAKING THE TRIUMPHANT CHOICE

Kristin Thorson, 39, a chemical engineer in Bakersfield, California, developed fibromyalgia in 1983. The disease forced her to choose between having a career and having children. Children won, and now she has two. This is her story.

I used to be a runner. My neighbors would kid me, "How many hours are you going to run today?" because I just felt like I was a butterfly and I would just go and go and go. And the only constraint I had was how much time I had to run before I had to get dinner on.

Then one day I woke up with a 102° fever. I hurt like I never hurt before. My buttocks were sore. I couldn't be touched. I had this burning sensation. My pants rubbing against my knee when I moved were so painful that I could hardly walk. I had a very heightened sensitivity, triggered by what was later thought to be some viral infection.

I stopped doing everything. I was so lethargic that I shut down everything unless it was absolutely necessary. All I did was eat, sleep and go to work. I mean that was it. Except to see doctors.

There's a tremendous loss of self-esteem after you've seen 20 doctors and they have all told you, "Well, Ms. Thorson, why don't you just go home and think happy thoughts?"

I've been told that a lot. I was pushed out the door and told to go home and think happy thoughts even though I never said I wasn't happy. I had a wonderful husband and a career—I had everything going for me.

So I kept thinking, I'm going to hang in there till I get a diagnosis. Then the doctors are going to give me a magic pill and I'm going to be fine. But finally the doctors said, "Well, the good news is, we know what you have: Fibromyalgia. The bad news is, we don't know what to do about it."

I stayed on my job for another three months. But by that time I was 30, and my husband and I wanted to have a baby. But I knew there was

kind of wife and mother you'd like to be—they'll begin to develop some insight.

      TAKE CONTROL. Re-evaluate the goals you set for yourself before you developed fibromyalgia. Throw out those that are no longer possible, revise others and make new ones that you're certain you can achieve.

---

no way I was going to be SuperMom—have a baby and a very demanding career. So I decided, well, I'm just not going to have a job right now.

I was very fortunate because this is not a decision that everyone can make. But the result was two beautiful children.

How do I make it through the day?

It's like I wake up to a body that has run a marathon and it doesn't want to do anymore. It took all the years that I've had this disease to realize that when I get out of bed I should try to do only the simplest of things, like eat breakfast, scan the newspaper, get my hands in warm water. If I just do nonthinking movement-type things, my body eventually does come alive. Then I can do stretches.

If I'm still feeling lousy at 10:00 A.M., I'll go back and take a nap. That little bit of extra sleep is better than any pill. I still want to be up by noon, because I don't want it to interfere with my normal sleep cycle.

Naps have been very important, although it's difficult sometimes for my family and friends to understand why I took that nap when I look great. They think, "Oh, that lazy thing went back to sleep," you know?

I started attending a support group in Los Angeles, a three-hour drive away. But the group leader was burning out. So I filled in. Then I got together with the four or five other group leaders in Los Angeles, plus the group I started in my hometown of Bakersfield, and we'd have speakers—doctors, nutritionists, people who speak on relaxation techniques. But I thought that with all these speakers coming and giving us all this great information, we should put something in writing so that everyone could share it. So I volunteered to do a newsletter, which today goes to 25,000 people all over the country.

Some days are good; some are bad. But after coping with the disease for so long, I know I always come out of it. I know I'm going to make it through.

Food Allergies

WHEN YOUR BODY JUST SAYS NO

It's one thing to make rules for yourself about food. It's another to have your body make them for you.

But that's what happens to women who have a food allergy or food intolerance, two health problems that are often mistaken for one another.

With both conditions, the body decides that certain foods should be off-limits. Through hives, rashes and a variety of other physical reactions, your body suddenly says "Nope. Can't handle that food. Time to give it up." And eating goes from being pleasurable to being problematic.

While it can be easy to confuse food intolerance and food allergy, there are important distinctions between them. While food allergy involves the immune system, food intolerance is generally a digestive problem. And while some symptoms of both disorders resemble each other, others do not.

The Allergy Label

Food allergy is often what people think they have when they have trouble with a particular food. Some folks truly do have an allergy. Researchers don't really know for sure how many Americans, let alone how many women, have food allergies, but estimates are that about 35 million people, or between 1 and 2 percent of the population, are affected. Others have allergy-like symptoms that are caused by something other than an allergy.

Research indicates that the public's perception of food allergies is actually quite different from reality, says Daryl Altman, M.D., an allergist and immunologist and director of Allergy Information Services, an allergy consulting service in Lynbrook, New York. In a study, Dr. Altman and her colleagues found that 13.9 percent of 3,700 U.S. households reported that at least one person in the household had a food allergy.

Anatomy of an Allergy

When you develop a food allergy, there's an actual shift in the functioning of your immune system. Your body starts treating food like the enemy. The immune system, designed to fight off foreign invaders like bacteria, starts attacking different types of food proteins. Researchers aren't sure why or how, but somehow the body starts to see what would normally be innocent, nutritious elements as harmful. "It treats it like an invader," says Michael McCann, M.D., a clinical allergist and immunologist at Kaiser Permanente Medical Center in Parma, Ohio.

When an allergic person is exposed to an offending food, the body produces a series of chemical reactions that result in the release of histamine. Histamine in turn causes many of the physical symptoms of allergy—itching, hives, runny nose or watery eyes. While food allergy can start off mildly, in some people it has the potential to progress into a more severe reaction called anaphylaxis, a life-threatening condition in which the throat swells and closes, blood pressure drops and the body goes into shock.

With food intolerance, there is no shift in the immune system. Instead, a number of things can be happening. Sometimes you have trouble digesting and metabolizing food because certain enzymes are lacking or not functioning right, says Dr. Altman. Symptoms can vary, depending on the food, but you can experience stomach and intestinal problems. You may also experience intolerance to certain foods because of the nature of the foods themselves. Some contain vasoactive amines, natural chemicals that constrict the veins and arteries in the head, she says. When you eat these foods—coffee, chocolate and hard cheeses—the vasoactive amines provoke migraine headaches.

Name That Food

There is a range of foods that trigger allergies or intolerance. The most common food allergen is milk, says Rosemarie Bria, Ph.D., director of nutrition at Allerex, a Greenwich, Connecticut, company that advises food companies about adverse reactions to food.

There are at least 20 protein components in milk that can lead to the production of food-fighting IgE antibodies. Two of the proteins, casein and whey, are sometimes found in other foods, so it's important for individuals with milk allergy to check labels. Casein is found in some brands of tuna even though it's not always listed on the label, so if you have a life-threatening allergy, consider calling the company that makes the brand of tuna you like to ask about the ingredients.

Milk allergy can be confused with lactose intolerance, a digestive problem in which individuals experience discomfort from dairy products because they don't have the right amount of the digestive enzyme—lactase—to digest milk sugar, or lactose. While these individuals can drink milk supplemented with lactase, this enzyme-treated milk will not work if you have a milk allergy, says Dr. Bria.

Other common foods that trigger allergies are soy, eggs, wheat, nuts and seafood.

Chicken eggs contain several common allergens. The white of the egg generally causes more allergies than the yolk. Cashews, Brazil nuts, almonds, pecans, hickory nuts, pine nuts, pistachios, walnuts and hazelnuts have been found to cause anaphylactic reactions in some individuals. The food responsible for the most allergy-related deaths is peanuts, experts say.

Seafood can also cause allergy, including anaphylaxis. People may be allergic to mussels, snails, oysters, scallops, clams, squid, octopus, lobster, shrimp, crab and prawns. However, some studies have shown that some individuals who are allergic to fresh tuna or salmon are able to eat canned forms of those fish.

Wheat is another food that may cause allergy, and often this sensitivity goes hand-in-hand with an allergy to rye and barley.

Food Allergies and Our Bodies

Women with allergies are often worried that their children will inherit them, says Stephen Wasserman, M.D., professor of medicine at the University of California School of Medicine at San Diego.

Babies may be exposed to allergens in problem foods like eggs, peanuts, wheat and milk either in the womb or after birth, through breastfeeding. If a woman with allergies avoids such foods during pregnancy or while nursing, she can decrease her child's risk of food allergy, Dr. Wasserman says.

Some studies show that such a strategy is most useful from pregnancy through the first year of a child's life, says Dr. Wasserman. Pregnant or nursing moms who are avoiding calcium-rich dairy products, however, must take calcium supplements, he cautions.

Avoiding certain foods during pregnancy or breastfeeding is not necessary for all women, says Dr. Wasserman. But in highly allergic families—where either the mother, the father or both are allergic—it may be something to consider, he says. A pregnant woman considering this should consult with her doctor before deleting foods from her diet.

Living with Food Allergies

There's no way for women to prevent food allergies, says Dr. Altman. But there are effective ways to cope with them. Here's how.

MAKE IT OFFICIAL. If you suspect that you have a food allergy, it's important to be diagnosed by a doctor, says Dr. Altman. If you have symptoms, don't assume it's a food allergy. For referral to an allergist, call the American Academy of Allergy and Immunology's Physician Referral and Information Line at 1-800-822-2762.

GET TESTED. Your allergist can test you to see if the physical discomfort you experience after eating certain foods is indeed food allergy, says Dr. Bria. The most accurate test is called the double-blind, placebo-controlled test. For this test, your doctor will instruct you not to eat the suspected foods for one to two weeks. Then she will have you eat samples of foods that contain the suspected foods and others that do not. She'll observe your reactions as the dose is increased.

Other tests that are used but are less accurate are blood tests, which measure certain antibodies in the blood, and skin-prick tests, which involve pricking the skin, exposing it to the suspected food and watching for a red, puffy reaction. For the most accurate diagnosis, ask your doctor for the double-blind, placebo-controlled test.

WORK WITH A DIETITIAN. If you have a diagnosed food allergy, work with a registered dietitian to figure out what to eat, says Dr. Altman. She'll help you replace the nutrients you give up when you stop eating some foods, she says.

KEEP IT SIMPLE. When you're dining out, try not to get too fancy. Stick to dishes in which you can easily identify the ingredients, says Dr. Altman. Steer clear of fancy sauces that might have hidden ingredients you're allergic to.

BE BLUNT. If you have a severe food allergy and you're eating out, be direct with the restaurant staff, says Dr. Altman. "You have to say, 'I am severely allergic to peanuts and if I eat even the slightest little bit of peanut, I can die,' " she says.

USE SEPARATE UTENSILS. "If someone is severely allergic to a particular food, get a special set of utensils for that food," says Dr. Altman. Use the utensils with that food only and don't use them for other dishes. This will prevent the food from accidentally being transferred into foods that the allergic person might eat.

Also, don't be afraid to ask a restaurant to cook your meal in a pan separate from that being used to cook other people's meals, says Dr. Altman. This will prevent any traces of the food you're allergic to from accidentally getting on your plate.

WATCH THE FRUITS. If you've got latex allergy or suspect you might, be careful about eating bananas and avocados. Some individuals with latex allergy have also been found to be allergic to these foods.

KEEP YOUR MEDICINE WITH YOU. If you've got a severe allergy that can throw you into anaphylactic shock, you should carry injectable adrenaline, called epinephrine (EpiPen), with you, says Dr. Altman. "It does not help if the medicine is at home," she says. The injectable adrenaline comes in pen-size units and is easy to carry. It's a good idea to get several of these prescription devices so that you can keep them in different purses and jackets and in your gym bag and briefcase.

Foot Pain

If the Shoe Fits—Wear It

The best advice about avoiding foot pain comes from Cinderella: if the shoe fits, wear it—and if it doesn't, *don't!* Women have four times the foot problems men do, largely because of the design of our shoes.

Squeezing toes, which are roughly semioval, into unyielding leather triangles causes the corns, calluses, blisters and bunions that prompt Americans to spend nearly $5 billion on specialized foot-care treatment.

In one study of 356 women by Carol Frey, M.D., associate clinical professor of orthopedic surgery at the University of Southern California at Los Angeles, 80 percent of the women's feet hurt, which is no wonder, since 88 percent of them wore shoes that were too small. The reason for this may be revealed in another survey, conducted for the American Podiatric Medical Association: 98 percent of the women interviewed agreed that having healthy feet is important, yet 32 percent of them reported having shoes that were uncomfortable but looked good.

There are more than 300 foot ailments, which is not surprising considering that your two feet have 52 bones, 230 ligaments and 38 muscles. Though a tendency toward some foot problems like bunions and ingrown toenails is hereditary, they may not appear until you tempt Fate with ill-fitting shoes or gain weight. There's really no reason for this, since modern materials require little breaking in, and you don't always have to sacrifice comfort for style if you get the right fit.

Don't ignore problems with your feet, says Bruce Lebowitz, D.P.M., director of the podiatric clinic at the Johns Hopkins University School of Medicine/Francis Scott Key Medical Center in Baltimore. The consequences of doing that can be serious. People whose feet hurt carry themselves differently to avoid pain, but this can throw joints out of alignment and lead to problems in the ankle, knee, hip and back. Besides, when your feet hurt, you can't think of anything else.

Corns: Banish the Bumps

If shoes chafe, the body responds by thickening the skin over the bones. Hard corns usually appear on the little toes, and soft corns occur between toes.

KEEP TOES LOOSE. Avoid corns by wearing shoes that are loose enough but still fit properly. Avoid tight shoes without a high toebox at all costs, advises Terry Spilken, D.P.M., adjunct faculty member of the New York College of Podiatric Medicine in New York City and author of *The Dancer's Foot Book*. You can treat hard corns yourself by rubbing a pumice stone or podiatry file over them, he says. You may also use over-the-counter nonmedicated corn pads, unless you have diabetes or poor circulation.

Moisture irritates soft corns, so keep your feet dry. Put lamb's-wool between your toes to absorb moisture and prevent toe-to-toe pressure.

Bunions: Coping with a Curving Joint

Bunions occur when the big toe angles toward the little toes instead of straight forward. A bump forms on the large joint of the big toe. It can rub against the shoe, causing pain and swelling. Although the bone structure that predisposes people to bunions is inherited, women get them at four to five times the rate men do, mainly from wearing high heels with pointed toes, Dr. Spilken says. Bunions are also irritated by tight shoes. According to a study of 2,100 foot surgeries by Michael J. Coughlin, M.D., a Boise, Idaho, orthopedist, 94 percent of the bunion surgeries involved women, many of whom wore tight shoes. Here's what to do about your bunion.

SHIELD IT. Many bunions are eased by comfortable footwear or bunion shields that you can buy at the drugstore, so try changing your shoes before taking stronger measures, advises Dr. Frey.

CONSIDER SURGERY. If walking and wearing shoes are too painful, corrective surgery to reduce the size of the protrusion or to straighten the toe may be necessary. But don't have it done unless you plan to change your footwear, says Dr. Frey, because if you go back to pointed shoes, you'll get another bunion.

Hammertoes: Straightening the Bend

Hammertoe, a deformity that makes the toe curl down, usually happens on the second toe, often to get out of a bunion's way. But more than one toe on a foot can curve in this way. Women with high arches are more susceptible to hammertoes because of the effect of the arch on the tendons. Here's how to fight back.

USE YOUR MARBLES. If the hammertoe is still flexible, you can strengthen the tendons by picking up 20 marbles with your toes three times a day, suggests Dr. Frey.

ASK ABOUT REROUTING. As a last resort, there is surgery to reroute the tendon or remove part of the bone to straighten the toe. Ask your doctor if this procedure is for you, says Dr. Frey.

Ingrown Toenails: Getting Rid of the Pain

Instead of growing straight out of the nail bed, ingrown toenails curve downward, into tender skin. The wounds that result open the door to bacteria, which can lead to painful—and potentially dangerous—infections.

While improper nail cutting and shoes that press on toes didn't start the problem, which is generally hereditary, both exacerbate ingrown toenails. Most people make matters worse by cutting their nails too short at the corners, leaving sharp edges that pierce the skin. Here's some advice for coping.

DON'T CUT CORNERS. "Resist the temptation to dig into the corners. You can round toenails with a file, but don't lift the nail," says Dr. Lebowitz. Some foot doctors advise people to soak their feet to soften the nail, then tuck a piece of soft cotton beneath the nail to "train" it to grow out straight. Others don't recommend this, fearing that if there's a break in the skin, you might push bacteria into an open wound, which can lead to infection—so be careful if you try this. Epsom salts baths can help, though, because the salts draw out infection.

TREAT INFECTION CAREFULLY. If an ingrown toenail becomes infected, wash it well, cover with an antiseptic ointment like Neosporin and cover it with a bandage, says Dr. Spilken. If the pain isn't gone overnight, see your podiatrist: An infection in your toe can

HOW TO BUY REALLY GOOD SHOES

You've heard that you should wear shoes that fit. But how do you do that? "Don't buy shoes and expect to break them in; usually the shoe breaks the foot in," cautions Terry Spilken, D.P.M., adjunct faculty member of the New York College of Podiatric Medicine in New York City and author of *The Dancer's Foot Book*. Use these guidelines to ensure a good fit.

DON'T GO BY THE NUMBERS. Even if you usually wear a size 7, if a particular shoe feels tight, try on the 7½, and if that feels comfortable, buy that size instead.

BUY LONG. Allow a thumb's width (about ½ inch) between the end of your *longest* toe and the end of shoe. This may not be your big toe: Twenty percent of the population has a second toe as long or longer than the first toe. Also buy for your larger foot.

BUY LATE. Buy shoes at midday (2:00 to 4:00 P.M.), when your foot has had a chance to swell from walking around all day. This way you'll buy a shoe to fit your feet at their largest.

BUY LARGER IF YOU'RE EXPECTING. If you are pregnant, your old shoes may not feel comfortable any more because your feet have swollen. Get a size larger for the last few months.

TAKE OFF EXTRA WEIGHT. Being overweight puts more pressure on foot tendons, ligaments and joints and can cause symptoms that wouldn't bother you if you weighed less.

REMEMBER, COST DOESN'T GUARANTEE GOOD FIT. Judge by the way a shoe feels on your foot, not how much it costs.

BUY MORE THAN ONE. If you find a pair of shoes you love, and they fit, buy a pair in every color you like. You'll thank yourself later.

spread up your leg, causing a serious problem. In severe cases, your podiatrist can perform minor surgery to cauterize the nail so it won't grow into the nail bed. This procedure can be done in the office. If you are diabetic or have poor circulation, see your podiatrist *immediately* if you have an infection; otherwise you could lose a toe or limb if gangrene sets in.

DON'T WEAR HIGH HEELS. A two-inch heel puts 57 percent more pressure on the ball of the foot than wearing no shoes. If you can't resist high heels, be sure to buy ones that are long and wide enough. Take your shoes off as much as possible.

TRACE YOUR FOOT. To ensure good fit in athletic shoes, stand on a piece of paper and have someone outline it. Then measure the widest part of the ball of your foot. When you're trying on shoes, pull out the sole liner and see if it matches your foot, advises Francesca M. Thompson, M.D., chief of the Adult Orthopaedic Foot Clinic at St. Luke's–Roosevelt Hospital Center in New York City. (You can get by with ½ inch narrower in a dress shoe.)

GET THE RIGHT SHOE FOR THE SPORT. If you play more than one sport, buy a different pair of shoes for each. For instance, tennis shoes accommodate side-to-side motion, running shoes accommodate heel-to-toe motion, and basketball shoes accommodate side-to-side motion, running and jumping. The manufacturers aren't just trying to get you to spend another $70 on shoes, Dr. Spilken insists. Look at it this way: The shoes will last longer.

SELECT SPORTS SOCKS. Like athletic shoes, sports socks match the sport for which they are designed by providing extra padding where the foot takes the heat. Sports socks tend to hold their shape, last longer and "wick"—that is, they draw moisture from the inside of the sock away from the foot. Natural fibers like cotton absorb moisture, which can amount to holding a wet washcloth next to the foot, so choose socks made of acrylic, which has wicking action.

Morton's Neuroma: Playing Down the Pinch

Morton's neuroma happens when two toe bones—generally between the third and fourth toes—rub together and pinch a nerve, which can then build up extra nerve tissue. Neuromas occur 90 percent more frequently among women, mainly from wearing tight shoes. To prevent neuromas, be sure your shoes don't cramp your toes. Here's what to do if you have one.

CUSHION YOUR FOOT. According to Dr. Frey, many patients get better after six months of conservative treatment. Ask your doctor where you can find metatarsal pads or Spenco sole liners, which cushion the foot so you don't pound on the nerve. The pads or liners can be fitted by your doctor.

TRY MEDICATIONS OR INJECTIONS. Serious neuromas that don't respond to liners or pads are treated with nonsteroidal anti-inflammatories (both prescription and nonprescription), cortisone injections to reduce swelling, and surgery, Dr. Frey says.

Plantar Warts: Cleansing Your Sole

The same group of viruses that causes warts elsewhere in the body—the papova viruses—lead to plantar warts, which appear on the sole of the foot. When you walk, the wart is compressed in the skin, which makes it very painful. Plantar warts don't cause cancer, nor do they grow into the muscle, but they can get larger and spread to other places.

Some people appear to be more susceptible to plantar warts than others, since, as Dr. Frey puts it, "that virus is everywhere!" Here's how to cope.

ZAP THEM. Methods your doctor will use to treat plantar warts include removing them with acid or a laser or freezing them. Surgery is also possible in severe cases, but there is a chance of scar formation, says Keith L. Wapner, M.D., director of the Division of Foot and Ankle Surgery at Thomas Jefferson University Hospital in Philadelphia.

DON'T GO BAREFOOT. Since the virus that causes warts thrives in warm, moist environments such as locker room showers and the decks of swimming pools, the American Podiatric Medical Association recommends wearing shoes to prevent contact.

Plantar Fasciitis: Relax the Pain Away

If you have plantar fasciitis, you'll feel pain under the arch or at the front inner part of the heel, often first thing in the morning or after you've been sitting for a while. This injury to the soft tissue that connects the heel bone to the bones of the ball of the foot happens to women who usually wear high heels and then suddenly stop—during summer vacation, for instance, when they spurn high heels for sandals. The heel tissue can't adjust to the difference in shoe height, so it gets injured. Walking on hard, flat surfaces can cause problems, too. Try these remedies.

RELAX YOUR FEET. Rather than making drastic changes in footwear, let the tissue relax by wearing moderate heels, an inch to an inch and a half in height, advises Dr. Lebowitz.

STRETCH AND MASSAGE. Stretch the Achilles tendon frequently and use ice massage for the pain, says Dr. Wapner. Since inflamed tissue tends to cause the foot to contract, he prescribes night splints that keep feet in a stretched position.

Pump Bumps: Relief Can Be a Lift Away

Women who wear high heels get "pump bumps"—pain and swelling on the heel near the Achilles tendon—when the heel bone rubs against the rigid back part (counter) of the shoe. Women with abnormal heel bones, such as those with Haglund's disease, are especially vulnerable, but anyone can have similar symptoms from wearing tight shoes. Here's what to do.

AVOID RIGID SHOES. Don't buy shoes that have hard counters, warns Dr. Lebowitz. You can also wear over-the-counter heel lifts or create a custom cushion for the back of your heel: Paint the bump with crayon or marker, then place a commercial heel cushion in the back of the shoe. Wear the shoe for five or ten minutes, then remove it and cut away the area of the cushion where the paint left an impression.

GET PROFESSIONAL HELP. If nothing helps, a foot surgeon may have to file down the heel bone, but some people have problems with Achilles tendinitis after this operation. Ask your doctor what your chances of a painless recovery are before an operation.

Getting Some Support From Orthotics

Many podiatrists recommend custom-made arch supports called orthotics for several foot conditions, including hammertoes, bunions and arch and heel pain.

Orthotics give the feet support and straighten them out, so they will sit properly in shoes. But some foot doctors question the expense—which can run over $300. Doctors also wonder whether they really help, since you can't use some of them in fashion pumps.

Gallstones

WHY THEY ARE A "WOMAN'S PROBLEM"

The chocolate Chambord birthday cake was a mistake. Duffy's boss had brought it to the picnic to celebrate her employee's 40th birthday. And everyone loved every bite of the dark, decadent chocolate—including Duffy. But half an hour after her last forkful, a sharp, stabbing pain began between her shoulder blades. Two hours later she could hardly breathe. Three hours later, she was in an emergency room and a surgeon was preparing to operate.

Not every woman reacts to a chocolate birthday cake by getting a gallstone stuck in the duct that leads from the gallbladder—where bile acids used for fat digestion are stored—to the upper intestine. But the fact is that women are more than twice as likely as men to complain of gallstones: Of the 971,000 Americans who report gallstones to the National Center for Health Statistics in Hyattsville, Maryland, every year, 666,000—more than two-thirds—are women.

Women at Risk

Why do women have more than twice the risk? In a word, hormones. Hormones that regulate our cycles and our pregnancies, along with oral or implanted contraceptives and hormone replacement therapy (HRT), put us at increased risk, says Henry Pitt, M.D., director of the Johns Hopkins University Gallstone and Biliary Disease Center in Baltimore.

Two factors affect gallstone formation, he explains. One is the amount of cholesterol that saturates the bile stored in the gallbladder; the other is how quickly the gallbladder fills with bile and how quickly it empties into the intestine. The more cholesterol in the gallbladder and the longer it stays there, the more likely it will thicken into the soft lumps that eventually solidify into gallstones.

The problem for women is that the two sex hormones—estrogen and progesterone—may affect the amount of cholesterol in bile. These hormones may also affect how the gallbladder fills and empties as well as the function of the sphincter between the bile duct and intestine. The result is the perfect incubator for stones.

Obesity, Smoking and Other Risk Factors

But increased hormone levels are not the only reason women form gallstones, says Dr. Pitt. Obesity, rapid-weight-loss dieting, diets high in fat and cholesterol and a family history of gallstones are other factors that put both men and women at risk. Fortunately, gallstones can frequently be prevented. Here's what Dr. Pitt suggests.

TAKE FISH-OIL SUPPLEMENTS. In several studies at Johns Hopkins, Dr. Pitt and his colleagues have found that the oils found in fish can prevent or at least reduce the formation of gallstones. Their animal studies indicate that fish oil prevents the formation of stones altogether. Their studies in people, which were limited to a two-week period before participants were scheduled to have their gallstones removed, indicated that 960 milligrams of fish oil—the amount found in one soft-gel capsule—taken three times a day alters the tendency to form stones. As a result, Dr. Pitt suspects that including fish oil in your diet will prevent the formation of gallstones.

KEEP YOUR DIET LOW IN FAT AND CHOLESTEROL. Both fat and cholesterol provide the raw cholesterol from which most stones are made, says Dr. Pitt. Reducing them will also reduce your risk.

EAT AT REGULAR INTERVALS. Some studies show that fasting for longer than 14 hours increases your risk of gallstones. The problem is that the gallbladder only empties significantly and squirts bile into the upper intestine when food is consumed. (It also releases bile at other times, but not in large amounts.) So if no food is consumed, the likelihood that cholesterol will have the time to thicken into

WOMAN TO WOMAN NEW SURGERY EASED RECOVERY

Linda Weinberger was a 42-year-old elementary school counselor and mother of two preteens in East Greenville, Pennsylvania, when she was struck with gallstones so severe that surgery to remove her gallbladder was the best option. Fortunately, it was at the same time that laparoscopic surgery, in which a telescopic device and surgical instruments are inserted through the abdomen to remove the gallbladder, was starting to be used. She became one of the first women in the country to have the procedure. This is her story.

As I recall, I was having a lot of stomach discomfort. But because it was happening near the end of the school year, I thought it was just the normal end-of-the-year stress kind of symptoms. I didn't even go to our doctor, but I had taken one of the boys to his office for something, and while I was there my stomach really hurt. So I said, "If you have time, could you check me out, too?"

So he did, and he said, "I think it's probably gastritis," which I've had before. So he said, "I'm going to prescribe this medication"—some kind of little pills—and he said, "Don't drink with them or you'll get really goofy. If anything gets worse, call me right away, but at any rate call me in about three or four days and let me know how this medication works."

We went out for dinner that night with friends and I didn't feel really good, but I didn't feel horrible. Then I had a baked potato with sour cream on it.

Well, I was so miserable, I thought, "This is how people die."

I remember not being very talkative on the way home. I just wanted to curl up in a fetal position and leave the earth. I was horribly nauseated.

lumps is increased. That's why skipping meals and fasting are not in your gallbladder's best interests.

MAINTAIN YOUR WEIGHT. Studies indicate that overweight women who are five feet four inches tall and weigh 175 pounds are twice as likely to form gallstones as women of the same height who weigh 145 pounds. That's why maintaining your weight makes it less likely that you'll develop gallstones, says Dr. Pitt.

We got home and I went to bed, but I couldn't sleep, and I thought, "I probably have cancer or something really dreadful," because I knew this was not gastritis.

In the morning I stuck my finger down my throat to force myself to throw up, thinking, "Maybe this will help."

It didn't. So that morning I went back to the doctor. By then the pain had localized on my right side, a little bit lower than my ribcage. The doctor's verdict was that I probably had a gallbladder problem.

He sent me for a sonogram. As I was lying on the table, the technician told me what she saw on the screen. "There are different sizes of grit that we can see when you have gallstones," she said. "They can be anywhere from the size of sand up to the size of boulders. And you've got rocks. Big rocks."

My doctor recommended a surgeon at Bryn Mawr Hospital. So I went to his office and he explained the procedure. My concern was that he couldn't do it until August 1. I had to wait two months—mostly living on this liquid stuff called Citrotein. Eating most foods caused me pain and discomfort.

I had the surgery at 5:00 P.M. on August 1. The next morning about 7:30, I jokingly said to the doctor, "Oh well, I'm ready to go home. When can I leave?" And he said, "As soon as you eat some breakfast, you can go." I had been there no more than 18 hours from admission to discharge.

I had a wonderful recovery. Within a few days I was back to normal. I remember two days after having surgery, I went to a barbecue at somebody's house. I didn't eat a whole lot, but I ate. The following day I was driving. Within a week I was totally recovered.

RECONSIDER TAKING CALCIUM SUPPLEMENTS. Animal studies at Johns Hopkins indicate that taking extra calcium—as many women do to reduce their chances of osteoporosis—may increase their risk of forming stones. Scientists aren't sure why.

"We're not saying 'Don't take calcium supplements' to everyone," says Dr. Pitt. "What we are saying is that if gallstones run in your family, you should talk to your family physician before you do."

THINK TWICE ABOUT TAKING HORMONES. Given hormones' involvement in making gallstones, women who know that gallstones run in their family should also be cautious about using oral contraceptives or HRT, says Dr. Pitt.

A study of more than 54,000 postmenopausal women at Harvard Medical School found that those who used HRT doubled their risk of having an operation to remove gallstones.

Ask your doctor to help you weigh the pluses and minuses of HRT and your own particular gallstone risk, says Dr. Pitt.

AVOID NORPLANT. Studies in prairie dogs—which have gallbladders that act like human gallbladders—indicate that using an implanted progesterone contraceptive like Norplant may increase your risk of gallstones over time, says Dr. Pitt.

SWALLOW BEAR BILE. Rapid weight loss in obese women is one of the major causes of gallstone formation. A review of studies by the National Institute of Diabetes and Digestive and Kidney Diseases in Bethesda, Maryland, reveals that 12 percent of 390 overweight people who went on 520- to 840-calorie diets for 8 to 16 weeks developed gallstones.

The cause? Their gallbladders didn't get enough food to stimulate the contractions that would allow it to empty. Cholesterol was allowed to build up and thicken, and gallstones were the result.

That's why anyone who's planning on using a super-low-calorie diet to lose some serious weight—say 40 or 50 pounds—should also take ursodeoxycholic acid, says Dr. Pitt. The acid—actually a form of bear bile that's sold by prescription as Actigall—will help prevent stone formation.

Rolling Away the Stones

Fortunately, 60 to 80 percent of those who have gallstones will probably never even know they have them. The stones will either stay in the gallbladder or remain so small that they'll pass through the duct between the gallbladder and intestine without causing a problem. And their owners will never experience the pain—located in the right side of the chest below the breastbone or sometimes between the shoulder blades—that occurs when a stone gets stuck in the duct.

But if a stone does gets stuck, you have only one option, says Dr. Pitt: Gallbladder and stones must go.

"The treatment of choice today is a laparoscopic cholecystectomy," says Dr. Pitt. It's a procedure in which the surgeon makes four tiny punctures in and around the navel. Through one puncture he inserts a thin, telescope-like instrument through which he can see the gallbladder, then he inserts surgical instruments through the others. The gallbladder is cut away from surrounding tissue and removed.

A study of 294 women and 86 men at the University of Kansas School of Medicine in Wichita indicates that the procedure carries little risk. The procedure took approximately two hours to complete, and most patients were sent home the next day—though some needed more hospital time for recovery. Only 3 percent experienced any complications.

Moving from a laparoscopic procedure to open surgery is something for which every woman who undergoes gallstone surgery should be prepared, says Dr. Pitt. If the surgeon peers through the laparoscope and finds that he or she cannot adequately see the gallbladder or duct or finds that there is an inflammation, bleeding or scarring from prior disease or surgery—all of which increase the risk of injury during laparoscopic surgery—the surgeon will simply remove the laparoscope, make a standard surgical incision across the abdomen and remove the gallbladder that way.

Studies indicate that this type of surgery—called an "open" cholecystectomy—usually requires a 5- to 12-day hospital stay and heavy-duty postoperative painkillers. The complication rate is a whopping 35 percent—primarily involving respiratory difficulties and infection.

Gender Discrimination
HOW TO HANDLE HARASSMENT

In 1994, women earned 76 cents for every dollar men earned. More than half had been sexually harassed on the job or knew someone who had been.

In 1993, one in four women in a national poll said she was "talked down to" by doctors. One in six was told a medical condition was "all in her head." One in ten said she had been sexually abused as a child. One in five had low self-esteem.

Editors of the *Journal of Women's Health* pointed out a huge gap: Women spend two out of every three health-care dollars in America, yet the bulk of medical research has focused on men. "Now," they said, "catch-up work must be done."

Sometimes, it seems, being female can be hazardous to your health and well-being.

Getting Mixed Messages

"Women must deal continually with society's mixed messages," says Georgia Witkin, Ph.D., assistant clinical professor of psychiatry and director of the Stress Program at the Mount Sinai Medical Center in New York City and author of *The Female Stress Syndrome*.

"We are most often expected to be sexy but not sexual," Dr. Witkin says. "To have a child but remain childlike; to be assertive but not aggressive; to hold a job but not neglect the home."

Gender bias? You bet. And it's more than just a hot topic for the TV talk-show circuit.

Subtle or blatant, unequal treatment can take a psychological and physical toll on any woman—whether she's just discovered she earns less than a male colleague or is a working mom who's rushing home to start the "second shift," caring for a family and household. And many women feel a nagging suspicion that dealing with a male auto mechanic, banker or boss might be a little easier if she were one of the guys. Dr. Witkin says these strains are "hidden stresses that distress, distract and deplete us." The impact? Bias contributes to unhealthy levels of stress, poor self-esteem, depression rates that are twice as high among women as among men, and the fear of failure. With all these can come physical difficulties ranging from stomachaches to insomnia, from panic attacks to skin rashes, from headaches to anorexia.

"The good news is, you can retrain yourself," says Dr. Witkin. "You can treat yourself well and boost your self-esteem. You can take risks and satisfy your desire for accomplishment. You can change things."

Rooted in Our Pasts

Psychologists trace gender bias and its impact to childhood, a time when Dr. Witkin says some girls learn "nonassertiveness." When University of California psychologists followed 91 young people through their teens and early twenties, they saw girls lose self-esteem while boys gained it. Why? Perhaps because girls are given less autonomy as they mature. "In crasser terms," they wrote, "females are socialized to get along in society and males are socialized to get ahead."

Girls who are self-confident and outspoken at age 7 become unsure of themselves by 15 or 16, and less willing to discuss their feelings and observations. The American Association of University Women's landmark report "Shortchanging Girls, Shortchanging America," notes that while 60 percent of elementary school girls told researchers they were "happy as I am," just 29 percent of high school girls felt that way.

"Moving from 'young girl' to 'young woman' involves meeting unique demands in a culture that both idealizes and exploits the sexuality of young women while assigning them roles that are clearly less valued," says Susan Bailey, Ph.D., a social scientist and director of the Wellesley College Center for Research on Women in Massachusetts. Her report charges that schools don't do enough for female students, who take fewer advanced math courses and for the most part see few women role models in their textbooks.

It struck a chord in grown women. "Everyone I talked to had a story of her own," Dr. Bailey says. The stories concerned "either being discouraged from pursuing math and science, confronting sexual harassment or finding it suddenly was not okay to be a tomboy anymore."

Where We Stand in Medicine

From a family doctor who says "it's all in your head" to medical research that has historically focused on men, bias in the medical profession can influence the quality of your health care, doctors say.

"Medical school doesn't prepare doctors for women patients," says Lila A. Wallis, M.D., clinical professor of medicine at Cornell University Medical College in New York City and director of the American Medical Women's Association's advanced curriculum on women's health.

"Historically, women have not been treated kindly by the established medical profession, either as health-care consumers or as health-care providers or as subjects of medical research."

In fact, when researchers looked at diseases affecting both men and women, many studied only males and later applied the results to women.

Heart disease, for instance, kills 250,000 women a year, yet major studies of heart attack prevention excluded women—including the 1989 Physician's Health Study of the effects of low-dose aspirin, which focused on 22,071 male doctors.

AIDS is the fifth leading cause of death among women of childbearing age, but fewer than 10 percent of the participants in large, government-funded studies between 1987 and 1991 were female.

Many researchers omitted women because of concerns that fluctuating hormones would compromise test results. But it's precisely those fluctuating hormones, along with other factors, that influence the health, course of illness and response to treatment in a woman, says Dr. Wallis.

This lack of research means that women's unique symptoms are often overlooked.

"I had a woman come to me with a terrible yeast infection. She had been to three gynecologists and had a bag full of pills," says Dr. Wallis. "None realized she had a systemic disease. It turned out to be AIDS. Often, AIDS in women is not diagnosed because it manifests itself differently than in men, and the differences have not been studied much."

ILLEGAL AND UNWANTED

Suggestive comments. Sexual advances. Unwanted touching. In the workplace, sexual harassment is more than offensive. It's against the law.

Under the Civil Rights Act of 1991, unwanted and repeated harassment is illegal if it creates a hostile work environment or if you have to tolerate it to keep your job. Here are steps that you can take to end it, suggested by 9 to 5, the National Association for Working Women.

SAY NO CLEARLY. Make it plain—in writing if necessary—that the behavior is offensive.

DOCUMENT IT. Record each incident, including your response and the date, time and place it occurred. Keep a copy at home in case you file a lawsuit.

GET EMOTIONAL SUPPORT. Sexual harassment is not your fault. Tell friends or family what's happening.

DOCUMENT YOUR WORK. Keep performance reviews and memos that attest to your work's quality. The harasser may question your job performance to justify his behavior.

LOOK FOR WITNESSES AND OTHER VICTIMS. Two accusations are harder to ignore than one. Ask around—you may find someone to support your charge.

EXPLORE IN-HOUSE CHANNELS. Use company grievance procedures. If you're in a union, tell the shop steward.

FILE A COMPLAINT. Contact the federal Equal Employment Opportunity Commission (EEOC); it's listed in your local telephone directory under U.S. Government Offices.

FIND A LAWYER. You don't need an attorney to file a sexual harassment claim, but you may get useful advice from legal services or a private-practice lawyer who specializes in employment discrimination.

Hope for the Future

While doctors disagree as to whether there has been gender bias in the treatment of heart disease, there is evidence that women receive less care than men. In a University of Tennessee study, men with heart disease were twice as likely as women to have had bypass surgery. In 1991, Harvard University researchers found that for 80,000 cardiac patients in Massachusetts and Maryland, the odds of undergoing certain medical procedures were 27 to 45 percent higher for men.

But the research gap may be closing. In 1991, the National Institutes of Health in Bethesda, Maryland, launched a 14-year, $625-million Women's Health Initiative to study prevention of osteoporosis, cancer and heart disease in postmenopausal women. In 1993, the federal government pumped $5 million into a large-scale investigation of women with HIV.

But to beat the odds and get the best health care, Dr. Wallis suggests that women choose family doctors and internists who understand the whole female body and can perform medical checkups that include gynecological exams.

"A woman who is sophisticated enough to know that she exists not just from the waist down but that she has a head, a heart and lungs, knows she needs her whole body considered," Dr. Wallis says.

A Woman and Her Doctor

Should that doctor be a woman?

Probably.

"While there are some male doctors who are better than some female doctors at listening and communicating, taken as a whole, female doctors appear to be doing a better job," notes Debra Roter, Dr.P.H., professor of health policy and management at Johns Hopkins School of Hygiene and Public Health in Baltimore.

Dr. Roter analyzed audiotapes from office visits to 100 doctors—half male, half female—with men and women patients. The women physicians spent more time taking patient histories, got more information from patients and seemed to draw patients further into a partnership to meet their medical needs.

"Women doctors gave women patients the most time, and men doctors gave women patients the least," she says. "So gender does make a difference. Female doctors also asked more often what was going on in other parts of a patient's life." A woman who appreciates the connection between her daily routine, her feelings and her physical health "may do better with a female doctor," says Dr. Roter.

When Minnesota researchers looked at care received by 97,000 women in 1990, they found that those who saw female doctors were more likely to have regular Pap smears and mammograms. "Women doctors often feel they are advocates for women patients," notes Dr. Wallis, "and have honed their skills to serve them."

In the doctor's office, at home or on the job, doctors say the following tips can help you take control.

CONSIDER YOUR BODY. Ask your doctor how a treatment or drug affects a woman's body. For instance, will a medication have an impact on fertility or bone density? Could a treatment cause birth defects now or in the future? Will a prescribed drug interact with birth control pills?

PAY ATTENTION TO YOUR CYCLE. Some drugs used for migraines, depression, hypertension and insomnia have different effects at various points in the menstrual cycle. Ask if the dose can be tailored to your needs.

ASK WHAT MEN GET. Researchers say women may not be tested as aggressively as men for problems like heart and lung disease. Find out what tests are available for your health condition and ask if they're appropriate.

DISSOLVE DENIAL. "Many of us deny the truth of our painful experiences as much as possible," says clinical psychologist Ellen McGrath, Ph.D., executive director of the Psychology Center in Laguna Beach, California, and author of *When Feeling Bad Is Good*. "But denial robs us of our energy." Look into your past for signs of emotional, economic, physical or sexual abuse. Write them down.

SAFELY RELEASE ANGER. Releasing feelings can repair emotional damage. Dr. McGrath suggests ripping the pages of a telephone book or smashing a pumpkin. "Think about the person you're angry at while you do this," she says. "Any time you can make it more real by doing it, you've got more power over your situation."

DO A REALITY CHECK. You were passed over for a promotion; a male co-worker got it. Was it bias? "Get the facts, and try not to take it personally," says Dr. Witkin. "I tell women, at all times, 'see yourself as someone in business for yourself. Your company is your client. Take necessary action to right what is wrong. Be forceful and tactful—but don't overreact.'"

Gum Disease
What Comes between You and Your Teeth

To lose a lover or even a husband or two during the course of one's life can be vexing," the sagacious Madame Armfeldt observes in *A Little Night Music*. "But to lose one's teeth is a catastrophe."

It's true. Unlike men, teeth are virtually impossible to replace. With teeth, nothing fits or works as well as the original article.

The secret to keeping your teeth is caring for your gums. The proof? Well, gum disease is the leading cause of tooth loss in people over 35. Since it usually arrives without warning, you've got to be on guard against it.

"It's a very subtle disease," says Susan Karabin, D.D.S., assistant clinical professor of periodontics at Columbia University in New York City. "There's not much pain, so patients are often unaware. The only signs are a little bleeding or sensitivity when they brush their teeth, and patients tend to ignore that."

The Part Hormones Play

About 70 percent of women 35 and older have some degree of gum disease, estimates Marjorie Jeffcoat, D.M.D., chairman of the Department of Periodontics at the School of Dentistry at the University of Alabama in Birmingham.

Gum disease doesn't seem to be any more common in women than in men. But women do tend to get worse cases during menstruation, pregnancy and possibly menopause, Dr. Jeffcoat says. At those times hormonal changes make gums more sensitive to bacteria.

Researchers have known for years that bacterial infections cause gum disease. But they're still not sure why gum disease first makes an appearance once you've reached your midthirties. Some speculate that its arrival follows years of damage to the gums.

Even the most committed brushers and flossers can get a mild form of gum disease called gingivitis. With gingivitis, your gums may bleed a bit when you brush, but that's all the warning you'll get. If you don't take care of it—by brushing and flossing daily and seeing your dentist for professional cleanings at least once every six months— gingivitis can open the door to periodontitis. A particularly nasty form of gum disease, periodontitis can quietly destroy the tissues that hold your teeth in place.

Who Gets It?

Research suggests that some people inherit a predisposition to gum disease. In one study, scientists at the Medical College of Virginia in Richmond compared the mouths of nearly 5,000 sets of identical and fraternal twins and concluded that genes "make an important contribution to periodontal disease." The researchers found that identical twins, who have identical genes, were twice as likely to have nearly identical levels of gum disease as fraternal twins, who have different genes.

Medications for epilepsy, depression, heart disease and allergies can also make you more vulnerable to gum disease. So can Type I, or insulin-dependent, diabetes and immune system disorders like AIDS, which weaken your ability to fight invading bacteria.

While some prescriptions hurt, others may help. Estrogen replacement therapy (ERT) seems to offset some symptoms of gum disease in postmenopausal women. Dental researchers at the State University of

New York at Buffalo found that postmenopausal women who were getting ERT had about 20 percent less gum bleeding than those who weren't on the therapy.

The most important elements of any prevention plan, though, are brushing, flossing and regular visits to the dentist. Nearly 95 percent of cases of gum disease can be controlled or prevented, says Dr. Karabin.

The Problem with Plaque

The idea of brushing and flossing is to get rid of plaque. That's the film of bacteria, food particles and mucus that collects between your teeth and under your gumline. If you don't brush and floss it away, plaque hardens to form calculus, or tartar, which then has to be scraped away by your dentist or dental hygienist. You can't get rid of tartar yourself.

Plaque and tartar aren't simply an aesthetic liability. Even if your immune system is in top form, some of the bacteria they harbor produce toxins that irritate and damage your gums. Your immune cells can fight the bacteria, but with limited success. While battling the bugs, some of the cells inadvertently damage your gums as well, and they become swollen and tender. That's gingivitis.

During menstruation and pregnancy, the problem gets worse because progesterone and estrogen levels fluctuate, prompting immune cells in your gums to launch a more aggressive attack. This leaves your gums even more swollen, Dr. Jeffcoat explains. You end up with a very bad case of gingivitis.

If you have gingivitis but don't realize there's a problem, or you ignore it, there's a possibility your inflamed gums can start to pull away from your teeth. Gaps, or pockets, form between the tooth and gum. This is periodontitis. Unchecked, bacteria-laden plaque move into the pockets, infect and damage more gum, then do a job on the connective tissue anchoring your teeth to your jawbone—and ultimately the bone itself. Your teeth get loose and fall out.

What You Can Do

Up to the very end, you may not suspect anything's amiss. You can't see the bacteria attacking your gums, of course, and you can't see the periodontal pockets that are forming. They're too small. That's why you have to visit the dentist regularly for checkups. Between visits, here's what you should do to hold on to your teeth.

BRUSH, BRUSH, BRUSH. Do it at least twice a day with a soft toothbrush and a fluoride toothpaste. A hard brush can irritate your gums, so you don't want that, says Joan Otomo-Corgel, D.D.S., adjunct assistant professor at the School of Dentistry at the University of California at Los Angeles. The fluoride is for cavity protection. Researchers aren't sure whether fluoride fights the bacteria that hurt your gums, says Dennis Mangan, Ph.D., director of the Periodontal Diseases Program at the National Institute of Dental Research in Bethesda, Maryland. But they know it strengthens the teeth, making it harder for acids produced by bacteria to erode the tooth enamel.

To get the most out of brushing, follow this advice from the American Dental Association (ADA): Hold your toothbrush beside your teeth horizontally, with the bristles at a 45-degree angle to your gumline. Move the brush back and forth in short strokes several times before starting on a new section. Brush both the outer and inner surfaces of every tooth. To clean the inside of your front teeth, hold the brush vertically and make several gentle up-and-down strokes with the front bristles. Move on to the chewing surfaces, brushing them with back-and-forth strokes. Finish by brushing your tongue.

AND BRUSH AGAIN. Make it three times a day if you've got braces, crowded teeth, a bridge or a family history of gum disease; if you take medications that aggravate gum problems; or if you're menstruating, pregnant or going through menopause, says Dr. Otomo-Corgel.

FLOSS DAILY. A toothbrush can't clean between your teeth and under your gumline. That's where floss fits in: It can slip through every crevice. To use it like a pro, the ADA suggests this approach: Take an 18-inch piece of floss and wrap it around both index fingers. Guiding the floss with your thumbs, slide it between your teeth. Curve the floss into a C-shape against one tooth and gently slide it into the space between the gum and the tooth until you feel resistance. Hold the floss against the tooth and gently scrape the side, moving the floss away from the gum. Move on to the next tooth, and don't forget to floss the back side of your last molar.

PICK AT IT. If you can't floss, clean your teeth with a toothpick. Gently run one around the neck of each tooth. Don't stab! "A toothpick won't do as good a job as floss, but it'll help," Dr. Jeffcoat says.

TRY A RINSE. "In my opinion, Listerine, which has the American Dental Association's seal of approval, is the only over-the-counter rinse that's proven its mettle against plaque," says Dr. Karabin. Try it. Or ask your dentist about rinses containing chlorhexidine, such as Peridex. These also have the ADA's approval but are available only by prescription. The jury is still out on other over-the-counter "anti-plaque" rinses like Plax. So far, there's no scientific evidence that they work.

BUILD YOUR BONES. Finnish researchers studied 227 postmenopausal women and concluded that those with strong bones were more likely to keep their teeth than those who'd lost bone density to osteoporosis. To protect your bones and teeth, eat calcium-rich foods like low-fat yogurt, skim milk, low-fat cheese, sardines and canned salmon (with the bones), says Kendra Kaye, M.D., clinical assistant professor of medicine at the University of Pennsylvania School of Medicine and attending physician at Graduate Hospital, both in Philadelphia. Shoot for at least 1,000 milligrams of calcium daily. Make it 1,200 milligrams if you're pregnant and 1,500 milligrams daily if you're past menopause and not on ERT. Take a calcium supplement if you don't get enough from the foods you eat.

And remember to exercise, Dr. Kaye says: It helps keep bones strong. You don't have to join a gym. You can walk the dog, ride your bike around the neighborhood, jump rope in the backyard—whatever it takes to get at least 30 minutes of exercise at least three times a week.

HIT A HIGH C. Vitamin C helps keep your gums healthy, says JoAnne Allen, D.D.S., a dentist in Albuquerque. So make sure you have a least five servings of C-rich foods—like citrus fruits, tomatoes, strawberries, green and red peppers and broccoli—daily.

STOP SMOKING. Tobacco delivers a triple whammy to your teeth and gums. "Smoking removes calcium from the bone and suppresses the immune system," Dr. Allen says. "It also decreases blood supply to the mouth, so if there's anything that needs healing, there's less blood to do it." If you chew tobacco, quit that, too.

RELAX. Stress can take a toll on your immune system, which needs its strength to fend off bacterial invaders, Dr. Jeffcoat says. To beat stress, soak in a warm tub, go for a walk, listen to soothing music or just breathe deeply.

SEE THE DENTIST. Go at least once every six months. "Even the best tooth cleaners, after three to four months, get to the point where they can't keep things clean anymore," says Douglas Hall, D.D.S., a periodontist in Edmond, Oklahoma.

If your gums look inflamed or bleed when you brush, head for the dentist even if it's been less than six months since your last visit.

And go every three months if you're pregnant or have other risk factors for gum disease. During pregnancy, make sure you schedule a visit before your third trimester, Dr. Otomo-Corgel says. In the last trimester, you shouldn't lie flat on your back as you would for a dental cleaning. In that position, the baby will put too much pressure on the major veins in your midsection, which could restrict blood flow and make you pass out, she explains. If you must see a dentist during the last trimester, ask the dentist or hygienist to let you sit in a semi-reclining position.

LEFT TO YOUR OWN DEVICES

Various gadgets promise to help you keep your teeth and gums in shape. Are they as good as their word? Here's the verdict from the experts.

Electric toothbrushes. If you have limited dexterity or you just like things with motors, these are a good investment, says T. F. McNamara, Ph.D., professor of oral biology and pathology at the State University of New York at Stony Brook. Choose one with soft, rotating bristles, like the Interplak or Braun Oral B Plaque Remover, says Douglas Hall, D.D.S., a periodontist in Edmond, Oklahoma.

Oral irrigators. These shoot an intermittent, pulsating stream of water—or mouthwash-and-water combination, if you choose—between the teeth and under the gumline. (Don't use straight mouthwash or you can gum up the machine, advises Dr. Hall.) The Water-Pik and other irrigators are a particularly good buy if you've got braces or a partial bridge. Dr. Hall suggests you use it on a medium setting, no higher, and keep it moving over the sides of your teeth. Even if you use an irrigator, though, you still have to floss. Only floss can slip into the really tight spots.

Floss holders. Reminiscent of slingshots, these are Y-shaped plastic handles strung with dental floss. The American Dental Association recommends these if you have a hard time handling floss.

Rubber tip stimulators. Some toothbrushes come with little rubber points attached at the end. Although the rubber tips that come with the toothbrush generally aren't that well-made, the ones you can buy separately are worth the price, says Joan Otomo-Corgel, D.D.S., adjunct assistant professor at the School of Dentistry at the University of California at Los Angeles. You can run the tips under your gumline to gently wipe away plaque.

GET CLEANED. In the office, your dentist or hygienist should scrape away the hardened tartar between your teeth and under your gumline, Dr. Otomo-Corgel says. When you get home, you should redouble efforts to brush and floss plaque away before it hardens to form more tartar.

SAY "PERIODONTAL EXAM, PLEASE." Make sure you get a periodontal exam with every checkup. Your dentist or hygienist should look for and measure pockets using a periodontal probe, which looks like a tiny ruler. She should also take periodic x-rays to determine whether you're losing bone, Dr. Otomo-Corgel says. A full-mouth x-ray every two to three years is sufficient if you've had little trouble with cavities or gum disease in the past, Dr. Jeffcoat says. If you have chronic trouble, once a year may be best for you.

What to Do When You've Got It

A diagnosis of gum disease isn't the prelude to an elegy to your lost tooth. Periodontists (gum specialists) have the know-how to save even loose teeth these days. Here's a rundown of your options.

GET TO THE ROOT OF THE PROBLEM. If you've got periodontal pockets between the tooth and gum, you probably need more than just the regular cleaning at your dentist's. A scaling and root planing may be in order, says Dr. Otomo-Corgel. This is a more intense version of the cleaning you usually get. After scraping away the tartar above and just below the gumline, your dentist reaches farther down below the gumline with her instruments and scrapes clean the roots of each tooth.

ASK ABOUT ANTIBIOTICS. If scraping and planing still don't close the pockets, you may have some particularly truculent bacteria in your mouth. Antibiotics may fix that, says Sebastian Ciancio, D.D.S., professor and chairman of the Department of Periodontology at the State University of New York at Buffalo. Your dentist or periodontist can prescribe oral antibiotics. Or she can slide antibiotic-saturated fibers into the pockets, wait ten days, and then remove them after the antibiotics have had a chance to rout the bacteria, Dr. Jeffcoat says.

REBUILD TOOTH AND GUM. Your mouth isn't a lost cause even if gum disease has progressed to the point where you've lost bone and gum tissue. It's possible to stimulate regrowth of both bone and gum. Your periodontist first cleans away all tartar, then inserts small meshlike pieces of fabric in each pocket between the tooth and gum. These fabric barriers create space into which bone can grow. Since gum regrows faster than bone, you need the barrier to reserve some growing room for the bone. After several weeks, the periodontist removes the fabric barriers. "Some dentists will place a bone graft under the material to stimulate regeneration of lost bone," says Dr. Jeffcoat.

Some periodontists prefer to use newer dissolving barriers, which don't have to be removed because your body absorbs them after a few weeks.

RECLAIM A LOST TOOTH. If you lose a tooth, you still have options. Your dentist can replace the tooth with a fixed bridge—a false tooth attached to wires that loop around the remaining teeth on each side. Or she can put in a removable bridge, a less expensive alternative to a fixed one.

For something closer to the original article, she can give you a dental implant. To do this, she implants a titanium screw in your jawbone. After the bone grows into the implant, which can take eight weeks to six months, she can top the screw with a crown.

Hair Loss

FINDING THE PERFECT COVER-UP

The way you style your hair—whether you bob it or braid it, sculpt it into peaks or dye it purple—can say a lot about you.

Women have always made personal statements with their hair, and that's one of the main reasons that hair loss can be so traumatic, says Marietta Lynn Baba, Ph.D., professor of anthropology at Wayne State University in Detroit, who has studied the significance of hair in various American subcultures.

"People get really uptight when they lose hair because they lose this identity marker," explains Dr. Baba. "Hair is also a signal of one's health and vitality. And having hair, for a woman, is a sign of her sexuality. It's a gender marker."

Losing hair can be just as tough for a woman to deal with as it is for a man. In fact, when researchers at Erasmus University in the Netherlands interviewed 58 women with permanent hair loss, they found the loss contributed to low self-esteem in three-quarters of the group.

More Common than You Think

Bald men are a more familiar sight than bald women. But hair loss in women is more common than you may think. Generally their hair thins, but not to the point where they've got recognizable bald spots.

"In men, it's easier to see," says David A. Whiting, M.D., director of the Baylor Hair Research and Treatment Center in Dallas. "Women don't go totally bald, even if their hair loss is severe. They get a thinning on their heads but they retain an intact frontal hairline, so it's not so obvious."

Although some women inherit a genetic predisposition to lose hair more or less permanently, most lose it only temporarily.

Lots of things can lead to temporary thinning, says Harry L. Roth, M.D., professor of dermatology at the University of California at San Francisco. Surgery, fevers, anemia, nutritional deficiencies and rapid weight loss can do it. Emotional stress can cause temporary hair loss, as can an underactive thyroid, anemia, menstrual irregularities and severe cases of psoriasis, dandruff and eczema. Pregnancy can set the stage for temporary loss, and chemotherapy drugs, certain blood pressure medications, birth control pills, high doses of vitamin A and the acne drug Accutane can also cause it, Dr. Roth says.

It can take three months before things like stress, a new medication or an illness cause hair loss. So if your hair starts thinning, ask yourself whether you got a new prescription or went on a crash diet a few months earlier. Keep in mind that it often takes another three months before the hair you lost grows in again.

Are You Really Losing It?

Every day, the average head sheds 100 to 125 hairs. During an initial active stage, which lasts two to six years, the hair grows. Then comes a two- to three-month resting stage, after which hair gets pushed out by up-and-coming replacements. Finding 100 to 125 hairs in your comb, bathtub and towel every day, therefore, does not mean your hair is thinning. It means it's reached old age, and usually each hair is replaced.

If you're shedding more than the usual number and wonder if something is amiss, Dr. Roth suggests a simple test. Grab a small tuft of hair in your fingers and gently pull your hand through it. If you get more than one or two hairs per pull, you're losing more than average.

The good news is that if you're losing this much hair all at once, you're probably losing it only temporarily, Dr. Roth says. Permanent hair loss tends to be more gradual, confirms Laura Sears, M.D., a dermatologist in Dallas.

Avoiding Temporary Loss

You can prevent a lot of temporary thinning by taking care of your hair—and the rest of yourself. Here's how.

SHAMPOO. Contrary to popular belief, frequent shampooing won't make your hair fall out. And if psoriasis, seborrheic dermatitis or eczema is causing your hair loss problem, washing with a medicated shampoo should help solve it, according to Dr. Sears.

CHECK OUT THE COSMETOLOGIST. Permanent waves and dye jobs won't cause hair loss either—if they're done properly. An inexperienced stylist who leaves perm solution on too long and then uses it with a peroxide dye could damage your hair so much that it breaks off near the roots, Dr. Roth says. Choose an established salon

---

WOMAN TO WOMAN A RARE CONDITION LEFT HER BALD

Mary Ann Monson, a retired administrative assistant, works as a travel agent in California. She's one of the 2.5 million Americans who have alopecia areata, a condition that causes varying degrees of hair loss. A founding member of the National Alopecia Areata Foundation, she was the organization's past national support group coordinator. This is her story.

When I was 21, all my hair fell out. That was hard because I was married and I'd just had a baby the year before.

Everyone is different with this condition. It is devastating to each person in their own way. With me, I tried to hide it. I was embarrassed and ashamed. You think to yourself, "What did I do I to be punished like this?" I didn't accept it and went into denial for years.

At that time doctors said it was caused by nerves. When they're telling you it's nerves and not to worry, you're so worried because you think you've caused it. It's a big relief to find out it's nothing you've done. I took cortisone and got my hair back. But once I quit taking it, my hair fell out again. You can't take cortisone forever because it has side effects.

My family knew. My children, they just grew up with me having alopecia areata. But you kind of go into withdrawal. I didn't want to go out. I didn't want anyone to laugh. When I got a nice hairpiece, I went out again. I pretended I didn't have alopecia areata. But when people would say, "You have real nice hair," I'd go to pieces, because it wasn't my hair. I

rather than a beauty school and ask friends to recommend a stylist.

WAYLAY A FEVER. If you get an illness—like strep throat—that brings on fever, see a doctor right away, Dr. Roth advises.

EAT RIGHT. Avoid fad diets and the nutritional deficiencies that go with them. Eat at least five servings of fruits and vegetables, two servings of low-fat milk, yogurt or cheese, a few small portions of protein-rich foods and plenty of whole grains daily, says Dr. Roth. Hold fat consumption to 25 percent of daily calories and exercise more to lose weight. A daily multivitamin is okay, but avoid megadoses, particularly big doses of vitamin A, since too much A can cause hair loss.

GO EASY. Don't pull your hair into tight ponytails or braids. The constant tension can make it fall out, says Dr. Roth.

---

was married at the time, then divorced. My new husband has never known me with hair. He is a big support to me.

As far as saying, "I'm not going to let this interfere with getting a job or having friends," I didn't. I just pretended I didn't have it. This caused a lot of distress. You should let people in. People want to help you and I shut them out. I was too scared that I was going to lose friends so I didn't tell them. They knew anyway—you could tell it was a hairpiece—but they didn't say anything. They waited for me to say something.

There weren't organizations back then saying, "So and so has it, talk to them," like there are now. In 1981, the National Alopecia Areata Foundation and support groups started. Now that word is getting out, it's not that hidden and we've gotten together.

At the support group meetings, you're among people who are in the same situation. It helps just being able to talk with someone understanding. At a meeting, they may have a speaker talking about coping, or someone coming in with hairpieces or giving a medical update—telling what's happening in the field. And each person gets a chance to tell their story and help one another.

Not hiding it and reaching out helped me to see it was okay, that I didn't do anything wrong. I do wear a hairpiece still. There are people at our annual conferences who go without wearing a hairpiece in their daily lives. This is good. It's what people are comfortable with.

Accentuate the Positive

Whether the thinning is temporary or permanent, you can enlist all sorts of cosmetic techniques to camouflage it. Try these.

GO SHORT AND CURLY. Cut your hair short or perm it, and it will have more volume. That means it'll do a better job of covering your scalp and masking loss, Dr. Sears says.

GIVE EYE SHADOW A NEW VENUE. If your scalp is reflecting light and drawing attention to itself, dust it with eye shadow that matches your hair color, Dr. Sears suggests. Your scalp won't be as noticeable and your hair will look thicker.

When Loss Is Lasting

If your hair loss doesn't ease up after a month, have a doctor check it out, Dr. Roth says. You may have a thyroid problem, a menstrual cycle irregularity, anemia or a severe case of psoriasis, seborrheic dermatitis or eczema. Tumors on the adrenal glands or ovaries and adrenal gland irregularities can also cause continued hair loss, he says.

If the hair is falling out in patches, the cause could also be an auto-immune disorder. Researchers speculate that an immune system glitch causes this patchy hair loss, known as alopecia areata. It's estimated that 2.5 million Americans have it. Some lose only small swatches of hair on their scalps. Others lose even their eyebrows and eyelashes. The hair may regrow and fall out repeatedly or never regrow at all. Cortisone treatments can help bring it back.

Most often, however, permanent hair loss is genetic. According to estimates, more than 20 million American women carry the gene or genes for hereditary hair loss, also known as androgenetic alopecia.

You can inherit this legacy from your mother's and/or your father's side of the family, says Howard Baden, M.D., professor of dermatology at Harvard Medical School.

In this type of alopecia, genes seem to make hair follicles more sensitive to dihydrotestosterone, a form of the male sex hormone testosterone, Dr. Sears explains. Under the influence of dihydrotestosterone, follicles stop doing their job.

Medical Options

Both men and women produce testosterone. But men produce much more, which explains why hair loss is more common in men. Women also produce more of the female sex hormone estrogen, which usually offsets testosterone's effect on hair follicles.

"Most women are protected by production of a sufficient level of estrogen until they hit menopause and the estrogen level drops," says Walter Unger, M.D., associate professor of dermatology at the University of Toronto. Depending on their genetic heritage, though, some women start to see hair loss as early as their teens.

Even if your hair loss is permanent, you've no reason to throw in the towel. See your doctor. She may suggest one of these treatments for you.

RUB IN MINOXIDIL. The most commonly prescribed treatment for hair loss—and the only one with the Food and Drug Administration's seal of approval—is minoxidil (Rogaine). It's a clear, nonoily lotion you rub into your scalp twice daily.

In a study, researchers at the University of Texas at San Antonio tested minoxidil on 308 women with androgenetic hair loss. One group used 2 percent minoxidil twice a day. The other group used a placebo. After 32 weeks, 13 percent of the minoxidil group had moderate hair growth and half had minimal growth. By comparison, 6 percent of the placebo group had moderate growth and 33 percent had minimal growth. Apparently the drug works equally well in both men and women, Dr. Baden says. It usually takes a couple of months for minoxidil to show results, Dr. Whiting notes, and you have to use it regularly. If you stop, the hair you gained will fall out again. And you shouldn't use minoxidil if you're pregnant, Dr. Whiting says.

ASK ABOUT ANTI-ANDROGENS. Anti-androgen drugs can sometimes slow hair loss by blocking male sex hormones (androgens) and prevents the shrinking of hair follicles that leads to hair loss, Dr. Whiting says. The most commonly prescribed anti-androgen is spironolactone. A newer drug called Proscar, originally used for prostate disease, may be even more effective. "In some people Proscar not only stops hair from falling out, it encourages extra growth," he says.

If you're pregnant, you shouldn't use antiandrogens. Going off the medication doesn't necessarily mean you'll start losing hair again, but it could happen. The changes in hormone production that accompany pregnancy may counter the hair loss somewhat, Dr. Baden says.

CONSIDER BIRTH CONTROL PILLS. An extra dose of female sex hormones may also slow hair loss. "Birth control pills can bring in a little more estrogen to counteract testosterone," Dr. Sears explains.

THINK ABOUT HORMONE REPLACEMENT THERAPY. By the same token, hormone replacement therapy may slow loss after menopause, Dr. Sears says. Talk over the pros and cons with your doctor.

Headache
TAKING CONTROL OF THE PAIN

It's been an especially busy week, so you've been skipping meals and missing sleep. Not only that, you're a few days away from your period and you're feeling run-down.

Don't be surprised if you get a headache, since these are just a few of the contributing factors that may bring on those nagging or disruptive pains that just about everybody gets at one time or another.

While your brother or your husband may complain about their headaches, researchers have found that women get headaches more frequently than men and experience more severe pain.

Egilius L. H. Spierings, M.D., Ph.D., director of headache research at Brigham and Women's Hospital in Boston, says 80 percent of his patients are women, generally between the ages of 20 and 50.

"Headaches are not a 'female problem,' " he says, "but headaches in women are generally more intense." That's because the female hormone estrogen is "among the most potent chemicals to cause headaches," says Dr. Spierings. Estrogen regulates the makeup of the endometrium, the mucous lining of the uterus, Dr. Spierings explains. The estrogen builds up during the first half of your menstrual cycle, falls during ovulation, rises further and falls once more when your period begins. "It's not known exactly how estrogens cause headaches, but they do have an effect on the blood vessels," Dr. Spierings says.

The most common type of headache is the tension, or muscle-contraction, headache, described as feeling as if a rubber band were being tightened around your head. In addition to this pressure, you may also feel painful knots in your neck or scalp. Eighty-eight percent of women and 69 percent of men studied at San Jose Medical Center in California said they had experienced at least one such headache within the previous year.

About 18 percent of women and 6 percent of men also suffer from migraine, one type of neurovascular headache in which vessels become inflamed and expand. In women prone to migraine, serotonin, one of the chemicals that normally regulates pain messages by carrying nerve impulses from your head and face back to your brain, may misdirect those impulses to blood vessels in the brain's protective covering and scalp. This causes them to swell, then send a pain message back to the brain.

Migraine is a throbbing or pulsating headache, usually felt on one side of the head. It may be accompanied by nausea and sensitivity to light or noise. Migraines often occur for the first time when a teenager begins to have menstrual periods or when a woman starts using birth control pills.

A cluster headache, sometimes mistaken for a migraine, is a particularly excruciating form of pain. At its worst, the cluster headache feels like a red-hot poker in the eye, and it can last up to three hours. Cluster headaches are much more prevalent in men—particularly heavy smokers and drinkers—than in women.

Another kind of headache, an organic headache, is triggered by a tumor or an abnormality in a blood vessel in the brain. This type of headache is rare, occurring in fewer than 5 percent of men and women.

The Origins of Headache

Why do women get headaches?

Let's start with the fact that we're female. "It is always important to see if headaches are related to your cycle," says Dr. Spierings. Migraine attacks, for example, occur around the time of menstruation in 60 percent of women who have them.

Migraines are associated with falling estrogen levels, but any changes in your estrogen levels—such as increases after menstruation— may bring on migraines. If you are using estrogen replacement therapy, you may also begin to suffer from migraines. Postmenopausal women using such therapy should take as low a dosage as possible on a daily basis, recommends Dr. Spierings.

Oral contraceptives can also lead to migraines for some women, again because they act by changing the level of estrogen in your system. "Headache is the most common side effect of the Pill," Dr. Spierings says. "Often headaches appear during the week when you are off the Pill." If that's the case for you, Dr. Spierings says you should discuss other birth control options with your gynecologist.

Another primary headache trigger is stress, and women may be hit harder than men. "For most headache sufferers, the incidence of headaches increases with significant stresses like divorce and loss of a job, as well as milder stresses like dinner guests and sick children," says Joan Miller, Ph.D., a clinical psychologist in Marietta, Georgia, and author of *Headaches: The Answer Book*.

Generally speaking, says Dr. Miller, women internalize their stress, as well as fear and anger. When you hold in any intense emotion, eventually your body will alert your system to the buildup of pressure.

"A headache is part of your feedback system telling you something needs to be changed," Dr. Miller says. "A headache sufferer needs to adjust both externally and internally in a way that's less difficult on her system."

When you're feeling stressed, you may sleep less, and this too can bring on a headache. Fatigue makes it difficult for the muscles to relax, so they stay tight and may go into a painful muscle contraction, says Dr. Spierings.

Another factor is diet. Caffeine is a well-known trigger. The drug—found not only in coffee and tea but also in cola, chocolate and pain relievers—works to constrict blood vessels, contributing to the onset of a tension headache.

If you are susceptible to migraines, the chemical tyramine, found in red wine, aged cheeses and yeasty products such as freshly baked bread and beer, may bring them on. Tyramine is another blood vessel constrictor.

What's Ailing Me?

The list of possible headache triggers, it turns out, is indeed a lengthy one. "You can usually identify at least ten," Dr. Spierings says. "Some you can't do anything about—like changes in the barometric pressure or your menstrual cycle. Look for the ones that you can do something about, like getting enough sleep and eating right." For example, he suggests, if you've missed some sleep, try to nap later. And eat at regular intervals so that you are not caught hungry, which in turn will lead to fatigue and possibly a headache.

When headaches begin to interfere with your life, no matter what their frequency, you should contact your physician or internist. A headache clinic may be the answer if your headaches don't respond to over-the-counter analgesics or are chronic or long-standing, according to William G. Speed III, M.D., director of Speed Headache Associates and associate professor of medicine at Johns Hopkins University School of Medicine in Baltimore.

How to Take Control

Once you know what's bringing on your headaches, you can set about preventing them. Perhaps most crucial is maintaining moderation in your daily life, says Patricia Solbach, Ph.D., a headache specialist and director of the Menninger Center for Clinical Research in Topeka, Kansas. "If your period is about to begin and you've worked a 60-hour week and you've had some glasses of red wine with the girls on Friday night . . . well, that probably wasn't the best thing to do," Dr. Solbach advises. Here are some other strategies for taking control.

MAINTAIN A HEADACHE DIARY. Dr. Miller says that learning about your personal headache triggers is a key to preventing them. Keep a journal for two or three months, recording events prior to attacks. Keep a record of your food and alcohol intake and your menstrual cycle. Also note the type and location of each headache, how long it lasts and whatever action you take to relieve it—such as medication or relaxation. Then note the results of these actions. Look for patterns so you can check whether a certain food brings on a headache and whether you get one when you're feeling tired or stressed.

VENT YOUR ANGER. Journal writing, talking over problems with a friend, changing your expectations and shifting into problem-solving mode are all proactive ways of handling stress and thus warding off headaches, suggests Dr. Miller.

STAY REGULAR. Three meals a day, enough sleep and

regular exercise to beat stress will go a long way toward keeping headaches at bay, Dr. Solbach says. Any disruption in your normal patterns, from a missed meal to sleeping late on the weekends, may wreak havoc with your head.

Regular meals and adequate sleep are especially important during the week before and during your period. Women are more easily fatigued at these times in their cycle, says Dr. Spierings.

GO MOBILE. Many of us live sedentary lives—on the job and at home. Dr. Miller suggests that when you're sitting at a computer keyboard or hunched over a sewing machine, you occasionally shift position, rotate your head, massage your shoulders or stand up for a while to avoid bunching up muscles. And Dr. Solbach emphasizes the importance of getting regular exercise to relieve stress and improve sleep. In addition, the endorphins released during a physical workout may help you to better withstand pain when it occurs.

CUT THE COFFEE HABIT. Cutting your caffeine consumption gradually, by a half-cup at a time, will help the withdrawal process go more smoothly, says Dr. Miller. You can replace coffee, tea or cola with a variety of decaffeinated drinks. Avoid all sources of caffeine, including chocolates, colas, teas and pain relievers that contain it.

BE AWARE OF OTHER TRIGGERS. The artificial sweetener aspartame (NutraSweet); monosodium glutamate, often found in Asian dishes, soups and meat tenderizers; and sodium nitrate, which is added to hot dogs, bacon, salami and ham, all contain chemicals that act upon the nervous system and can cause headaches, says Dr. Spierings. If your journal reveals regular patterns of headaches after consuming these things, cut them out.

SEE YOUR DOCTOR. If you are having menstruation-associated headaches, consider asking for a prescription for an anti-inflammatory prophylactic medication, such as Syntex, to use during the week before your period, says Dr. Solbach, especially if headaches occur like clockwork—10 migraines out of 12 cycles, for example.

Make the Pain Go Away

If, despite your best efforts, you do develop a headache, you can act to reduce your suffering. Here's how.

GO OVER THE COUNTER. In most cases, over-the-counter pain relievers, such as aspirin, ibuprofen, acetaminophen or nonprescription-strength naproxen (Aleve), are all you need if you are experiencing a tension headache, says Dr. Speed. But be careful not to get into a cycle of overusing them. After a while they'll no longer ease the pain, so you'll increase your dosage and become dependent on them. "You should not take pain medications on the average more often than once or twice a week," says Dr. Spierings. "If you are taking them more often, you should do something good for your body, like using a heating pad or trying some relaxation exercises to relieve the headaches."

Studies and physician experience have shown a decrease in headache intensity and frequency following withdrawal from pain relievers, so Dr. Spierings recommends an abrupt withdrawal from such medications for those caught in the cycle. "Don't get scared by the withdrawal headache you may get," he says. "It is better to just tough it out for one or two days—you will be relieved from the perpetual headache."

GET A PRESCRIPTION. Ergots and ergotamines (Ergostat) have traditionally been used as therapy for migraine attacks, but these prescription drugs may exacerbate nausea and vomiting. Sumatriptan (Imitrex) has not shown any side effects and is extremely fast-working, says Dr. Solbach. Ask your doctor about it.

Most anti-migraine medications work by altering serotonin levels to block pain messages. Some also constrict swollen blood vessels.

TURN ON THE HEAT. To reduce muscle fatigue and turn back a headache, Dr. Spierings suggests you use a heating pad on your neck and shoulders every night for 15 minutes or so.

RELAX AND VISUALIZE. Because so many headaches are caused by fatigue, practicing progressive relaxation exercises can help, says Dr. Spierings. Tense and release your muscles in groups, first the feet, then the calves and so on up the body. But avoid contracting the muscles in your head, face or neck, which could make the headache worse.

Biofeedback maneuvers such as visualization may also help you relax your muscles—and make the pain disappear. The next time you feel a tension headache coming on, imagine the tight band loosening and continuing to slacken until the pain is gone. Or lie back and picture yourself in a peaceful place such as a deserted beach or an untouched forest. More than anything else, these moves give you back a sense of control. And ridding yourself of the frustrating sense of helplessness that so many women feel when they suffer recurrent headaches is an important aid to achieving a clear head, says Dr. Miller.

Hearing Loss

AVOIDING THE SILENT TREATMENT

Most of us take hearing pretty much for granted. A bird sings and we feel good. A child calls and we come. A boss yells and we feel like running the other way.

But the actual act of hearing—the complex process that begins with sound waves entering our ears and vibrating through a complex channel of sensory hairs, fluids and structures to the brain—is something that we do without thought—until something interferes.

The major causes of hearing loss in women under the age of 45 are loud noise; degenerative diseases such as lupus, a chronic inflammatory disease that affects the skin, joints, kidneys, nervous system and mucous membranes; and otosclerosis, a condition in which bone grows over a tiny structure in the middle ear, according to Douglas Mattox, M.D., chairman of otolaryngology at the University of Maryland in Baltimore. Infections, trauma, tumors and Meniere's disease can also cause hearing loss, although they're less likely to do so.

Some scientists say that our ears were made for a primitive world in which the loudest sound might be a twig snapping underfoot, so just the normal cacophony of the twentieth century may be something of a challenge to our ears.

But add an extra 105 decibels—the pounding music in an aerobics class or from a portable tape player—and you have a good chance of having a significant hearing loss, says Edwin Monsell, M.D., Ph.D., director of the Division of Otology and Neurotology in the Department of Otolaryngology at Henry Ford Hospital in Detroit. And if you are in an aerobics class, keep in mind that at least one researcher suspects that the physical impact of aerobics on your inner ear may also cause hearing loss.

For the most part, however, how long it takes for these noises to damage your hearing probably depends on how your ear is built and how much noise it's been exposed to throughout your life. As a general guideline, scientists agree that if you listen to a sound at 85 decibels for eight hours, 88 decibels for four hours or 91 decibels for one hour, you are at risk for hearing loss, says Dr. Mattox.

Decibels are the units that are used to measure loudness of sound. The sound you hear when you're standing next to a running diesel truck engine is 84 decibels, and what you hear when you're standing 1,000 feet away from a revving propeller aircraft is 88 decibels.

The point is that the louder the noise, the less time it takes to cause a hearing loss, says Dr. Monsell. A 140-decibel gunshot can instantly tear apart a single sensitive organ in your ear, resulting in immediate and permanent hearing loss.

Dr. Monsell adds that most noise-induced hearing loss is related to factory work, loud motors and firearm discharges. He says it's very unlikely that women would be at risk from typical noise volumes in the office or at home.

The Quiet Zone

Fortunately, there are several simple ways to prevent noise-induced hearing loss.

LIVE QUIETLY. Leaves rustling in the forest register only 20 decibels. Whispers register 30. Normal conversation registers 50, and busy traffic registers 70.

Clearly, no one who lives on a mountaintop will ever experience noise-induced hearing loss. But neither will those who live in city apartments, if they learn to keep their windows closed and televisions, radios and voices at a low volume.

KEEP NOISE LEVELS BELOW A SHOUT. If you have to shout when you're standing four or five feet away from someone, the surrounding noise is loud enough to damage your hearing, says Dr. Mattox.

WEAR PROTECTION. Wear ear protectors whenever you know you'll be exposed to loud noise, says Dr. Mattox. The decibel level inside a subway car is 95. Standing beside a lawnmower, it's 96. A live rock concert can reach 130 decibels.

Earplugs that fit into the outer ear canal will reduce your exposure to noise by anywhere from 6 to 35 decibels. Look for the noise reduction rating (NRR), which provides a rough estimate of effectiveness, listed on the package of any earplugs you buy to figure out which pair is best for you. Some earplugs are premolded, while others are soft

TINNITUS: THE SOUNDS OF SILENCE

Clang. Pop. His-s-s, bz-Z-z-t- . . . h-u-m-m-m-m-m.

If you have tinnitus, the clanging, popping, hissing, buzzing and humming that are common to high-voltage wires or an electric generating plant are likely to be what you hear instead of silence.

The sounds affect some 40 million men and women in the United States. Ten million have serious difficulty living with the condition, researchers say, while another million say that they can no longer live a normal life. Some, in fact, attempt suicide.

Temporary tinnitus may be caused by something as simple as earwax or as complex as a drug. Caffeine and aspirin, as well as indomethacin (Indocin), carbamazepine (Atretol), propranolol (Inderal) and levodopa (Atamet)—drugs prescribed for pain, heart disease, high blood pressure and Parkinson's disease—can cause the problem.

Chronic tinnitus may be triggered by "crosstalk" between nerve transmissions to and from the brain, a mistake in nerve cell transmission, an imbalance in the electrical charges normally found within the inner ear, or something no one's thought of yet, researchers say.

And it frequently occurs with hearing loss and hearing-related diseases such as otosclerosis and Meniere's syndrome.

Although tinnitus can sometimes be "masked" by other

enough to be molded to the shape of your outer ear canal.

Protective earmuffs that fit firmly over the entire outer ear to form a seal will reduce the sound level by 14 to 29 decibels. They are available from industrial supply houses. Whichever kind of protective device you use, make certain you use it correctly.

Experts recommend that earplugs and earmuffs be worn together when the surrounding sound level exceeds 105 decibels—about the sound level you hear in an aerobics class.

AVOID CERTAIN DRUGS. Antibiotics such as streptomycin, some diuretics, salicylates such as aspirin, and anti-cancer drugs such as cisplatin (Platinol) are known to damage sensitive structures within the ear and may cause permanent hearing loss, doctors report.

---

sounds such as radio static or running water, there is no medication or surgery that will cure it, says Douglas Mattox, M.D., chairman of otolaryngology at the University of Maryland in Baltimore.

Surgery to knock out nerves that may be involved in transmitting the sounds has had varied results. In a study of 72 men and women at the University of Pittsburgh School of Medicine, only 18 percent of those who had surgery experienced total relief of symptoms—at least for a while. Twenty-two percent reported "marked" improvement, 11 percent had "slight" improvement, and 49 percent reported no improvement at all.

Women had a slightly higher response to the surgery than men. Of the 31 women who had it, nearly 29 percent experienced total relief of tinnitus.

But other treatments—including antidepressant and anti-epileptic drugs or tranquilizers such as benzodiazepine (Valium)—can achieve similar results, says Dr. Mattox.

That's why researchers at the University of Maryland's Tinnitus Center are taking this approach to the problem. In place of trying to eliminate the source of tinnitus, researchers are stopping the signal from reaching a level of awareness or perception through sound retraining techniques. Since tinnitus normally can't be stopped, the idea is to train your brain not to hear it.

Anytime a drug that falls into one of these categories is suggested by your physician, you might want to ask your doctor or pharmacist what the odds are that it will affect your hearing.

If you are thinking of becoming pregnant, you also need to know that exposing your baby to various drugs during pregnancy can cause a congenital hearing loss. Ask your doctor which drugs to avoid.

LISTEN TO YOUR EARS. If you've ever walked off a plane or out of a concert and felt a ringing in your ears as though your hearing were muffled, you've probably experienced a temporary threshold shift. The threshold is the quietest sound you can hear; when it shifts, it means that you've lost some of your ability to hear.

WOMAN TO WOMAN IN THE NO-SILENCE ZONE

Teresia Guinn is a dentist's receptionist in Gibson, Tennessee. She can no longer hear most of the high-pitched sounds that surround us, but she loves the sound of a dentist's drill because it obliterates the sounds of tinnitus. This is her story.

I don't ever hear quiet anymore.

I had someone tell me one day that she noticed the first thing I did when I came home was turn on the TV. She said, "You know, my kids are all grown and gone from home like yours. Wouldn't it be nice to just not turn on the TV and have everything quiet?"

"Well, that would be nice," I told her, "but I can't." I could turn off everything that was making any kind of noise in this house and I'd never have quiet.

What I hear is like a high-tension wire, a voltage wire. It's between a ringing and a hum. It started out real low and quiet three years ago, but then it got louder. And every once in a while I'll get a real high-pitched squeal, a real whistle sound almost. It lasts just a few seconds and it dies back down. But it just terrifies me because—God!—if I have to listen to that the rest of my life!

Sometimes it sounds like what you hear when you're watching TV, flipping from channel to channel. Once in a while it'll come across and, for some reason, that noise agitates me so much. It's like people are shouting and screaming and it just really tears my ears up.

My tinnitus eventually got so bad that my doctor prescribed tranquil-

The loss is probably temporary. But it may become permanent if you repeatedly expose your ears to noise levels that cause the shifts, doctors warn. That's why you should take your ears' hint and avoid any type of noise that causes this effect, doctors agree. Or at the very least, make sure you're wearing ear protectors the next time you're exposed.

HAVE YOUR HEARING CHECKED. Check with your doctor if you're beginning to miss things in conversation, says Dr. Monsell. If you have to switch ears on the telephone to hear clearly, or if you have to ask people to repeat what they've said, you should have your hearing tested. Getting your doctor to work on the problem may prevent further hearing loss.

---

izers. That terrified me. "Yes," I told him, "Yes, okay, give them to me. And if I have such a bad day I can't make it, I'll take them."

But I got the prescription and I just sat down and I thought to myself, "There's got to be something else. There's got to be another way to deal with this." So I started looking for a support group.

I called the American Tinnitus Association and I told them where I lived, and a woman said, "Let me look in the computer and see what we have in Tennessee." Well, she came back on the line and said, "Sorry, there's not one."

So later I discussed it with my friends and they said, "Why don't you start your own?" And I did.

How do we cope? Well, the majority of people in my group all said the same thing: You can mask tinnitus with certain kinds of sounds, like when you hear running water—a waterfall, or dishwater running in the sink.

So I got a tape recorder, then went into the bathroom and turned on the cold water. I set the shower nozzle at a certain angle and recorded for about 45 minutes to an hour.

Now I take a portable cassette player and headset everywhere. And when things are slow in the office—it really drives me crazy because it gets really quiet—I put it on and just turn it up to where I can just lose this other sound. After about 30 minutes, I noticed, the tinnitus will quiet down and stay that way for hours at a time.

Then I can smile.

Heartburn

HELP TO COOL THE FIRE

That late-night indulgence tasted so good: pepperoni pizza, cola and a bowl of mint chocolate chip ice cream. But now it's midnight, and you hurt so much it's as if your chest's on fire.

Small wonder—you consumed the perfect heartburn meal: late, large and laden with fat.

"What people eat and when they eat it are the usual causes of heartburn," says Malcolm Robinson, M.D., a gastroenterologist at the University of Oklahoma Health Sciences Center in Oklahoma City and director of the Oklahoma Foundation for Digestive Research. "And often, a change in habits can prevent it."

Heartburn is really just a teaspoon or two of stomach juices back-washing up from the stomach and into the esophagus—the tube that carries food from your mouth to your stomach. Laced with harsh hydrochloric acid, the juices burn the tender lining of the esophagus. Acid reflux, as it's known, can carve deep ulcers, lead to narrowing or even obstruction of the esophagus and cause bleeding. In rare cases, frequent reflux leads to a precancerous condition called Barrett's esophagus.

For 75 million Americans, feeling this unwelcome burn is a once- or twice-a-month experience. Another 14 million get heartburn every day, which fuels $2 to $3 billion in antacid sales every year.

The Causes of Heartburn

Usually, women and men are equally prone to heartburn. If you're pregnant, the odds are as high as 50-50 that you will experience acid reflux by your third trimester. Pregnancy, in fact, is a double whammy for heartburn—higher hormone levels relax the muscle that's supposed to keep stomach acid where it belongs, while your growing baby presses upward on your stomach.

"I've had women who end up sleeping in recliner chairs to try to control heartburn," says Deborah Gowen, a certified nurse-midwife with the Harvard Community Health Plan in Wellesley, Massachusetts, and Brigham and Women's Hospital in Boston. "And some get heart- burn eating even the smallest thing. It can be tough." Luckily, it usually subsides after childbirth.

Symptoms of acid reflux—a burning sensation, chest tightness and a feeling of warmth sweeping upward into the throat—can mimic a heart attack. In fact, doctors say you should visit the emergency room, pronto, if the pain is new or especially intense. Forget what you've heard about heart attacks happening mostly to men.

"Women, like men, should go to the hospital with any strong chest pain," says Frank Hamilton, M.D., director of the Gastrointestinal Diseases Program at the National Institutes of Health in Bethesda, Maryland. "We're seeing more and more females who have increased risk factors for heart disease, so this isn't something to take lightly."

If it's just heartburn, your own habits and tastes could be the cause. Fat, alcohol, smoking and even mints and chocolates can weaken the muscle, called the lower esophageal sphincter (LES), that controls the opening between your stomach and esophagus. Carrying extra weight around your midsection and wearing tight clothing can also make the LES work less efficiently.

Meal size and timing also play a role. Gobbling hefty portions and dropping into bed is an invitation to heartburn. A full stomach puts pres- sure on the LES, while lying flat makes it easy for acid to flow backward.

But lifestyle doesn't always explain heartburn. Aspirin, prescription drugs, a stomach ulcer or straining to cough or have a bowel movement can also be the cause.

How to Smother the Flames

"For quick relief, nothing beats an antacid," says Dr. Robinson. "That's the best way to neutralize the acid burning inside your esophagus. But it's not a long-term solution."

Pharmacists recommend seeing your doctor if you've been popping antacids for more than two weeks. She will likely recommend changes in your lifestyle and eating habits.

For stubborn heartburn, treatment may include a prescription drug to slow the production of stomach acid. "In about 90 percent of cases, that's enough," says Dr. Hamilton. "But some people need surgery to strengthen the LES muscle. Surgeons actually pull part of the stomach up and wrap it around the lower esophagus."

There's plenty you can do to cope with heartburn at home. Here are some tips.

REACH FOR THE RIGHT ANTACID. Which one? There are caplets and liquids, chewable tablets and even lozenges. But researchers at the Oklahoma Foundation for Digestive Research found that because antacids actually perform their acid-neutralizing routine most effectively in the esophagus—not in the stomach—chewables or thick liquids may be best.

"The kind that work best are the ones that stay in the esophagus as long as possible," says Dr. Robinson, who led the study. Even pregnant women can take antacids, says Gowen. "I would take one with calcium in it, like Tums, and avoid those with aluminum," she says. "Aluminum is a heavy metal that can be toxic."

CHOOSE FOODS WISELY. Foods and beverages that make reflux worse should be avoided. Among the bad guys are onions, chocolate, peppermint, spearmint and any fatty foods, which actually relax the LES and promote reflux. Citrus juices and fruits, tomatoes and tomato juice, spicy dishes and coffee—either decaffeinated or regular—irritate the esophagus and make the burning sensation more intense, says Dr. Robinson.

BE AN EARLY BIRD. Sitting down to supper three to four hours before bedtime ensures that your stomach will be empty by the time you go to sleep. "So often, people with heartburn tell me they get home late from work, eat a late dinner and fall into bed," Dr. Hamilton says. "They awake hours later with terrible burning pains.

When you lie down, stomach acid flows more easily into your esophagus. If your stomach's empty, there's less acid there."

GO SMALL AND FREQUENT. Gowen tells her pregnant patients to eat four or five small meals a day instead of three big ones. The advice can work for anyone, however. "There's less pressure to cause reflux that way," she says.

PICK A PAPAYA. This tropical fruit contains papain, an enzyme that soothes the stomach, Gowen says. If fresh papaya isn't available, try chewable papaya tablets, available at health food stores. "Dried papaya has the enzyme, too, but since it also contains a lot of concentrated sugar, your best choice is the tablets," she says.

HOLD YOUR HEAD UP. Raising the head of your bed on cinder blocks or 6- to 12-inch wooden blocks puts gravity on your side in the nighttime battle against heartburn. Sleeping on such an incline will make it harder for stomach juices to fight gravity and climb uphill into your esophagus, says Dr. Hamilton.

Or try one of the wedge-shaped foam pillows available at stores that sell home health-care products. These pillows are long and gradually taper from a height of about six inches at your head to an inch or less below your hips. "These are good if your partner doesn't want the whole bed raised or if you sleep on a waterbed, which you cannot raise," says Dr. Robinson. "You can even take them traveling with you."

But shoving an extra pillow under your head is less effective—chances are you'll be bent in the middle and put extra pressure on your abdomen, which can cause reflux.

LIE ON YOUR LEFT. If you must lie down after a big meal but are prone to heartburn, try lying on your left side. Studies at Thomas Jefferson Medical College in Philadelphia measured how long reflux lasted in 15 people who consumed a high-fat meal and then hit the hay—or at least the sofa. Reflux time was "significantly greater" among those resting on their right sides. Researchers speculate that lying on the right side puts the junction of the stomach and esophagus lower than the gastric pool in the stomach, making it easier for acid to seep into the esophagus.

DEFLATE YOUR SPARE. "Even a reduction of five to ten pounds can significantly alleviate heartburn," says Dr. Hamilton. Extra weight around the midsection acts like a belt or a too-tight skirt, squeezing the esophagus and making the LES relax. "So when the muscle should be turning off the flow of acid, it's really ineffective," he says. "It can't shut as tightly as it should."

BANISH THE BUTTS. Smoking weakens the LES, so "smoking can be a significant cause of reflux," says Dr. Hamilton. "When patients review their habits and work on lifestyle changes to control heartburn, a stop-smoking program is something that's always important."

DENY THAT DRINK. Alcohol can also make the LES work inefficiently, in addition to irritating an esophagus that's already burned by stomach acids. Those are two good reasons that limiting—or eliminating—beer, wine and mixed drinks is usually one of the first actions a doctor will ask you to take to control heartburn.

LOOSEN UP. Girdles, tight belts and constricting waistbands increase the pressure on your abdomen and weaken the LES, doctors say.

CONSIDER YOUR MEDICINES. Searching for the true cause of your heartburn? Don't overlook aspirin, as well as the prescription anti-asthma drug theophylline, anticholinergic medicines used to treat bowel spasms, heart medications like calcium channel blockers, and antidepressants. All can weaken the LES and cause heartburn, doctors say. Try to cut down on aspirin, and ask your doctor about dosages of the other drugs.

Heart Disease
LISTEN TO THIS
IMPORTANT MESSAGE

You're 40. You've got a high-pressure job that demands intense concentration, a quickgrasp of complex subjects and an obsessive devotion to deadlines. You've also got a propensity for cheesecake, a husband who smokes and an exercise program that stops with taking out the trash.

You know it's not a heart-healthy lifestyle, but so what? You're a woman. And women don't have heart attacks.

Wrong. Nearly one of every two fatal heart attacks happens to a woman. Nearly half a million women die of heart disease every year. After age 45, heart disease affects one woman in nine. By age 65, it affects one in three. It kills twice as many women as all cancers combined and four times as many women as the next three most common causes of death combined.

A Woman's Special Protection

Although the clogged, hardened arteries that set the stage for heart disease begin with the first ice cream cones of early childhood, heart disease doesn't manifest itself in most women until their estrogen levels drop at menopause (unless they have their ovaries removed during a hysterectomy).

Until one of these events occurs, estrogen literally coats a woman's heart with protection. It keeps her arteries supple, increases substances that sweep cholesterol from the bloodstream and enables other substances in the body to actually dilate blood vessels and slow the formation of maverick blood clots that can trigger a heart attack.

But once estrogen's protection is withdrawn, heart disease hits women hard—harder, some doctors say, than it hits men. Women are more likely than men to die from a first heart attack. Even if they survive the first, they are more likely than men to have a second attack within a year. Clot-busting therapy, or thrombolysis, which is commonly used to fight an attack, is more likely to result in stroke for women. And most women who are candidates for such aggressive treatment are less likely to be offered lifesaving interventions like thrombolysis, catheterization or heart bypass surgery because of "gender bias," says Marianne Legato, M.D., associate professor of clinical medicine at Columbia University College of Physicians and Surgeons in New York City and author of *The Female Heart*. Awareness of such bias among heart disease specialists, however, is bringing significant improvement in the treatment of women, Dr. Legato adds.

Measuring the Odds

What puts women at risk for heart disease? Cigarette smoking, high blood pressure, overweight, abnormal blood fats, a sedentary lifestyle and poor diet, says JoAnn Manson, M.D., co-director of women's health at Brigham and Women's Hospital in Boston and co-principal investigator of the cardiovascular component of Harvard University's Nurses' Health Study. This is a comprehensive, ongoing research project begun in 1976 and involving more than 100,000 women.

But the effects of almost every risk factor can be turned around, she adds.

"I think a key point for younger women to understand is that we largely control our own destiny in terms of heart disease," Dr. Manson says. "We control the most important risk factors such as whether or not we smoke, whether or not we exercise, whether or not we keep our weight under control, whether or not we eat a healthy diet. Except in the very rare person, unchangeable risk factors such as genetics are just not as important." Here's how a woman can prevent heart disease.

BEGIN BY AVOIDING CIGARETTES. "Cigarette smoking is, without question in my mind, the number one risk," says Dr. Manson. "Among women in the Nurses' Health Study who were 30 to 55 years old at entry, smoking was the cause of over *half* of all heart attacks."

Even environmental smoke—in restaurants, workplaces and cars—can be a danger. In a study at the University of California at San Diego, for example, researchers followed 695 nonsmoking women. After ten years, the researchers found that women married at one time or another to smokers were two and a half times more likely to die from heart disease than women who lived in smoke-free homes.

MONITOR YOUR BLOOD PRESSURE. High blood pressure beats up your arteries and overworks and weakens your heart. Keep an eye on it, says Dr. Manson, and if it starts creeping up, work with your doctor to get it back down. You can reduce your risk of a heart attack 2 to 3 percent for every point you reduce the bottom or top number of your blood pressure reading. (For tips on reducing blood pressure, see page 276.)

DROP EXTRA POUNDS. Overweight plays a major but indirect role because it contributes to high blood pressure, diabetes and abnormal blood fats, says Dr. Manson. "It also increases the workload of the heart."

In the Nurses' Health Study, Dr. Manson and her colleagues found that every extra pound weighs on the heart. Even women who were mildly to moderately overweight—15 to 30 pounds or so—had a risk of heart disease 80 percent higher than their leaner counterparts.

GET OUT THE TAPE MEASURE. How can you tell if your extra pounds are particularly likely to put you at risk?

"The key here is shape," says Michael Miller, M.D., director of preventive cardiology at the University of Maryland Medical Center and assistant professor of medicine at the Johns Hopkins Medical Institutions, both in Baltimore. "Apple-shaped women are more likely to get heart disease than pear-shaped women."

To find out which you are, get out the tape measure and wrap it around your waist, then your hips. Divide the waist measurement by the hip measurement. If the result is 1 or above, you're an apple—and in trouble. If it's 0.8 or below, you're a pear—and probably okay.

This is not just a game of numbers, adds Dr. Miller. Apple shapes seem to metabolize fat and cholesterol differently. For one thing, they're more likely to have high triglycerides—a particularly nasty type of blood fat that can cause heart disease. They also have low levels of HDL cholesterol—the "good" kind that puts a half-nelson on bad, artery-clogging LDL cholesterol and flips it to the liver for disposal.

How are "high" and "low" measured? In a study of 140 women who were tracked over a 15-year period, Dr. Miller and his colleagues found that women who had triglyceride levels of 171 or more were nearly three times more likely to die of heart disease than women who had levels of 115 or less. Women who had HDL levels of less than 45 also had triple the risk.

Apple shapes also seem to have increased resistance to insulin, says Dr. Miller. This can lead to Type II, or non–insulin-dependent, diabetes, which increases the risk of dying from heart disease fourfold.

Together, this clustering of risk factors—apple-shaped obesity, high triglycerides, low HDLs and insulin resistance—has been nick-named syndrome X.

MOVE IT. "The cornerstone of prevention is exercise," says Dr. Miller. It zaps all four risk factors at once. It can help control weight, lower triglycerides, increase HDLs and prevent the insulin resistance that leads to diabetes. Exercise also decreases your body's ability to form the blood clots that can lead to a heart attack.

Start exercising three times a week at a pace that keeps you moving but is not so strenuous that you can't hold a normal conversation, says Dr. Miller. And whether it's walking, swimming, cycling or some other aerobic sport, keep moving for a good 20 minutes.

A Heart-Healthy Diet

A major factor in reducing the risk of heart disease is learning what you should—and should not—eat.

LOAD YOUR PLATE WITH FRUITS AND VEGGIES. In the Nurses' Health Study, "we found that women who had the high-est combined intake of vitamins C and E plus beta-carotene had a 46 percent lower risk of heart disease than women who had the lowest in-take," says Dr. Manson.

"I think it's premature to recommend over-the-counter supple-ments, but I think it would be prudent for everyone to increase their intake of fruits and vegetables," she says.

As a result of her research and that of other investigators, says Dr. Manson, "I try to eat at least five servings a day of fruits and vegetables."

Not only do many fruits and vegetables—such as mangoes, spinach, broccoli and carrots—contain the healthful nutrients that seem to protect the heart, they also form the nucleus of a low-fat, low-cholesterol, high-fiber diet, adds Dr. Manson. And there's plenty of evidence that suggests such a diet can reduce the risk of heart disease.

SKIP THE MEAT. A study at Loma Linda University in California found that eating meat as little as three times a week actually increases a woman's risk of death from heart disease by 25 percent. And with every added bite, the risk escalates. "I try to avoid eating any red meat at all," says Dr. Manson.

GARNISH WITH GARLIC AND ONIONS. Substances that are released when raw garlic and onions are cut or crushed seem to make platelets less likely to clump together to form the artery-blocking clots that trigger heart attacks, reports Eric Block, Ph.D., professor of chemistry at the State University of New York at Albany.

An occasional meal heavy on cooked garlic and onions probably won't do very much, he adds. But regularly chopping raw garlic into your salad dressing or slicing an onion into salads probably will.

ADD NUTS. Researchers at Loma Linda University who are studying 26,000 Seventh-Day Adventists have discovered that eating the equivalent of a handful of nuts five times a week may reduce the risk of heart attack by 50 percent.

Nuts contain a potent relaxing factor that may inhibit spasms in arteries, explains Gary Fraser, M.D., Ph.D., professor of medicine and epidemiology at Loma Linda, who headed the study. They also contain monounsaturated fats, vitamin E, fiber and magnesium—all of which may protect the heart.

Which nut is best? The jury's still out, says Dr. Fraser, but the men and women in his study ate peanuts, almonds and walnuts.

DITCH THE STICK MARGARINE. Given the artery-clogging fat content of butter, it seemed to make good sense for doctors to suggest that people use margarine instead. But since those suggestions were first made, Dr. Manson and her colleagues have found that women in the Nurses' Health Study who ate even four teaspoons of margarine a day—either as a spread or in baked goods—increased their risk of heart disease by 66 percent.

The culprits, scientists suspect, are the trans-fatty acids that allow vegetable oils to solidify into the stick form that people expect.

"I don't think people should return to using butter," cautions Dr. Manson. "But the research does suggest that people should consider moving more toward olive oil and the softer, tub margarines." Olive oil is free of the trans-fatty acids in stick margarine that sabotage the heart, and tub margarine contains less of them than stick types. Dr. Manson also warns that, along with margarines and baked goods, fast-food french fries are one of the most common sources of trans-fatty acids.

SKIP THE HEAVY MEALS. Scientists have known for years that a high-fat diet will gradually clog the heart's arteries and set the stage for a heart attack. But researchers in London and Chicago have discovered that dietary fat may pose an even more immediate threat—clots.

The problem is a substance called factor VII. When stimulated by an influx of dietary fat, factor VII may lead the body to form the clots that can cause a heart attack. Even a single fatty meal ups the factor VII ante for a short time and puts you at increased risk, researchers report. But a habitually fatty diet sustains that risk.

DRINK IN MODERATION. Several studies—including the Nurses' Health Study—have found that consuming a moderate amount of alcohol daily reduces the risk of heart disease. (A moderate amount is considered to be 12 ounces of beer, 5 ounces of wine or a drink with 1½ ounces of hard liquor.) In the Nurses' Health Study, the risk declined by 40 percent.

In a study of 81,825 men and women at the Kaiser Permanente Medical Care Program in San Francisco, however, researchers discovered that wine appears to be most beneficial against heart disease and that women who drank white wine had a slightly lower risk of heart disease than women who drank red wine, beer or anything else.

Beat the Sudden Stress Syndrome

Stress is not usually considered a major risk factor for heart disease in women. Yet in a study at Harvard, approximately 40 percent of all heart attacks were preceded within two hours by a psychologically stressful event, says psychologist Sue C. Jacobs, Ph.D., who was a member of the study's research team and is now associate professor of counseling psychology at the University of North Dakota in Grand Forks.

What caused the stress? "For some it was having a son come home from the Gulf War," Dr. Jacobs says. "For others it was winning the lottery." For still others, it was losing a job. It made no difference whether the stressful event was good or bad, says Dr. Jacobs. Either way, the event increased the risk of a heart attack nearly 15-fold.

A stressful event causes the body to secrete "fight or flight" chemicals so we can react quickly in an emergency, explains Dr. Jacobs. The problem is that in addition to giving us fast reactions, these chemicals also trigger substances that can form blood clots.

If you were indeed in a battle, particularly one in which you were wounded, that might be helpful. But for a woman in twentieth-century America, those clot-forming substances are more likely to cause a heart attack than patch a wound.

Here are some ways to deal with stress before it becomes dangerous.

WATCH OUT FOR SIGNS OF STRESS. Before you can eliminate the stresses that can cause a heart attack, you need to know when your body's actually experiencing stress, says Dr. Jacobs. Watch for

SEPARATE AND UNEQUAL TREATMENT

Recognizing a heart attack in women is more difficult than it is in men. The symptoms are just different enough to confuse medical specialists—who are further handicapped by what has come to be called gender bias.

One study indicates that doctors are ten times less likely to refer a woman for needed cardiac treatment and three times more likely to diagnose a woman's chest pain as being "in her head."

As a result, 35 percent of all heart attacks in women go unrecognized, undiagnosed or unreported.

Early signs of a heart attack include an uncomfortable pressure, fullness, squeezing or pain in the chest, usually for longer than two minutes. Pain may radiate to the shoulders, neck, jaw, arms or back. You may also feel dizzy, faint, short of breath, nauseated or weak. You may break out in a sweat.

But there are several variations on that particular scenario. Some women feel pain just in their arms, jaw or back. Some women feel as though they're inhaling cold air. And some women don't feel anything at all.

Obviously, if you have any of these symptoms, you need to see a doctor immediately. But to guard against a "silent" heart attack in which there are no symptoms at all or symptoms go unrecognized, doctors suggest that all women over 45 have yearly checkups in which they are screened for heart disease.

sweaty palms, increased heart rate, shallow breathing, headache, muscle aches, stomachache, insomnia and mind chatter that just won't stop.

DEVELOP A RELAXATION RESPONSE. When you find yourself reacting this way to a particular event, take a deep breath, exhale and begin to consciously tense and relax muscles all the way from your toes to your head. Or visualize yourself doing something that makes you relax. "I'll picture myself jogging on the beach with my attention focused on the rhythm of my steps," says Dr. Jacobs.

RETHINK YOUR ROLES. A study at the University of Stockholm indicates that the multiple roles women play may increase their risk of a heart attack, says Margaret Chesney, Ph.D., professor at the University of California, San Francisco, School of Medicine.

In a study of managers at the Volvo plant in Sweden, a Swedish researcher found that the levels of stress chemicals increased throughout the day in both male and female managers until 5:00 P.M. At that time, the levels of stress chemicals started to drop in male managers and continued to decline into the evening. But for female managers, the levels either stayed high or continued to rise until 11:00 P.M.

What caused the difference? "We think the men were unwinding. They were home and would relax," says Dr. Chesney. "Women were home and started into their second shift." They didn't sit down. They prepared dinner, cleaned up the kitchen, did the laundry and supervised the kids' homework.

It's not that men weren't helping, she adds. Some were. But what they weren't doing was taking the responsibility for getting things done. As a result, the women's managerial responsibilities never stopped until they dropped.

The key to reducing this type of role-related stress is twofold, says Dr. Chesney. First, women have to learn how to delegate not only chores but the responsibility that goes with them. For example, "I know someone who delegated the dry cleaning to her husband. It became his responsibility, since he had the most to be cleaned anyway. She puts out her clothes that need to be cleaned, then doesn't worry about them."

Women also have to lower their expectations of themselves. "For example, I'm not a good cook," says Dr. Chesney, "so I've given up on entertaining. Instead of four-course meals, we'll go Dutch with another couple to a restaurant. Maybe we'll start out with hors d'oeuvres at our house. Or we'll pick up dessert and go back to our friends' house." But either way, says Dr. Chesney, the only expectation she has of herself is to have a good time.

Estrogen Forever?

Estrogen naturally protects women from heart disease until menopause, when the body stops producing it. Now scientists are finding that estrogen replacement therapy (ERT), in which women take a synthetic form of the hormone to offset the side effects of menopause or of having their ovaries removed, offers some protection. ERT reduces the risk of heart disease by 44 percent, the Nurses' Health Study indicates.

"Women's tissues are estrogen sensitive," explains Trudy Bush, Ph.D., professor at the University of Maryland School of Medicine and adjunct professor of epidemiology at the John Hopkins Medical Institutions, both in Baltimore. "And when estrogen is withdrawn, we're just not as healthy."

ERT is particularly beneficial if you have a number of risk factors for heart disease, she adds. No one is quite sure how it protects the heart, but researchers have discovered that it reduces LDL cholesterol levels while increasing HDL cholesterol (HDL molecules clear LDL cholesterol from the blood). ERT may also prevent arteries from going into spasms, which can choke off blood to the heart or brain.

The effects of oral contraceptives, which also contain estrogen, on heart disease are not quite as clear, according to Dr. Bush. "The old high-estrogen formulations actually promoted blood clots, but the new low-dose estrogen formulations don't.

"My best guess right now is that the new low-dose estrogen pills are safe for women right up to menopause—as long as there are no other risk factors," she says. She cautions, however, that women at any age who smoke should not use oral contraceptives.

But ERT is not without controversy. For one thing, it is not recommended for women at risk for certain cancers.

The Aspirin Advantage

Studies have indicated that as little as 325 milligrams of aspirin (usually one tablet) every other day can help reduce the risk of a heart attack in men. But what about women? "The Nurses' Health Study indicated that one to six aspirin per week was associated with about a 25 to 32 percent reduction in heart attack risk in women," says Dr. Manson. And although more studies are needed to clarify just whom aspirin is most likely to help, women at high risk of heart disease should ask their physician about the benefits and risks of starting aspirin therapy, she says.

Heart Palpitations
GETTING BACK THE BEAT

Betty Hughes, a 45-year-old homemaker from Wilkes-Barre, Pennsylvania, looked toward the store entrance. Her husband was supposed to pick her up, but his car was nowhere in sight.

She began to tap her foot in annoyance, her heart skipped a beat, and then she dropped dead.

Very rarely do the heart's occasional flutters, skips, flip-flops, leaps or pounding rhythms indicate a serious problem in women under 45 unless they have underlying heart disease, such as coronary artery disease, a previous heart attack, serious valvular disease, problems with the heart muscle or rare congenital syndromes.

But every once in a while someone like Betty Hughes, who had a history of heart palpitations, gets into trouble. The heart's electrical system short-circuits, the heart quivers frantically, and the person drops dead.

That's why any heart palpitations that are accompanied by dizziness, shortness of breath or chest pain—all indicators of underlying diseases that can turn simple palpitations into a life-threatening condition—should be checked by a doctor, says Marjorie S. Stanek, M.D., director of the Cardiac Stress Laboratory at Einstein Medical Center in Philadelphia. And so should any palpitations in which the heart begins to race and flatly refuses to stop.

When Hearts Flutter

Serious rhythm disturbances are more likely if you have had previous heart problems or if there is a family history of fainting or sudden unexplained death (particularly if it occurs at a relatively young age). If you have any concerns, discuss them with your doctor, who can prescribe treatments to stabilize your heart rhythms.

Palpitations that are unaccompanied by the symptoms described above, stop almost instantly or happen only once in a while can often be ignored, adds Dr. Stanek. However, if your palpitations annoy you, see your doctor. You can have a checkup to rule out serious conditions and get medication to relieve your symptoms.

Palpitations—which are really nothing more than a forceful pulsation of the heart, an irregular rhythm or a faster-than-normal heartbeat—occur in 20 percent of all adults during any given 24-hour period. There's also a condition called arrhythmia in which these palpitations may not be felt.

In younger women without underlying heart disease, heart palpitations are usually caused by stress, over-the-counter medications, caffeine, cigarette smoke or alcohol, explains Dr. Stanek.

Occasionally they're caused by thyroid disease or by any activity that is particularly exciting or anxiety-provoking, including sex.

Three's the Charm

Most of these palpitations are caused by premature contractions, says Dr. Stanek. The heart beats once, then beats a second time prematurely. That gives the heart a split second longer to fill up with blood before the third beat, so when that beat comes, the increased blood in the heart makes it contract more forcefully. And although most people describe the feeling as a "skipped beat," says Dr. Stanek, it's that third, extra-forceful contraction that actually grabs their attention. Palpitations are also felt when the heart beats faster than normal or if its rhythm is irregular.

Frequently palpitations can be prevented simply by avoiding circumstances that are known to encourage them, says Dr. Stanek.

READ THE INGREDIENT LABEL. Two flutter-triggering substances (which are frequently tucked away in unexpected places) are epinephrine in over-the-counter nose drops, cold remedies and allergy medicines and caffeine in coffee, chocolate and aspirin compounds.

Alcohol, which can be found in a cough syrup as well as a wine glass, also encourages palpitations, adds Dr. Stanek. So do prescription diuretics that flush out potassium along with excess fluid.

If your doctor has prescribed any type of medication to help eliminate excess fluid, says Dr. Stanek, check with her to see whether you need to supplement your diet with potassium.

"I THINK I'M HAVING A HEART ATTACK"

Sarah Dunn is a working mother from Fountain Hill, Pennsylvania. She has experienced paroxysmal tachycardia—a rhythm in which the heart beats twice as fast as it should for short periods of time—for 13 years. This is her story.

It's a very frightening experience. The first time it ever happened— I can remember this so clearly—it was a Sunday morning during my freshman year in college.

I was lying in bed and for some reason my room was full of people. And all of a sudden I felt my heart just start to beat really hard.

For no reason.

So I said to my roommate, "Oh, my God! I think I'm having a heart attack!" and everybody laughed and I said, "No—somebody come and help me!"

And one of my friends came over, put her hand on my chest and said, "Oh, my God!" and the palpitations ended.

I don't think it happened ever again in college. But then it happened two or three times within six months—one time in an elevator in Atlantic City—so I went to a cardiologist.

The cardiologist took a videotape of my heart—which was incredibly cool; I did the treadmill and all that stuff. They found a slight heart

STAY IN SHAPE. If you have been forced to sit or lie around for a while, chances are that your body will become deconditioned and any activity will require your heart to work harder, which may cause palpitations, says Dr. Stanek.

"I had one patient who was pregnant. She was worried about losing the pregnancy because she'd had lots of miscarriages in the past," she says. "So she was confining herself to bed. She wasn't even getting up to turn the television on. Then one day she got up to walk—to go to the doctor's office or the store or something—and she had terrible palpitations."

The cause? Flabby muscles making the heart work harder, says Dr. Stanek.

The key here is to stay in shape if at all possible, she says. Even if you're in the hospital, do your best to stay active. If your doctor allows

---

murmur. Then they told me I had paroxysmal tachycardia.

How does it feel? Well, when it first hits I try to catch my breath. I try to breathe. But I feel like I can't take a deep breath, you know? Then I realize that my heart is pounding.

It feels like one of those strong beats like when you're frightened—like when a car cuts you off on the highway and your heart starts pounding and you can feel it pounding through your whole body.

Not a boom-boom pounding. A hard flutter. And it goes so quickly that you can't even count it.

I also get the feeling that I'm light-headed, that I'm flushed.

Usually what I do is stop and put my hand out to steady myself because I do a kind of brown-out—a screen comes across my vision, things fade in and out, and I hear a buzz.

The brown-out goes away first. Then the pounding. Then I feel like I can breathe again.

I usually just wait for it to go. I guess it lasts only about a minute—maybe it's a little less—but it seems like an eternity.

Anyway, I'm glad I was diagnosed because now I don't have to worry every time that I'm having a heart attack.

I can just get on with my life.

it, walk up and down the halls, back and forth to the bathroom or around your bed if that's what it takes to keep your heart in shape.

KEEP CALORIES ABOVE 1,000. Many doctors are concerned that very-low-calorie diets—typically, diets of less than 1,000 calories a day—may cause the life-threatening irregular heartbeats that you may be trying to prevent with a weight-loss diet, says Janis S. Fisler, Ph.D., associate research cardiologist at the University of California at Los Angeles. Commercial diet programs such as Jenny Craig, Weight Watchers and Nutri-System that keep your calories above 1,000 are all fine, says Dr. Fisler. Dieting on your own is fine, too, she notes, as long as you check with a doctor first and keep that 1,000-calorie marker firmly in mind. And, adds Dr. Fisler, weight loss should never exceed one to two pounds per week unless you are under the supervision of a physician.

Beating at Double Time

One type of palpitation that appears commonly in young women with no heart disease is paroxysmal supraventricular tachycardia, a condition in which the heart slams into double-time.

"These episodes may last from minutes to several hours," says David J. Wilber, M.D., professor of medicine and director of the electrophysiology lab at the University of Chicago. "While these episodes are rarely life-threatening, they are very uncomfortable and may be associated with dizziness and fatigue."

There are several simple maneuvers that can be performed to cut off these attacks. Squatting, coughing, breath-holding, or "bearing down" as during a bowel movement are often effective. Occasionally other measures, such as gagging or splashing cold water on the face, may help. If the attack continues despite these measures, and particularly if you feel light-headed or short of breath, you should seek prompt medical attention. A simple injection of medication, either in the emergency room or your doctor's office, is virtually always effective in stopping these more recalcitrant episodes.

It is important to consult your doctor to confirm that a heart rhythm problem is responsible for your symptoms. If these attacks are frequent or troublesome, there are several oral medications that can be taken on a daily basis to prevent further episodes. There is also a non-surgical procedure that can permanently cure the rhythm disturbance. In this procedure, called catheter ablation, a catheter is used to cauterize the tiny area of heart muscle that's causing the rhythm problem.

Hemorrhoids
SOOTHING A SORE SITUATION

The trouble started when we stood up, got a good look around and discovered things like steak au poivre and crème brûlée.

If we were still walking on all fours and eating roots and berries the way our forerunners did, we'd probably never have problems with hemorrhoids. But we'd also never enjoy the view from more than three feet off the ground or celebrate special occasions with anything more festive than tubers.

According to the National Institutes of Health in Bethesda, Maryland, 10.4 million Americans a year suffer from hemorrhoids—but fewer than one-third of these people seek professional treatment. They either ignore them or try treating the problem at home.

Nearly 60 percent of those with hemorrhoids are women, many of whom develop them during pregnancy. Both men and women can inherit a predisposition for hemorrhoids, says Sidney Wanderman,

M.D., a retired New York City proctologist and author of two books about hemorrhoids.

What's in a Vein?

Despite all the bad jokes, hemorrhoids are nothing to blush about. One theory is that they're simply swollen blood vessels, like varicose veins. Instead of being in your legs, these vessels are in your rectum and anus, the last two stops in your digestive tract.

Called hemorrhoidal blood vessels, these veins are particularly prone to swelling with blood because they lack the tiny valves found in most veins that help channel blood back toward the heart.

Researchers speculate that we didn't need valves in our hemorrhoidal blood vessels when we were down on all fours. In that position, blood traveling through the vessels didn't have to fight gravity to get back to the heart.

Standing upright changed all that. Now any additional pressure on these vessels can make them swell and turn into hemorrhoids.

Another theory speculates that hemorrhoids aren't swelling veins but actually sagging, blood-filled cushions. These cushions have two major functions. First, when engorged they help with continence, and second, they support the anal lining during a bowel movement. Elastic tissue holds the cushions in place. But due to aging, the constant downward pressure from chronic straining and the passage of hard stools, the tissue loses its elasticity, allowing the cushions to sag. Then you have hemorrhoids.

Whether they're swelled veins, sagging cushions or a combination, there's plenty we can do about hemorrhoids, short of returning to our old quadruped ways. Although they can be distressing and sometimes very painful, hemorrhoids are relatively easy to treat and largely avoidable.

What's behind Them

Though some hemorrhoids can be excruciating, many who have them are oblivious—at first, says Steven Wexner, M.D., chairman of the Department of Colorectal Surgery at the Cleveland Clinic–Florida in Fort Lauderdale. But pain and bleeding can crop up if people persist in the habits that started the hemorrhoids in the first place.

If you carry extra weight—because you're overweight or pregnant—you'll increase the pressure on your hemorrhoidal vessels. If you're constipated and strain to defecate, you'll do the same. The result? Hemorrhoids.

Since we left our original high-fiber, roots-and-berries diet behind for a more refined, low-fiber menu, constipation has become uncomfortably widespread. In fact, most people who have hemorrhoids are simply eating too little fiber, which we need to make stools easy to pass.

There are two kinds of hemorrhoids, internal, which appear inside the rectum, and external, which are visible at the end of the anus. Both types can bleed, but internal hemorrhoids tend to bleed without the associated pain or discomfort. This can happen when you pass hard feces that irritate the swollen blood vessels, explains Philip E. Jaffe, M.D., assistant professor of medicine in the gastroenterology section at the University of Arizona College of Medicine in Tucson.

When internal hemorrhoids bleed, you may notice blots of bright red blood on toilet tissue or in the toilet. Internal hemorrhoids usually don't hurt, since your rectum is free of pain-sensing nerves. But they will hurt, keenly, if continued straining pushes them through the anal opening.

External hemorrhoids bleed if you scratch them or wipe too hard with toilet tissue. They can be excruciatingly painful if the blood inside them forms clots. This happens when pressure builds up to the point where blood can barely move through the hemorrhoid and the blood congeals. The pain usually subsides after a week or so, after the body absorbs the clot, says John J. O'Connor, M.D., chairman of the colon and rectal surgery section at Suburban Hospital in Rockville, Maryland. But the pain may be so intense that it sends you to the doctor, who can drain the clot in the office.

When It's Something Serious

Hemorrhoids are rarely life-threatening. But some people have so much bleeding that they become anemic. In rare instances infection may set in, and hemorrhoids may become gangrenous, Dr. Wexner says.

It's worth seeing a doctor, because you may have an infection and because anal discomfort can be a sign of all sorts of things—some more serious than hemorrhoids. A persistent itch may mean the skin around your anus is allergic to something you're eating—caffeine and citrus fruits are prime culprits—or to the dye in your toilet tissue. Pain may signal a tear in the anus.

Bleeding can be a warning sign of colon or rectal cancer, as well as inflammatory bowel disease, such as ulcerative colitis or Crohn's disease. Though they're relatively uncommon in women in their thirties and forties, colon and rectal cancer are possibilities nonetheless. That's why it's important to see a doctor to be evaluated if you have any bleeding, Dr. Jaffe says.

How to Get Rid of Them

Treat your hemorrhoids right and, after a week or two, the swelling usually subsides and the discomfort passes, says J. Byron Gathright, Jr., M.D., professor of surgery at Tulane University in New Orleans and past president of the American Society of Colon and Rectal Surgeons. The hemorrhoids are still there—and they'll remain unless a doctor removes them surgically—but they're no longer causing you trouble. The same things that soothe hemorrhoids also help prevent new ones from forming. Here's how to take care of them.

EAT LIKE A NEANDERTHAL. High-fiber foods, like the tubers our prehistoric predecessors subsisted on, are kind to sensitive hemorrhoidal blood vessels. They make for bulky and soft stools, which move quickly through your digestive tract and keep you from straining. You don't have to get by on raw roots and berries, but you do need to add high-fiber foods—fresh fruits and vegetables, cereals and other whole grains—to your diet. Dr. Wexner recommends 25 grams of fiber a day, minimum.

Add fiber and you may also lower your risk of colon and rectal cancer, both far more prevalent in countries with low-fiber, high-fat diets, like ours.

DRINK UP. Remember to drink a lot, too. You need both fiber and fluid for bulk. But avoid alcohol and beverages that contain caffeine, since they have a diuretic effect. Eight to ten eight-ounce glasses of nonalcoholic, caffeine-free fluids a day are essential, Dr. Wexner says. Water is best.

ADD BULK. Over-the-counter products, such as Metamucil, that contain an insoluble fiber called psyllium will also make your stool bulkier and easier to pass. Try those, but pass on the laxatives, Dr. Gathright advises. They're too harsh for your digestive tract. "There's no particular reason for America's fascination with laxatives," he says. "Eating a diet with sufficient bulk, most people should have normal bowel function. Normal is anywhere from three bowel movements a day to one every third day."

GO IMMEDIATELY. Take a lesson from Holly Golightly, who was always excusing herself to use the powder room in *Breakfast at Tiffany's*. It was perfectly polite, and very healthy. When you feel the urge, you must go. If you don't, the feeling of urgency will fade and so will your ability to defecate with ease. Then, when you do make time to use the bathroom, you may find yourself straining on the toilet, putting excess pressure on your sensitive hemorrhoidal blood vessels, says Dr. Wanderman.

DON'T LINGER. Don't read or ponder the meaning of life on the toilet. "Maintaining a sitting position is thought to increase the risk of hemorrhoids because of the effect it has on blood flow in the pelvis," Dr. Jaffe explains. It's believed to cause pooling and congestion of blood in the hemorrhoidal blood vessels.

WORK OUT. Regular exercise helps to move feces through your body, Dr. Wanderman says. Walking, running, doing yardwork or playing sports are all good things to try. Do whatever it takes to get in at least 30 minutes of continuous exercise three times a week. If you sit or stand all day on the job, remember to take a break every hour or so and walk around a bit. And take the stairs.

SOAK IN A SITZ. A 20- to 30-minute soak in a very warm bath two to three times a day may help ease the pain of hemorrhoids while you're waiting for the swelling to subside, Dr. Jaffe says. There is no need to add anything to the bathwater. If a bath is inconvenient, or if you're pregnant, use a hand-held shower, Dr. Gathright suggests. Hot soaks are out during pregnancy because the heat can harm a fetus.

SOOTHE WITH MILD LOTIONS. Emollient lotions like over-the-counter Balneol will also temper the pain, Dr. Wexner says. But avoid products that contain witch hazel and alcohol, since they're too harsh for the skin around your anus. He suggests you also steer clear of petroleum jelly and other oil-based lotions, which will trap irritating sweat and mucus near your skin, and cortisone creams, which will thin the skin.

Commercial hemorrhoid preparations like Preparation H are no better than cheaper all-purpose emollient lotions, Dr. Gathright says. According to Dr. Wanderman, suppositories aren't particularly useful either, since they often slide too high up in your rectum to help hemorrhoids that are lower.

Hepatitis

PREVENTION IS YOUR BEST DEFENSE

Country-western singer Naomi Judd was near tears. She and her daughter Wynonna had just finished their signature song "Love Can Build a Bridge" at Murphy Center in Murfreesboro, Tennessee, in front of 10,000 screaming fans. But as the two stood on the stage holding hands and waving to the audience during the concert's final moments on that December night in 1991, mother and daughter were clearly reluctant to leave.

Tonight, Naomi Judd, 45, was not just leaving the stage until her next performance. She was leaving it for the last time—forced into retirement by hepatitis C, a virus that attacked her liver, sapped her strength and ended her career.

There are five different forms of the hepatitis virus that have been identified, says Francisco Averhoff, M.D., an epidemiologist with the

Centers for Disease Control and Prevention (CDC) in Atlanta, and they attack men and women in about equal numbers.

Hepatitis A, which is transmitted most commonly by food and water, affects an estimated 100,000 to 200,000 people every year in the United States. It's occasionally passed along when infected restaurant employees forget to wash their hands after going to the bathroom. It accounts for 30 percent of all cases of hepatitis in the United States.

Hepatitis B, which can be transmitted through sexual intercourse, affects 200,000 to 300,000 people in the United States every year, says Dr. Averhoff. It is also spread by sharing razors, needles and toothbrushes with carriers and is passed from infected mothers to their newborn infants. It is responsible for half of all reported hepatitis cases in this country every year.

Hepatitis C may also be transmitted through sexual intercourse and shared needles, but the cause is unknown in 40 percent of cases. It affects approximately 150,000 people in the United States and is a particular problem among health-care professionals: A moment's carelessness when disposing of a syringe can cause a needle-stick injury that transmits the virus.

Most—But Not All—Recover

The other two hepatitis viruses, D and E, are rare, says Dr. Averhoff. Hepatitis D is transmitted primarily among drug users already infected by the hepatitis B virus, and hepatitis E occurs mostly in India.

People often recover completely from hepatitis within a few weeks or months, says Dr. Averhoff. The flulike symptoms—malaise, muscle aches, mild fever, abdominal pain and nausea—disappear, although the infection may flare up once in a while until the virus is gone forever. And in some cases, particularly with hepatitis B or C, people who are infected will have such mild symptoms that they won't even realize they've been infected, even though they are still carrying the virus and are able to infect other people.

People with hepatitis B or C may go on to develop chronic disease, says Dr. Averhoff. Approximately 5 percent of those with hepatitis B and 50 percent of those with hepatitis C—like Naomi Judd—will develop a chronic liver disease that can lead to cirrhosis of the liver, a condition in which the liver becomes scarred. It can eventually lead to liver failure and the need for a liver transplant.

"Hepatitis B and C are probably the most serious forms of hepatitis because they can go on to cause chronic disease," says Dr. Averhoff.

"Hepatitis B kills 5,000 people a year and hepatitis C about 10,000. With either form, many people don't even know they have it until they're diagnosed with cirrhosis."

Since there are no reliable cures for hepatitis, the best way to handle the virus is to prevent it, experts agree. Here's how.

WASH YOUR HANDS. Washing your hands, and teaching your children to wash theirs, will go a long way toward preventing hepatitis A, says Dr. Averhoff.

PRACTICE SAFE SEX. "Any woman who is sexually active with multiple partners is at risk for hepatitis B," says Miriam Alter, Ph.D., chief of the epidemiology section at the CDC's hepatitis branch. "So if you're sexually active, practice safe sex." Use condoms every time you have intercourse.

GET A SHOT. A vaccine is available for hepatitis B. If you are sexually active with more than one partner or are a health-care worker, doctors caution, you should talk to your doctor about getting the vaccine.

PROTECT YOUR LIVER. "If you get chronic hepatitis, don't drink and don't take drugs—not even over-the-counter drugs—without consulting a doctor," says Dr. Alter. Both can significantly damage a liver that's already been hurt by hepatitis.

High Blood Pressure
A WOMAN'S PROBLEM, TOO

You feel fine. You look fine. But if you're one of those stoic types who has to be sick as a dog before she'll see a doctor, you could be walking around with a life-threatening medical condition without knowing it.

Long called the silent killer, high blood pressure can lead to heart disease and stroke—conditions that kill more women than all other diseases combined. The tragic part is that while it's easy to detect and control, most women don't even know they have high blood pressure unless they have it checked at the doctor's office during a routine visit.

Estrogen Protection

Until menopause, we have a natural advantage over men when it comes to matters of the heart, thanks to the sex hormone estrogen. Besides regulating the menstrual cycle, estrogen keeps our cholesterol in check, reduces the formation of artery-clogging plaque and generally keeps our hearts running smoothly.

It also keeps our blood pressure down. One in ten women between 35 and 44 has high blood pressure, compared with one in five men.

But knowing we've got such a powerful ally can give us a false sense of security. If you think high blood pressure is a man's problem, something women don't have to worry about, consider this statistic: By age 45, one in nine women shows signs of cardiovascular disease, a condition that kills half a million women a year. By the time we're in our fifties, we're just as likely to have high blood pressure as men are.

Once it strikes, high blood pressure damages the heart in two ways: It enlarges and weakens the organ and contributes to atherosclerosis, clogging your blood vessels with plaque and setting the stage for a heart attack.

The sooner high blood pressure is detected and controlled, the less time it has to wreak havoc. Once your blood pressure is brought down to normal—either with medication or through weight loss, exercise or cutting your salt intake—your risk of heart attack approaches that of a person whose pressure has always been normal.

Playing by the Numbers

A blood pressure reading consists of two numbers: The top one, for systolic pressure, indicates the maximum pressure in your blood vessels, which occurs when your heart contracts. The bottom one, for diastolic pressure, represents the minimum pressure while your heart is resting between beats.

Normal blood pressure for women is usually between 110/65 and 140/90, though it may vary depending on the time of day. It's normal for blood pressure to go up when you're stressed or excited, but it should return to normal quickly. A consistent reading of 140/90 or above is considered high.

Keeping on top of blood pressure is simple. Have it checked at every doctor's visit, which should be at least once a year, suggests James Reed, M.D., professor of medicine at Morehouse School of Medicine in Atlanta. "Once a year is fine if you've always had normal blood pressure. If you've had high readings in the past or are on high blood pressure medication, your doctor will want to see you more often."

Regular screenings are particularly important for women with a family history of high blood pressure, since the condition has a genetic link.

Researchers don't know why, but African American women are far more likely to develop high blood pressure than white women and tend to experience more severe complications.

Being overweight—even by as little as ten pounds—can also contribute to high blood pressure.

The Stress Factor

While many doctors believe that stress plays a role in high blood pressure, the relationship is difficult to prove. "The problem is defining what you mean by stress," says Peter Schnall, M.D., assistant professor of public health at Cornell University Medical Center in New York City, who's been studying the relationship for 15 years.

Dr. Schnall's research focuses on a particular type of stress at work known as job strain, typically experienced by workers in demanding jobs who have little control over their work environments. "Job strain is greatest in women who must work at a rapid pace set by someone else, with little say over how the job gets done," says Dr. Schnall.

No matter what the cause, once it's detected, high blood pressure is easily controlled. And reducing blood pressure even a little can add years to your life. For each point you shave from the top or bottom number of your blood pressure reading, your heart attack risk drops 2 to 3 percent, says JoAnn Manson, M.D., co-director of women's health at Brigham and Women's Hospital in Boston.

While blood pressure can be controlled with medication, a growing body of research shows that nondrug approaches like weight loss, regular exercise, cutting back on sodium and reducing or eliminating alcohol also can be effective.

In fact, studies show that if you're overweight, achieving and maintaining a normal weight may be enough to get your blood pressure under control.

Your doctor will also recommend reducing the amount of salt in your diet. A high-sodium diet causes the body to retain more water, which increases the volume of blood traveling through blood vessels and adds to the burdens on the heart and kidneys.

Excess sodium doesn't cause high blood pressure, but it does aggravate the problem in about half of all patients, according to W. Dallas Hall, M.D., professor of medicine and director of the Division of Hypertension at Emory University in Atlanta. To find out if it's a problem for you, cut back on salt for several weeks and then have your blood pressure tested.

Going the Medicine Route

If your blood pressure is very high (over 105 diastolic) or doesn't improve with lifestyle changes, your doctor will prescribe medication to bring it down. The most commonly prescribed blood pressure drugs fall into four categories: diuretics, beta-blockers, angiotensin converting enzyme (ACE) inhibitors and calcium channel blockers.

Diuretics have been used since the late 1940s to reduce blood pressure by increasing the excretion of excess salt and water, leading to reduced blood volume and less work for the heart. Beta-blockers reduce blood pressure by slowing the heart and central nervous system. ACE inhibitors stop the body from producing angiotensin, a chemical that tightens the arteries and increases blood pressure. Calcium channel blockers relax the arteries, easing blood flow and reducing pressure in the blood vessels.

Each type of drug comes with its own benefits and risks, says Dr. Reed. Your doctor will want to see you regularly to judge the drug's effectiveness and guard against possible side effects.

How to Get It Down

Doctors agree that there's a lot you can do to prevent or control high blood pressure. Here are some suggestions.

LOSE A LITTLE WEIGHT. "Almost any overweight woman who successfully loses weight will see her blood pressure come down," says Dr. Hall. Your doctor can help you determine a healthy weight for you and offer tips to help you get there. Even a small weight loss—as little as ten pounds—can have a beneficial effect on blood pressure.

GET OFF THE COUCH. "It takes about six months of a regular exercise program—15 to 45 minutes a day three to five times a week," says Dr. Hall. "If patients stick with it, they can expect a decrease similar to what we see with sodium restriction: about seven points off the top figure and seven points off the bottom," says Dr. Hall.

BE CAREFUL WITH SODIUM. It's not enough to swear off the salt shaker. Up to 80 percent of the sodium in the American diet comes from processed foods. Cheese, lunch meats and snack foods, as well as canned soups and vegetables and vegetable juice, are often very high in sodium. Check food labels for sodium content, and look for lower-sodium versions of foods you can't do without. Try to limit your intake to 2,400 milligrams a day, says Patrick Mulrow, M.D., chairman of the Department of Medicine at the Medical College of Toledo in Ohio and chairman of the American Heart Association's Council for High Blood Pressure Research.

CUT BACK ON ALCOHOL. Exactly how it works isn't clear, but even moderate drinking can raise blood pressure in some individuals, says Arlene Caggiula, Ph.D., associate professor of nutrition and epidemiology at the University of Pittsburgh School of Public Health. Reduce or eliminate alcohol and see if your blood pressure comes down.

INCLUDE MINERALS. Potassium and magnesium may help keep blood pressure down, according to researchers. Try to get 3,500 milligrams of potassium and 350 milligrams of magnesium a day, says Dr. Caggiula. Good sources of potassium are potatoes, spinach, bananas, orange juice, corn, cabbage and broccoli. Nuts, spinach, lima beans, peas and seafood are high in magnesium. You can usually achieve adequate levels through a good diet, so don't take supplements of either mineral without consulting your doctor.

GET OFF THE PILL. Oral contraceptives containing estrogen, like the majority of those sold in the United States, can sometimes cause an increase in blood pressure. And while progestin-only pills, the so-called minipills, aren't believed to increase blood pressure, their effect hasn't been thoroughly studied. "I would never recommend any oral contraceptive to a woman who already has high blood pressure," says Dr. Hall. "The best advice is to use another form of birth control."

SEEK SUPPORT. If you think job strain is sending your blood pressure through the roof, research shows that maintaining close, supportive relationships with co-workers may be your best bet for reducing the pressure and keeping it down. "Talking about your work experiences with other people actually acts as a buffer against the effects of job strain," says Dr. Schnall. "If you're in a demanding job and have nobody to talk to, you're in much worse shape."

AVOID DUELING PRESCRIPTIONS. Certain non-steroidal anti-inflammatory drugs (NSAIDs), such as those used to treat arthritis, can undermine the effectiveness of some blood pressure medications. To avoid drug interaction problems, be sure to tell your doctor about any medicine you're taking, whether it's a prescription or an over-the-counter drug, says Dr. Hall.

High Cholesterol

IT'S A NUMBERS GAME FOR WOMEN

Debbie was stunned. Standing in her office with the cholesterol report lying on her desk, she figured there had to be some mistake. The report showed she had a total cholesterol level of 255 mg/dl—about 45 points higher than the national norm and about 55 points higher than any doctor ever wanted to see it.

Yet Debbie, 42, followed a low-fat diet. She avoided liver and eggs. She ran four or five times a week.

How could her cholesterol be so high? And how dangerous was it?

Probably not half as dangerous as Debbie thought. Because, while studies indicate that high cholesterol predicts heart disease in men, what's high in men is not necessarily high in women.

"A lot of women are falsely worried about high total cholesterol levels," says epidemiologist Robert D. Langer, M.D., assistant professor of family and preventive medicine at the University of California, San Diego. "Largely based on data from middle-aged men, national cholesterol screening guidelines classify adults into three risk groups based on total cholesterol."

According to those guidelines, adults with a total cholesterol level of more than 240 mg/dl are said to have the most risk. And those with a total cholesterol of less than 200 mg/dl have the least. Those who fall somewhere in the middle have "borderline" risk.

Our Extra Bit of Protection

These evaluations of risk may be misleading for women, because total cholesterol is only part of the story. Total cholesterol is a combination of LDL cholesterol, the "bad" cholesterol that can clog arteries and set the stage for a heart attack, and HDL cholesterol, the "good" cholesterol that sucks up LDL and transports it to the liver for recycling. And although researchers are still trying to figure out why, women's HDL levels are usually at least 10 to 12 mg/dl higher than men's.

Debbie, for instance, found out that her HDL cholesterol was extremely high—93—and her LDL was low. So although her total cholesterol was high, her doctor told her that her risk for heart disease was almost nonexistent. The high HDL that women tend to have is added protection against heart disease. But it's also just enough to get them wrongly classified as "at risk" by the national guidelines if their doctors are only screening for total cholesterol.

In a study of 875 women, for example, Dr. Langer and his colleagues found that total cholesterol levels would have placed 31 percent of the women in a high-risk group if doctors used the national cholesterol screening guidelines. If doctors took HDL cholesterol into consideration as a second step in the screening process, fewer than 15 percent of the women were actually in the high-risk group.

In other words, more than half the women told by their doctors that they were seriously at risk for heart disease didn't need to worry about it—because their HDL was sufficiently high.

The same thing happened with the 47 percent of women in the study whose total cholesterol levels placed them in the "borderline" risk group. Once doctors looked at the HDL number, they found that fewer than 25 percent of the women were actually at borderline high risk.

As a result of ignoring the differences between men and women, researchers concluded, the national screening guidelines used by most doctors mistakenly identified at least three out of ten women as having cholesterol levels that put them at risk for heart disease.

How Much HDL Do We Need?

The value of HDL cholesterol cannot be underestimated. Some researchers say it actually "neutralizes" the effects of LDL cholesterol on the heart. And long-term studies of thousands of women here and abroad indicate that increasing HDL levels by 10 mg/dl can reduce the risk of heart disease anywhere from 42 to 50 percent.

How high should HDL be? Here again the standards are different for men and women because their average levels are different. In men, an HDL level of less than 35 is harmful. For women, an HDL level this low may be even *more* harmful, since "the average woman's HDL in the United States is between 55 and 60," says metabolic specialist Margo Denke, M.D., associate professor of internal medicine at the University of Texas Southwestern Medical Center in Dallas and a member of the National Institutes of Health panel of experts on HDL and heart disease. The panel sets the national standards for healthful cholesterol levels.

In a study at Johns Hopkins University in Baltimore, researchers found that women with HDL levels below 50 mg/dl were more than three times as likely to die of heart disease as women with higher levels. As a result, some researchers advocate that levels be kept as far over 50 as possible.

What You Can Do

The general rule is that you can reduce your risk of death from heart disease 5 percent for every point you increase HDL. How do you increase HDL? Here are the three strategies that have been proved to be effective.

DO NOT SMOKE. "The biggest cause of low HDL is cigarette smoking," says Dr. Denke. Studies indicate that HDL levels are 5 to 9 mg/dl lower in smokers than in their smoke-free friends.

JOIN A GYM. Scientists have found that regular exercise can raise HDL 10 to 20 percent. Weight training with exercise machines increased women's HDL by 5 percent in one study, while walking or running a total of six miles every week boosted HDL 3 mg/dl in another. And in a third study, researchers found that it didn't really seem to matter what kind of exercise you do as long as you burn off 1,000 calories a week—the equivalent of walking about 30 to 45 minutes three times a week.

"Exercise will increase HDL levels in some more than others," says Dr. Denke. And every movement counts. "If you exercise a small amount, it's a small increase. If you exercise a great amount, it's a great increase."

LOSE WEIGHT. "If you're more than 10 or 20 pounds overweight, your HDL can be depressed 8 to 10 mg/dl," says Dr.

THE TRIGLYCERIDE STORY

Triglycerides are the end result of all the fat-drenched foods you eat. Once through your digestive system, they're packed by the liver into cholesterol packets and transported through arterial highways to parking lots on your hips, thighs and belly.

They are known to increase your blood's tendency to clot, which can trigger a heart attack. And in women between the ages of 50 and 59, triglycerides double the risk of heart disease.

Although some doctors feel that measuring your triglyceride levels is not necessary unless you have other risk factors for heart disease—such as diabetes, obesity or high blood pressure—William Castelli, M.D., medical director of the Framingham Heart Study, which followed 5,000 Massachusetts residents for 40 years to assess their risk for heart attack, feels that anyone who's having their cholesterol checked should also have their triglyceride levels evaluated. Tell your doctor you want them checked.

International screening guidelines suggest that triglyceride levels over 200 mg/dl are a problem. But a 15-year study of 140 women conducted at Johns Hopkins University School of Medicine in Baltimore has shown that women who have triglyceride levels of 171 or above were nearly *three times* more likely to die of heart disease than women who had levels of 115 or less.

How can you lower triglycerides? Avoid too much alcohol, trim excess fat from your diet, exercise every day and eat plenty of fish, doctors suggest. A study at Oregon Health Sciences University in Portland found that eating the equivalent of seven ounces a day of fish reduced triglyceride levels by more than 50 percent.

Denke. Studies have shown that, in any group of people, those who are fattest will have HDL levels that are 10 to 15 percent lower than those who are leanest.

Defending Your HDL

Since cholesterol is essentially the transportation system throughout the body for any fat you eat, a low-fat diet has been the prescription to remedy high cholesterol for over a decade. The only trouble is, a low-fat diet lowers HDL as well as LDL. In a study of nearly 2,000 women at the University of California at Los Angeles, researchers found that three weeks on a strict low-fat, high-fiber diet that derived 10 percent of its calories from fat did four things: reduced body weight by 4 percent, lowered total cholesterol by 21 percent, lowered LDL by 19 percent and lowered HDL by 19 percent.

So what's the best way to get a healthful, low-fat diet without losing the benefit of HDL?

When it comes to cholesterol control, says Dr. Denke, research shows the best diet for women has 30 percent of calories from fat. This diet lowers LDL without affecting HDL, according to Dr. Denke. When a woman's diet gets below 30 percent of calories from fat, HDL begins to slide.

Does that 30 percent figure sound familiar? It should. A diet that derives no more than 30 percent of calories from fat is what is now recommended by both the American Heart Association (AHA) and the National Cancer Institute for optimal health. Here's your eating plan for hitting that goal.

EAT LEAN. Choose skim, ½ percent or 1 percent milk and nonfat or low-fat yogurt and cheese. Eat no more than six ounces of cooked lean meat, fish or skinless poultry a day.

PREPARE FOOD WITHOUT FAT. Use cooking methods that require little or no fat—steaming, sautéing, baking, broiling, grilling and microwaving, for example. Trim all the fat you can see from any meat or poultry before cooking. Drain the fat after browning.

USE NO MORE THAN TWO TABLESPOONS OF FAT A DAY. Use as little fat and oils in cooking, baking and salad dressings as possible. Consider two tablespoons your max. Replace saturated fats—the kind that raise cholesterol—with monounsaturated ones found in canola oil and olive oil—the kind studies show actually help bring cholesterol down. Chill soups and stews after cooking, then skim off the hardened fat and reheat before serving.

WATCH THE CHOLESTEROL IN FOODS. The watchword for cholesterol is this: Animal. Cholesterol is found only in animal foods, so if you want to cut down on your cholesterol intake, you need to limit your intake of meats, eggs and dairy products. These strategies should keep your dietary cholesterol to under 300 milligrams per day—the AHA's goal.

DRINK MODERATELY. No one wants to advocate alcohol use, so doctors are reluctant to say that alcohol boosts HDL. But research shows that women who drink moderately have HDL levels 6 to 18 percent higher than women who don't drink at all.

Obviously, common sense should prevail here. Since more than a glass a day of *any* alcoholic beverage can actually trigger other problems such as stroke or an increased risk of breast cancer, the fact that alcohol boosts HDL does *not* mean you should take up drinking if you've been a teetotaler all your life.

EAT CLAMS, OYSTERS AND CRABS. Once thought to escalate your cholesterol levels, these ocean dwellers have been found innocent of all charges.

The proof? In a study at the University of Washington in Seattle, a diet that included these three caused LDL cholesterol to sink 11 to 14 percent and HDL to rise 30 percent.

But don't try to extend the clean bill of health to other crustaceans. Although the study found that squid and shrimp had little effect on cholesterol levels, the researchers concluded that the amount of cholesterol in these two shellfish was still too high—280 milligrams in a 3½-ounce serving of squid and 157 milligrams in the same amount of shrimp—to be part of a heart-healthy diet.

EAT FOODS RICH IN VITAMIN C. Here's another reason that vitamin C is good for you: Studies have found that the vitamin C in oranges, cantaloupe, broccoli, brussels sprouts and other foods can help raise HDL.

But research also shows that if you have adequate vitamin C intake or are taking a supplement, taking more won't help. People with below-average vitamin C levels were the only ones whose HDL rose when they increased their vitamin C intake.

HIV and AIDS

BE SMART, BE SAFE

She was 32 and an executive with a small New England oil company. She had slept with only two men in her life: a guy in Alaska way back in the eighties and her husband.

The guy was a three-week fling while she was working on the Alaska Pipeline. She found out he used drugs and ditched him. But now she has found that the tryst was more than a mistake—it was life-threatening. Although she feels and looks good, she is infected with the human immunodeficiency virus (HIV)—the virus that causes acquired immune deficiency syndrome, or AIDS.

HIV destroys the immune system, leaving the body open to a wide range of infections that a healthy immune system could normally overcome. In the most advanced stages, HIV is diagnosed as AIDS. AIDS does not attack only gay men, as some thought when it was discovered in the 1980s. It is spreading throughout the heterosexual population, and it attacks anyone—male and female, young and old, regardless of race.

In 1992, AIDS was the fourth leading cause of death among U.S. women ages 25 to 44, behind cancer, accidental injury and heart disease.

It's believed that 100,000 American women are infected with the virus; in more than half of these adolescent and adult women, the infection has progressed to AIDS, report the Centers for Disease Control and Prevention (CDC) in Atlanta.

Yet even when the total number of women who died from AIDS more than tripled in one year—from 4,603 in 1992 to 16,417 in 1993—a national survey conducted for the American Medical Women's Association revealed that 70 percent of American women were not concerned about contracting HIV.

The Dangers for Women

Women who become infected with HIV usually get it through an exchange of blood or semen during sexual intercourse or when they share hypodermic needles with infected individuals.

Through June 1994, 48 percent of HIV-infected American women contracted the virus through intravenous drug use, 36 percent through heterosexual intercourse and 5 percent through blood transfusions or tissue transplants, according to the CDC. Eleven percent of women do not know how they acquired the infection.

In intravenous infection, the virus goes directly from the needle into the bloodstream and then to the lymph nodes, where it finds immune system cells to infect, says Charles Carpenter, M.D., associate director of the AIDS Program and professor of medicine at Brown University in Providence, Rhode Island.

With intercourse, however, the virus must work its way through vaginal secretions into cells that line the vagina, then get into the bloodstream and the lymph nodes. Infection occurs in roughly 1 of every 100 episodes of sex with an infected partner in which condoms are not used, says Dr. Carpenter.

But there are two ways during vaginal intercourse in which the virus can take a shortcut: One is to zip through a cut or abrasion in the vaginal wall and into the bloodstream. The other is to use the presence of a sexually transmitted disease, which increases the risk of transmission by at least three to five times, says Judith Wasserheit, M.D., director of the CDC's Division of STD/HIV Prevention.

STDs such as herpes or syphilis, which produce open sores, accelerate transmission the same way cuts or abrasions do. STDs such as gonorrhea or chlamydia, which do not have open sores, actually act as bait for the virus. Their presence draws immune system cells to the genital area. The virus can then attach itself to an immune cell and multiply.

Risks with Intercourse

HIV-infected semen is twice as likely to transmit the virus as infected vaginal fluids, doctors say. Not only does semen carry more of the virus than vaginal fluids, but the vagina provides more surface area for absorption than does the male urethra.

The risks go up sharply for women who have anal sex, which is practiced by an estimated 25 to 30 percent of women in the United States, Mexico and Canada. The risk of HIV transmission during anal sex is more than twice as great as the risk with vaginal sex. Among couples who participated in anal sex without condoms, 28 percent of uninfected partners became infected.

Besides abstinence, the best weapon in the fight against sexual transmission of the AIDS virus is the latex condom.

How effective are condoms? Well, just 1 percent of them break. But if you're counting on condoms, it's essential to use them all the time. In a study of 256 heterosexual couples in which one partner was HIV-positive, the European Centre for Epidemiological Monitoring of AIDS in France found that condoms prevented transmission in about 15,000 episodes of intercourse among couples who used condoms all the time. Among couples who used condoms at least half the time, nearly 13 percent of the initially uninfected partners were eventually infected. Among couples engaging in vaginal intercourse who refused to use condoms at all, 15 percent of initially uninfected partners contracted HIV.

Calming Your Fears

There have been worries over the years about HIV infection being passed through transfusions and operations, through equipment and needles at dentists', doctors' and electrologists' offices, and even at nail salons and tattoo parlors.

The American Red Cross and other blood banks say they test donated blood for the presence of HIV, and they have vowed that the nation's blood supply is without risk. Hospitals have also announced stepped-up safety precautions—from the use of latex gloves to more stringent monitoring of sterilization of equipment—to protect all patients and health care workers.

At medical offices, experts advise that you watch for signs of good hygiene and ask questions if you think there are dangers. When you have a blood test, tell the technician you want her to use a new needle (although she probably will anyway). Ask the dentist or dental hygienist to explain the office's disinfection procedures to you.

Although no cases of HIV infection have been traced to nail salons or electrologists' offices, experts advise you to take your own clippers, files, electrology needles and other equipment with you if you're concerned.

But remember this: It's nearly impossible for HIV to infect any human being unless it is in body fluid, adds Dr. Wasserheit. "Most organisms, including HIV, do not survive very long on surfaces." So even if the virus were present on food, dishes, towels, telephones, toilet seats or even tampons, the chance of transmission is just about zero.

Pregnancy and AIDS

Pregnant women who are infected with the AIDS virus have a good chance of giving birth without infecting their babies, especially if they take the drug zidovudine (AZT), reports the CDC. In a study conducted by the National Institutes of Health in Bethesda, Maryland, and the National Agency of Research on AIDS in France, researchers placed approximately 180 HIV-infected women on AZT when they were between 14 and 34 weeks pregnant. The drug was also given intravenously during labor and to each newborn every six hours for the first six weeks of life.

According to preliminary reports, the investigators found that 25 percent of babies born to HIV-infected mothers who did not take AZT were born with the AIDS virus. Eight percent of babies born to mothers who took the drug were infected at birth.

Doctors advise women to have an HIV test when they find out they're pregnant in order to safeguard their children, even though it isn't known if AZT causes birth defects, says Dr. Carpenter.

Protecting Yourself

AIDS is a threat to everyone. And studies of small groups of the general population—members of the Army Reserve, Job Corps candidates and urban residents—indicate that many adolescent females are being infected with HIV at the same rate as men are. Here's how to prevent transmission of the virus.

ALWAYS USE CONDOMS. Latex condoms are best, says Dr. Wasserheit, because they prevent transmission of HIV and STDs. Condoms should be worn during vaginal and anal intercourse and oral sex.

Female condoms are also an option, says Dr. Wasserheit. This type of condom, which resembles a clear plastic bread wrapper with a ring at one end to anchor it around the cervix, has been on the market since 1992. They haven't been popular, but they're the one condom that's under a woman's control.

WEIGH NONOXYNOL-9'S RISKS. Some years ago, the spermicide nonoxynol-9, found in contraceptive jellies, creams and foams, was touted as a means to prevent HIV transmission when used in conjunction with a condom. But a debate is raging about it. Some studies indicate that frequent use of nonoxynol-9 may actually cause inflammation that aids in HIV transmission, while at least one study indicates that nonoxynol-9 does in fact reduce the risk of transmission by 70 to 80 percent. "We currently don't know precisely where the cut-off is for safe and effective use of nonoxynol-9," says Dr. Wasserheit. Talk it over with your doctor.

LIMIT YOUR PARTNERS. "A woman should also give herself a chance to know her partner and his sexual behavior well before engaging in sex," says Dr. Wasserheit. Is he or was he a drug user? Is he bisexual? Will he use a condom? If not, rethink whether you want to have sex with him. (See page 472 for advice on how to raise these subjects with your partner.)

GET AN STD CHECKUP. Treating STDs can reduce your vulnerability to HIV, says Dr. Wasserheit. But since half of all STDs are without symptoms, it's important that you get checked for them by your health-care provider after having sex with any new partner. Even if you're in a long-term relationship, have your doctor test for STDs regularly, even in the absence of symptoms.

TEST BEFORE PREGNANCY. If you're thinking of getting pregnant, have your doctor check for HIV, suggests Dr. Carpenter. If the test is positive, discuss the situation with your family and health care providers to decide what to do.

Hysterectomy

GET THE FACTS FIRST

You know what a hysterectomy is.

It's a surgical procedure in which a woman's uterus, and sometimes her ovaries, are removed. And you probably know that a lot of women have the operation and that the surgery has a reputation for being performed unnecessarily.

But you may not know what you would do if your doctor said, "You need a hysterectomy."

Controversy and Confusion

Hysterectomies are the second most common operations performed in the United States, behind cesarean sections. From 1988 through 1991, an average of 564,000 hysterectomies a year were done. The surgery is performed most often on women in their early forties.

Controversy surrounds hysterectomy: Experts say about 25 percent of the operations are unnecessary. Gary Lipscomb, M.D., assistant professor in the Department of Gynecology at the University of Tennessee in Memphis, concedes that hysterectomies are sometimes performed when they're not medically warranted. In these cases, he says, doctors may err on the side of surgery instead of other approaches for a number of reasons.

"Part of it is the way we are trained. We are trained to be aggressive in managing disease," says Dr. Lipscomb. "Most of us, including myself, have surgical personalities. And doing surgery is an active approach to problems, instead of a more passive approach. There's an old adage among surgeons in general that a chance to cut is chance to cure."

Another reason some hysterectomies are done is that women who have heavy bleeding ask for the procedure as a way to stop it, says Dr. Lipscomb. Such hysterectomies may be medically unnecessary, but they may be appropriate as far as the woman is concerned, he says.

And some patients want treatment that will give them immediate results, so even when they are offered less invasive treatments that may take a while to be effective, they choose hysterectomy, he says.

Still another factor in the hysterectomy equation is money. "If you're in private practice, and you do surgery, it generates income," says Dr. Lipscomb—more income, in some cases, than less invasive treatments or more conservative surgeries.

Finally, some doctors may not offer alternative reproductive surgeries if they can't perform them as well, says Philip Brooks, M.D., clinical professor of obstetrics and gynecology at the University of California School of Medicine at Los Angeles. "Not all doctors are competent in all procedures," he says. So if a doctor is better at removing the uterus than he is at removing fibroids or the pelvic adhesions of endometriosis, he may offer hysterectomy alone.

A Big Decision

Deciding about hysterectomy is not easy. It's major surgery that involves incisions, a stay in the hospital, anesthesia and painful days afterward. It can also trigger physical, psychological and sexual changes, many of which doctors can't predict. If the ovaries are also removed, the surgery will cause a woman to have sudden, early menopause. And then there's the one definite consequence that's irreversible—the loss of the ability to bear children.

So women may wonder "Do I really need this procedure? Am I doing the right thing?" It's often hard to decide. And some women don't—they leave it up to their physician. "For some women who are having a lot of problems, they just want to get it over," says Linda Bern-hard, R.N., Ph.D., associate professor of nursing and women's studies at Ohio State University in Columbus. "It's like 'I just want to be done with it, I don't want to deal with this anymore, I'm so sick of it.' That puts women in a very vulnerable position to have some nice physician say, 'Well, we can fix you all up. We'll just take it all out, and then every-thing will be better.' "

But women can get involved, take control and make the decision that's right for them.

All about the Procedure

Hysterectomy is most clearly warranted when a woman has cancer or serious, life-threatening complications during childbirth.

Other conditions for which doctors might recommend or perform hysterectomies include fibroids, heavy bleeding, endometriosis, prolapsed uterus, pelvic pain and pelvic inflammatory disease, although when the surgery is necessary for these conditions is less clearly defined.

There are different types of hysterectomies. A total hysterectomy, for instance, removes the uterus and the cervix, while a partial hysterec-tomy removes only the uterus.

There are also different methods of doing a hysterectomy. In an abdominal hysterectomy, the uterus is removed through an incision in the abdomen. In a vaginal hysterectomy, the uterus is removed through an incision in the vagina. The surgery is less invasive, and recovery is eas-ier than with the abdominal procedure.

In the 1990s, new techniques have been developed using lapa-roscopy. During the procedure, a laparoscope, a surgical microscope at the end of a viewing tube, is inserted through an incision in the navel, allowing physicians to view the woman's reproductive area, says Dr. Lipscomb. They can then determine whether a vaginal procedure would be likely to be effective.

In cases where a traditional vaginal hysterectomy might prove dif-ficult to do, miniature operating instruments can be inserted through other small openings in the abdomen and the uterus removed vaginally under laparoscopic guidance. This is known as a laparoscopic-assisted hysterectomy.

In any of these procedures, doctors may recommend the removal of one or both ovaries in a procedure called an oophorectomy. Some doc-tors advocate removing the ovaries in women who have finished bearing children in order to prevent ovarian cancer, even though a woman's risk of getting the disease over her entire life span is only 1 in 80.

Other medical professionals recommend leaving the ovaries in as long as possible because they supply estrogen, which plays a role in preventing osteoporosis and heart disease, as well as androgen, which influences a woman's sex drive.

You Have a Choice

The thing to remember about hysterectomy is that a lot of times it's not the only possible treatment, says Paula Bernstein, M.D., Ph.D., attending physician at Cedars-Sinai Medical Center in Los Angeles. There are usually other treatment alternatives for fibroids, heavy bleeding, pelvic pain, endometriosis, prolapsed uterus and pelvic inflammatory disease.

Fibroids are the reason for about 30 percent of hysterectomies. Alternatives include leaving fibroids alone or removing them through myomectomy, which leaves the uterus in place.

Heavy bleeding, the problem that leads to 20 percent of hysterectomies, can often be treated with medication or a procedure called endometrial ablation, in which the lining of the uterus is removed but the organ is left intact. Endometriosis can be treated with drugs as well, or the diseased tissue alone can be removed through laparoscopy.

Fifteen percent of hysterectomies are performed for prolapsed uterus, in which the uterus literally starts to fall. It's believed that having a lot of children may contribute to prolapse because childbirth distends the birth canal and stretches and weakens the muscles and ligaments supporting the uterus, says Dr. Lipscomb. Aging can also play a role. As women grow older, the connective tissue that supports the uterus becomes weaker, says Dr. Lipscomb. Estrogen helps maintain the muscles and ligaments that support the uterus, so after menopause women who do not go on hormone replacement therapy may be at increased risk for prolapsed uterus, he says.

Women who develop a prolapsed uterus can ask their doctors about exercises called Kegels, which help to strengthen the uterine muscle. They can also ask about a pessary, a device that is inserted in the vagina—much like a diaphragm—and holds the uterus in place. An advantage of the pessary is that it is a nonsurgical way to relieve the symptoms—pelvic pressure, urinary incontinence and rectal discomfort—that can arise when a woman has a prolapsed uterus. The disadvantages are that sometimes it is uncomfortable and can cause an unpleasant odor and discharge.

Obstetrical complications, such as hemorrhaging during childbirth and gynecologic cancer, are the reasons for about 11 percent of hysterectomies. For these conditions, there's usually no alternative. "Those are the life-threatening reasons," says Susan Haas, M.D., assistant professor of obstetrics and gynecology at Harvard Medical School.

In other cases, though, whether a woman has a hysterectomy is ultimately up to her. "In my opinion, since the woman lives with all the risks and all the benefits, she's the one who makes the decision," says Dr. Haas. "We should term this 'elective hysterectomy.' That reinforces the concept that it's an option or a choice and that the final decision-making power lies with the woman. It also implies that she can make that decision at any point," she says.

Even in the case of cancer, if a woman feels she's not quite ready for the surgery, it probably can wait a day or two, says Marvel Williamson, R.N., Ph.D., professor of nursing and director of the School of Nursing at Park College in Parkville, Missouri. Meanwhile, women need to take the time to find out their options, adds Dr. Bernhard.

What You Need to Know

Hysterectomy may cause a woman to have an early menopause even if she does not have her ovaries removed. If you're a candidate for surgery and you're still in your childbearing years, consider the fact that you will no longer be able to have children. While this may seem obvious, Dr. Bernhard says that some women don't take it into account. "Most women seem to have all the negative symptoms and that's what got them into the surgery in the first place. And they want to get rid of the symptoms," she says. "In the process, feelings or thoughts about childbearing may get lost." Hot flashes and vaginal dryness, two other side effects of menopause, may also occur.

A study of 10,598 women, ages 39 to 60, in the Netherlands showed that the 986 women who underwent hysterectomy but kept their ovaries—especially those between the ages of 39 and 41—experienced more hot flashes and vaginal dryness than 5,636 menopausal women who had not had a hysterectomy. Women ages 39 to 41 who'd had the operation reported menopausal complaints one to three times more often than menopausal women who hadn't had a hysterectomy.

Women who undergo hysterectomy can also experience urinary tract symptoms such as frequent urination and urinary incontinence, as well as deepening of the voice and weight gain. These physical changes are the result of declining estrogen levels. In the Netherlands study, women ages 39 to 41 who'd had a hysterectomy but kept their ovaries reported about twice as many problems not exclusive to menopause— such as irritability, dizziness, tiredness, depression, forgetfulness, headache and muscle and joint pain—as did menopausal women who hadn't had the surgery.

Some studies indicate that women feel depressed after a hysterectomy, but whether the operation itself causes depression is unclear. "Our society still has this negative perception that hysterectomy is going to make you something less. If women internalize that, then they may feel depressed," says Dr. Bernhard.

Other studies show that depression after a hysterectomy may be no more typical than depression about bodily changes that can occur after other types of surgery. And some studies reveal that women are less depressed after hysterectomy than they were before, when they had to deal with problems such as heavy bleeding and pain.

Women may also experience a sense of loss after hysterectomy, says Dr. Bernhard.

Some women say they've experienced positive physical changes, reporting restored vigor because they're no longer bleeding heavily and having pain. The operation can often end anemia as well. "I've heard women say they just feel so much better. The physical improvement in their health is often the greatest reward," says Dr. Bernhard. The women are pain-free, are no longer hemorrhaging and no longer have to plan their life around their bleeding, she says.

While studies indicate that women have these positive responses in the short term, more study is needed on the long-term effects, says Dr. Bernhard.

Women may experience sexual changes after hysterectomy because they feel different about their bodies and have anxiety about resuming sex. For some women, the orgasm experience changes.

"The uterus elevates and contracts at the time of orgasm. Most women couldn't say, 'I know what that feels like,' but when the uterus is gone, it feels different," says Dr. Bernhard. "It's not that they don't have orgasms, they just are different."

What to Consider

If you are a candidate for hysterectomy, weigh your decision carefully. Here's some help.

FIND A DOCTOR YOU LIKE. Look for a doctor you can talk to, who understands what you're going through, answers your ques-

HYSTERECTOMY

tions and will do what you want, says Nancy Petersen, R.N., director of the Endometriosis Treatment Center at St. Charles Medical Center in Bend, Oregon. If your doctor tells you that you need a hysterectomy but it doesn't seem right to you, see another doctor. Hysterectomy is often overkill for endometriosis, she says.

ASK ABOUT YOUR OPTIONS. There are usually alternatives to hysterectomy, experts say. Ask your doctor what they are, says Dr. Williamson.

GET OTHER OPINIONS. Get a second, third, even a fourth opinion. "Don't let any one physician tell you this is what you should do," says Dr. Bernhard.

LEARN ABOUT THE PROCEDURE. Ask your doctor which particular procedure will be done and why, says Dr. Brooks. Find out how much experience your doctor has with the procedure she is suggesting.

DECIDE WHAT'S MOST IMPORTANT. Set your priorities, says Dr. Bernstein. Ask yourself "How debilitating is the pain?

QUESTIONS TO ASK THE DOCTOR

Deciding whether or not to have a hysterectomy is difficult. Explore all your options by asking questions. Here are some to begin with.

- Why are you recommending a hysterectomy?
- Is there an option other than hysterectomy?
- What are the pros and cons of a hysterectomy for my problem?
- Do you recommend removal of my ovaries? If so, why? What are the risks and benefits of keeping them? The risks and benefits of removing them?
- Why are you recommending an abdominal (or vaginal) hysterectomy?
- Are you planning to use a laparoscope? If so, how much of the surgery will you do with the laparoscope?
- How many procedures like mine have you done with a laparoscope?
- When you do the procedure, will there be another surgeon present who is experienced in using a laparoscope for hysterectomy?

How much is it interfering with my lifestyle? Do I want to have children? Would I feel comfortable about adopting?"

DON'T RUSH. Take time to make your decision, says Dr. Bernhard. "There's probably no rush," she says.

If You Go for It

If you decide to have a hysterectomy, ask your doctor whether the less invasive vaginal surgery is right for you. "If there is a choice, a vaginal is always the safer, more comfortable way to go," says Dr. Williamson.

Find out whether your doctor has experience using the laparoscope, since its use in hysterectomy is fairly new.

Keep in mind, though, that if you have ovarian cancer, an abdominal hysterectomy is usually the only option, says Dr. Lipscomb.

Here are some things you can do to make the surgery easier.

INVOLVE YOUR MATE. Studies show that men often view their partners differently after hysterectomy, so "we need to help him understand," says Dr. Williamson. "Don't be afraid to ask him 'What fears do you have about my hysterectomy? How do you think my surgery will affect our sex life?'" she says. You can start by expressing your own fears and see how he responds, Dr. Bernhard says.

GET SOME FEMALE SUPPORT. Talk to your friends or join a support group. "Sometimes women find talking about it with other women helps more than talking with just their partner," says Dr. Williamson. Ask your doctor or call a local hospital for support groups near you.

GRIEVE YOUR LOSS. "As for any loss, the grief process needs to be expressed verbally and emotionally. If women can't talk about it or cry about it, the feelings of grief will come out in some other way," says Dr. Williamson. "Give yourself permission to talk about it." Find someone, such as a friend or therapist, who will go through it with you, she says.

EXPECT A CHANGE. Women often feel different after hysterectomy, experts say. It's hard to know how you will respond, but be ready for something.

RESUME SEX ASAP. Try to have sex as soon as you can after the surgery, says Dr. Williamson. She recommends that women wait 10 to 14 days for the incision to heal. Part of the healing process after surgery is the development of scar tissue, and if women wait too long, the scar tissue in the pelvic cavity and around the vaginal incision can become very tough, making sex more uncomfortable, she says.

Having sex can minimize the scar tissue toughness, because the area gets increased circulation and expands during engorgement.

"We would like women to resume intercourse, gentle intercourse, between the two- and four-week period, if possible," she says. Women should try to have sex at least twice a week until the healing process is complete, she says, which can take as long as three months.

TAKE TIME ALONE BEFORE SEX. After surgery, women should start by "having their first orgasm alone," says Dr. Williamson. They should masturbate the first time so they can get used to any new sensations, she says. "It lets them know that everything still works and that it doesn't hurt to get turned on and have an orgasm."

START ALL OVER. With your partner, that is. When women who've had a hysterectomy are ready to start intercourse again, the couple needs to pretend it's their very first time having sex, says Dr. Williamson. "They need to allow her to be in control, to have as long a foreplay session as possible," she says. Many women are concerned that sex will be painful, so taking it slow can help, she says. And don't be afraid to use artificial lubricating jellies, she says. Products to consider for vaginal dryness include K-Y Lubricating Jelly and Replens, which are available in pharmacies.

VARY YOUR SEXUAL ROUTINE. Before the surgery, get in the habit of varying your sexual techniques, like the positions you and your partner use, because you probably will have to do so after the surgery, at least at first, says Dr. Williamson.

TRY KEGELS. Many women say the pleasurable feeling of needing to be filled that they experienced during sex is no longer there after hysterectomy, says Dr. Williamson. This may be due to vaginal scar tissue that does not engorge and stretch as well as other genital tissue. Or it could be because the woman's cervix has been removed, leaving her vagina shorter than before. Performing Kegels during sex can help women achieve that feeling, she says, because they help to lengthen and lift the vagina.

Normally Kegels can be done anywhere; you simply tighten your vagina as if you are trying to keep from urinating, hold it from two to five seconds, then release. After hysterectomy, do Kegels during sex. Besides strengthening the vaginal muscles, they will enhance the feeling of pressure on the penis, Dr. Williamson says. "What people describe to me is that the best feelings come when the muscles are contracted or tightened, and that it's held as long as possible," she says.

Incontinence
AGE IS NOT THE FACTOR

Do you leak when you sneeze or dribble if you jump?
What about that uncontrollable urge triggered by the sound of gushing water?

Quickly you cross your legs, clutch your gut and try to console yourself: "I'm not incontinent," you say. "I'm too young, too healthy. Besides, it only happens occasionally."

The truth is, age has nothing to do with this kind of incontinence. Doctors say that as many as half of all women younger than 45 know what it's like to accidentally wet themselves. The causes range from childbirth and smoking to everyday stress on weak pelvic or abdominal muscles.

You might think women in great shape wouldn't have a problem holding their urine. But many of them do.

Ingrid Nygaard, M.D., who does research on incontinence in young women at the University of Iowa in Iowa City, found leaking can be a real problem for female athletes. She says gymnasts especially report sudden, uncontrollable urine loss, and not only in the gymnasium.

Incontinence is also a problem for women who play basketball, tennis and field hockey and take aerobics classes, Dr. Nygaard says. These activities exert intense pressure on the pelvic floor muscles when the heels of a woman's feet hit the ground, she says.

If sports and working out don't make you incontinent, there is always a chance childbirth will. "Childbirth is a woman's biggest risk factor," says Dr. Nygaard.

It's not how many children you have but how your body reacts to the growing weight and pressure of a developing fetus or the trauma of vaginal delivery, says Joseph Montella, M.D., director of urogynecology at Jefferson Medical College in Philadelphia. He finds that a woman who's gone through ten births could have complete bladder control, while another develops incontinence after one child. The cause is usually a resulting weakness in the muscles that open and close the urethra, the tube that empties urine from the bladder.

"It could be a hereditary muscle weakness," he says, or an earlier muscle strain developed from sports, lifting or bending.

You seldom hear men complain about incontinence because they seldom leak until they reach their later years. Doctors offer a simple explanation: Men are designed not to.

"Males have a longer urethra. And they have thicker muscles to hold it shut," Dr. Nygaard says. And obviously, the physical stress of childbirth isn't a factor for men.

In both men and women, the bladder—when full—should hold around 12 ounces of fluid, enough to fill a soft drink can. A woman's ability to actually hold that much urine depends on the strength of the pelvic muscles around her bladder.

Why the Floodgates Open

Pelvic muscles help control the sphincter muscles at the spout of the bladder. You could think of the sphincter as a faucet. When the sphincter is open, liquid flows out. When the sphincter is closed, the bladder is shut. Sometimes the sphincter can't close all the way because the muscles surrounding it are stretched. It's like having a faucet that's never quite turned off. The result: Your bladder leaks, either constantly or at the slightest aggravation—a cough, a sneeze, a laugh.

When the muscles surrounding your bladder are causing your problem, you have what doctors call stress incontinence. It's the most common type of incontinence in women ages 30 to 50.

In older women, incontinence can be triggered by a stroke, medication, arthritis or depression. The most common form in older women is called urge incontinence.

"It's a sudden need to urinate that often can't be controlled," says Catherine DuBeau, M.D., an instructor at Harvard Medical School and a gerontologist at the Continence Center at Brigham and Women's Hospital in Boston.

National health officials report that some six to eight million women experience bouts of some type of incontinence every year. Urogynecologists—physicians who specialize in women's incontinence—say that up to 80 percent of all cases can be helped or cured with treatment or therapy. Once women begin behavioral therapy, they usually regain control of their bladders in 3 to 12 weeks, doctors say. Very few women require surgery.

Curing incontinence is usually not a problem. The problem is finding the women who need a cure.

WOMAN TO WOMAN HER BLADDER IS BACK IN CONTROL

Kim Stroud's undersize bladder meant she could never hold her urine as long as other girls. When the birth of her first son left Kim incontinent, the Spartanburg, South Carolina, mother was determined to regain control of her body. This is her story.

All teenage girls spend time in the bathroom, but I spent the most time there. Doctors said I had a pinch in my bladder. It made my bladder smaller. I had to use the bathroom three times an hour when I went on a date. My high school boyfriend married me anyway.

My first child weighed nine pounds, six ounces, and it was a difficult birth. After the baby I didn't feel a sensation of having to go at all. Suddenly, I would be all wet. I started carrying extra clothes with me.

Finally I went to a urologist. He barely started an internal examination when he looked up and asked if I ever saw my bladder poking out of my vagina. It had dropped so far, it emptied at will. The doctor said I

"It's socially unacceptable," says Kristene E. Whitmore, M.D., chief of urology and director of the Incontinence Center at Graduate Hospital in Philadelphia. "Women feel it's taboo to say they leak," even to a doctor.

When a woman finally decides to get medical help, it's usually after seven years of leaking, says Katherine F. Jeter, Ed.D., who founded Help for Incontinent People (HIP), a nonprofit information advocacy organization for people with incontinence, in Spartanburg, South Carolina.

"Many women really believe incontinence is their lot in life," says Dr. Jeter. "They think this is the price they must pay for having children."

Dr. Jeter estimates that her organization receives 3,000 letters and calls each month from women who have finally decided they don't have to live with incontinence. Most women tell her that for years they dealt with their problem by using sanitary napkins. It's a typical response to incontinence.

"About 38 percent of all menstrual products are used for incontinence," says Dr. Whitmore.

For many women, leaking becomes progressively worse after menopause, when they lose their natural estrogen supply. "Estrogen keeps muscles surrounding the bladder from drying out," explains Dr. Montella.

---

needed a hysterectomy and surgery to tack the bladder back.

I felt that I might want to have another child. A hysterectomy was out of the question. I called Help for Incontinent People.

They gave me a list of foods to avoid: Chocolate, artificial sweeteners, soft drinks with caffeine, coffee and foods with a tomato base, like ketchup. Smoking and even second-hand smoke aggravated my bladder.

Within a week I had cut my trips to the bathroom in half. The biofeedback program clicked in. I only went to the clinic for eight weeks. I started Kegel exercises that help you strengthen and control the muscles around your bladder. I still wore pads, but instead of eight a day, I was down to two a day.

Then I got pregnant with my second child. He was bigger than the first, but I kept doing Kegels. I haven't leaked for seven months, except for one slight accident, and I don't wear pads anymore except during my monthly cycle.

How to Overcome Stress Incontinence

When a sneeze might mean a sudden leak, Peggy Norton, M.D., a urogynecologist at the University of Utah Medical Center in Salt Lake City, who wrote a physicians' guide to incontinence, says that crossing their legs helps many women reduce leakage temporarily.

A more permanent cure calls for more effort.

"Incontinence treatment doesn't hurt," says Kathryn Burgio, Ph.D., a behavioral psychologist who is researching incontinence at the University of Alabama in Birmingham. "It's not even uncomfortable." Here are some suggestions.

PRACTICE YOUR KEGELS. Dr. Burgio recommends these exercises as the place to start. With Kegel exercises, you squeeze your internal pelvic muscles, hold for a slow count of three, then release. It feels like you are trying to start and stop the flow of urine.

Just make sure it is pelvic muscles that you are contracting. Test yourself when you are on the toilet. If you can stop or even slow the flow of urine, you are contracting the correct muscles.

Don't develop the habit of practicing Kegel exercises on the toilet, though, advises Dr. Montella. If you are constantly stopping and starting your urine flow, you may not completely empty your bladder, and that could compound your urinary problems.

"Do ten pelvic exercises three to five times a day," he says. If that seems like a lot, spread them out over the course of the day. Do Kegels every time you stop at a red light, for instance, or as you stand at the bus stop.

DON'T DROWN YOUR BLADDER. Your body only needs 50 to 70 ounces (between six and nine cups) of water a day, unless it is really hot outside or you're heavily exerting yourself, says Dr. Norton. But don't drink it all at once. A full bladder is a stretched bladder, and that could mean a leak.

HOLD IT IN THE SHOWER. If you start the habit of urinating in the shower, Dr. Norton says, you'll train your bladder to respond to the sound of gushing water. "It may explain why every time you hear water running you start to leak urine."

DOUBLE DO IT. To guard against leaks, some doctors suggest double-voiding. When your bladder feels empty, bend forward and push. Stand up, sit down and try to void again.

EAT AND DRINK WITH CARE. Avoid tomato-based foods, spicy foods, chocolate, citrus fruits and artificial sweeteners, which are acidic foods that irritate the bladder. Caffeine and alcohol are diuretics and may also stimulate incontinence, says Dr. Nygaard.

Try to eat more fiber, she says. Fiber fights constipation, and constipation can make your incontinence worse.

STAY AWAY FROM CIGARETTES. In a study of 606 women at the Medical College of Virginia in Richmond, researchers found that former and current smokers were more than twice as likely to suffer from stress incontinence as those who had never smoked. Nicotine irritates the bladder, plus smoke makes you cough—and a cough may make you leak. So stop smoking, and try not to inhale second-hand smoke.

GET INFORMATION. Call Help for Incontinent People toll free at 1-800-BLADDER. The organization mails out self-help packets that explain what causes the problem and how to begin getting help. HIP maintains an ever-increasing library about all aspects of incontinence. The Simon Foundation in Wilmett, Illinois, also offers advice on incontinence; call 1-800-23S-IMON.

LEND SUPPORT. Dr. Nygaard encourages women to use tampons or even a diaphragm. If women leak only during a workout, sometimes a tampon or diaphragm can help to support the bladder during an exercise session.

"It's okay to wear a tampon for a short term," says Dr. Nygaard. "Some women only wet during exercise." To alleviate some of the pressure on the bladder caused by exercise, Dr. Nygaard advises women to land on the balls of their feet instead of their heels, but that usually won't completely solve the problem.

Getting Professional Help

Sometimes you can regain continence only with the help of a doctor. Ask your family physician to refer you to a urogynecologist or a urologist. Help the doctor diagnose your problem by writing down what you eat, how much you drink and exactly when you leak. Give a good medical history and list all of the medicines you take.

Doctors have recently developed several types of incontinence therapy. Most don't require a hospital stay. The following therapies to help build muscle tone are usually done under medical supervision in an outpatient clinic or a doctor's office.

Vaginal cones. These tampon-shaped weights are inserted in the vagina, where they'll remain as long as you squeeze the right pelvic muscles. Cones come in various sizes. You start with the smallest and lightest, then once your muscles are able to hold onto the cone for at least 60 seconds, you move up to a heavier size, which will further strengthen your muscles.

Electric stimulation. This technique helps you identify the muscles you need to exercise. A low-grade electric current painlessly promotes contraction in the pelvic muscles. A stronger current brings on a stronger contraction. Several repetitive "shock" sessions can rebuild and strengthen pelvic muscles.

Biofeedback. This helps you gauge pelvic muscle development. Electric monitoring probes inserted in the vagina measure the strength of a pelvic contraction. Doctors often use biofeedback with electric stimulation.

Other treatments include collagen injections, which were first used by cosmetic surgeons to give women fuller lips. Urologists found this fibrous protein also causes swelling around the bladder, which stops leaks. Usually several injections, done under local anesthesia, are necessary.

Sometimes the muscles supporting the bladder are so weak that the bladder neck falls out of place. This allows urine to pour out of the body any time you make a sudden move. Surgeons can repair the fallen bladder neck by stitching it back into place, Dr. Whitmore says. But "surgery has a failure rate of 25 percent," she says. So it's always better to try behavior therapy first.

Infertility

REALIZING THE DREAM OF MOTHERHOOD

For years you took all kinds of precautions so you wouldn't get pregnant. But now that you're trying to, you can't.

For whatever reason—you're not sure what yet—it's just not happening. So every month you and your husband go through all the physical and mental gymnastics of scheduling sex, reading and charting early-morning body temperatures and going for test after test after test. And every month, instead of hoping that your period will come, the way you used to, you hope that it won't. You used to view your menstrual blood as the signal that you were fully a woman. Now when it comes it makes you feel as if maybe you're not.

There is a certain irony to it all, that what you once fought so hard to prevent—pregnancy—you're now trying so hard to create. But this isn't the kind of irony that makes you laugh. Instead you're frustrated, confused, angry, sad and worried.

The Infertility Frustration

Experiencing infertility is extremely painful emotionally for women, says Linda D. Applegarth, Ed.D., a psychologist for the In Vitro Fertilization (IVF) Clinic at the New York Hospital–Cornell Medical Center in New York City. It's an experience they never expected to go through, and many are left feeling inadequate as women. "It really strikes at a woman's identity as a woman," she says. While careers and work are often a large part of it, "the whole notion of being a mother is still very primary to who she is as a person," she says.

While infertility can be difficult for men, too, it's often more so for women, says Dr. Applegarth. Women tend to feel more stress about infertility, she says. "They worry about it more. It's usually never far from their thoughts. They're the ones who are reminded monthly of what's happening—or not happening—for them."

Women also are faced with having to shift their definition of what a family is, says Dr. Applegarth. They may have seen it as Mom and Dad and 2.5 children; now they have to get used to the idea that it might just be him and her, she says.

There's also a lot of fear and uncertainty about making decisions about other options, such as adoption, trying donor eggs or sperm or remaining child-free.

Sometimes you can be on a different track than your husband, says Dr. Applegarth. One partner may be more interested in pursuing a high-technology form of treatment, while the other may be ready to move to adopt, she says. This difference can often put additional stress on a relationship.

Infertility can bring a sense of loss on many levels, says Dr. Applegarth. There's the loss of not being able to pass on your and your husband's genes, as well as the loss of experiencing the birth process. Some women end up feeling that their bodies are letting them down, that they're defective, she says.

The Infertility Facts

Couples are considered infertile if they have been having unprotected intercourse for a year and no pregnancy has resulted. This happens to an estimated 10 to 15 percent of American couples. In 25 to 40 percent of cases the problem is related to the man and in 40 to 55 percent of cases to the woman, says Mark Hornstein, M.D., director of the In Vitro Fertilization Program at Brigham and Women's Hospital in Boston. In about 10 percent of cases the trouble is with both partners.

Understanding the Causes

There is a host of problems that can cause infertility in women. In an estimated 30 percent of infertile women, there is failure to ovulate. This can be caused by an imbalance of the hormones, including estrogen, that are required to mature an egg and release it from the ovary. Dr. Hornstein says low estrogen levels are often seen in women who have exercise-induced amenorrhea (in which periods cease), anorexia or dietary deficiencies or who are entering menopause. Other women have very high levels of the male hormone androgen, and as a result the eggs don't develop completely. A malfunctioning adrenal gland can lead to high androgen levels.

Age can also be a factor. "Most studies find a slight drop in the conception rates at age 35, a more pronounced drop at 37 and a dramatic drop by age 40," says Mary Martin, M.D., director of the In Vitro Fertilization Program at the University of California at San Francisco. And no one knows why.

"There's a barrier to conception at age 40 that we don't completely understand," explains Dr. Martin. "We don't understand it because many of the women who can't conceive will still be ovulating, they'll still be having regular menstrual cycles, and they appear healthy.

"But there is some change that occurs at some fundamental level within the eggs and the ovary itself—a change so significant that even if we stimulate the ovaries and take out the eggs to fertilize in the lab, the probabilities of pregnancy are much reduced.

"It isn't simply a question of not having eggs," adds Dr. Martin. "It's a question of egg quality."

Infertility can also result when the fallopian tubes are damaged or blocked, often as a result of pelvic inflammatory disease (PID) and sometimes endometriosis. Endometriosis, PID or cervical disease is the problem in about 50 percent of infertility cases.

Sometimes there are cervical problems, such as an infection, a lesion or small cervical size, which can lead to infertility. And some women produce antibodies to their husband's sperm.

Trying to Fix It

For many of us, finding out the problem behind infertility is not as important as fixing it.

The whole process usually begins with a medical history, says G. David Adamson, M.D., clinical associate professor at Stanford University School of Medicine. This involves taking a look at your age, how long you and your husband have been trying to conceive and whether you have been able to achieve a pregnancy before, either together or with other partners.

This is generally followed by a semen analysis to see if your husband is producing the quality and quantity of sperm necessary to fertilize an egg and a basal body temperature check to assess whether you are ovulating regularly. Doctors may also ask you to do a postcoital test, where a sample of your cervical mucus is examined several hours after intercourse. This test assesses the quality of the mucus and the sperm's ability to swim in it. To see if your fallopian tubes are clear, doctors may perform an x-ray screening test with dye, called a hysterosalpingogram.

"All couples should have answers to these questions within the first year," says Dr. Adamson.

If the problem lies with your husband's sperm, he should see a urologist, who may recommend medical treatment or, occasionally, surgery. There are also sperm-washing procedures that can be tried. This involves rinsing the ejaculate with a special solution and spinning it in a centrifuge so that the sperm are separated from the semen and become more concentrated. You can also consider artificial insemination, where sperm are collected and then deposited into the vagina or uterus.

If the problem is with ovulation, there are several medications you can take to try to stimulate it. Clomiphene citrate, sold as Clomid or Serophene, induces the pituitary gland to release the hormones that signal the ovary to produce follicles. Human menopausal gonadotropin (hMG), known as Pergonal, stimulates the ovary to produce more than one egg. Follicle-stimulating hormone (FSH), taken as a drug called Metrodin, is similar to Pergonal and helps the ovary ripen the follicle into an egg that can be released.

If there is damage to the tubes or pelvic cavity from endometriosis, doctors can remove endometrial adhesions and growths through a surgical procedure called laparoscopy.

Sometimes these techniques work right away, and other times it's necessary to keep trying a particular drug for months or to try several different approaches. The entire process can be time-consuming, expensive and emotionally trying.

If these early attempts fail, where to go from there often has to do with your age and how long you have been trying to get pregnant, says Dr. Adamson. A woman who has tried for more than three years to get pregnant should consider assisted reproductive technology—such as in vitro fertilization—very soon, he says. If the woman is in her midthirties, she should consider high-tech procedures after 12 to 18 months of trying unsuccessfully, he says. A woman in her late thirties or older may want to move to assisted reproductive procedures in 3 to 6 months, he says.

Coping with Infertility

The tests, the waiting and the uncertainty take their toll, both on your emotional health and on your relationship with your husband. Here are some tips that can help make coping a little easier.

UNDERSTAND THE TIMETABLE. "The general rules of thumb are that any couple that has not conceived after one year of exposure should see their physician. Couples should expect that after seeing their physician, they will have all the tests done and treatment initiated within four to six months, if not sooner," says Dr. Adamson. "Treatment following the testing should be for no more than an absolute maximum of 12 to 18 months before considering the assisted reproductive technologies. For older women, these time frames are all shortened significantly," he says.

FIND A REPRODUCTIVE ENDOCRINOLOGIST. "All couples, after 18 months of trying, should be referred to a specialist, a reproductive endocrinologist," says Dr. Adamson. "And they should be referred earlier if there are significant problems identified in the initial workup," he says. Write to the Society for Assisted Reproductive Technologies, c/o American Fertility Society, 1209 Montgomery Highway, Birmingham, AL 35216, for the names and numbers of reproductive endocrinologists in your area.

CALL FOR HELP. Resolve, an organization established to help couples dealing with infertility, can be incredibly helpful, says Dr. Applegarth. It has a hot line and support group listings. You can write to Resolve at 1310 Broadway, Somerville, MA 02144-1731.

SHARE WITH A FRIEND. "It might be important to tell just one friend or one family member," says Dr. Applegarth. Often women tell her that their husbands are supportive and that they are helping each other, she says. But that can lead to feelings of isolation and loneliness for the couple. You don't have to tell everyone, Dr. Applegarth says, but sharing your infertility experience with one other reliable confidant may help. Getting caring support from family or friends can often help couples cope at this difficult time.

TAKE 20. Couples who don't talk about the infertility problem are at a big disadvantage, says Dr. Applegarth. Communicating with your husband about infertility is important but difficult. So set a ground rule that you are only going to talk about it for 20 minutes each day or every other day, says Dr. Applegarth.

GET COUNSELING. Experiencing infertility can be emotionally difficult for couples, says Dr. Hornstein: "It's important for the couple to be supported through this." So consult a social worker, psychologist or psychiatrist for counseling. Ask your doctor for a referral.

Safeguarding Your Fertility Now

Perhaps you haven't tried to get pregnant yet but are concerned about preserving your fertility. While some problems can't be prevented, there are some things you can do now to prevent certain infertility problems.

PRACTICE SAFE SEX. One thing women can do to prevent infertility is protect themselves against sexually transmitted diseases (STDs), says Dr. Adamson. If you haven't already done so, have your doctor screen you for all STDs, since some can be present without symptoms. Ask your partner to get screened, too. If you have multiple partners or are having sex with someone whose history you're not sure of, use condoms. Latex condoms with nonoxynol-9 are the most effective in warding off most STDs.

FIND OUT YOUR FAMILY HISTORY. Your family's medical history may tell you whether you are at increased risk for infertility. For example, if your mother and sisters went through premature menopause or developed fibroids that interfered with their fertility, that's a clue that you might, too.

GET HIM TO STOP SMOKING. If your husband is a smoker, encourage him to cut back or quit altogether, since studies indicate that smoking can affect sperm quality.

DON'T OVERDO THE EXERCISE. Intense exercise can lead to amenorrhea, which is a sign that exercise has interfered with ovulation.

TRY NOT TO WAIT TOO LONG. Pay more attention to planning your reproductive life, suggests Dr. Adamson. It's important to realize that biology won't wait, he says. Women may want to wait till their job is on track or until they've moved, or whatever, he says. "There's always a better time to have a baby. But time marches on relentlessly." Just try to be realistic.

Inflammatory Bowel Disease

Dousing the Fire in the Belly

The pain shoots across your belly, prodding you into action even before you've opened your eyes.

You lurch out of bed, steady yourself on the nightstand and stumble toward the bathroom. You know there's not much time, because seconds after the pain begins, your body is going to turn itself inside out with the morning's bout of diarrhea.

The only thing that alters each morning's routine is how long it lasts. If the diarrhea stops within two hours, you can get to the office. If it lasts longer, your limp body won't be able to do anything but crawl back into bed.

Living with inflammatory bowel disease (IBD) is tough, says

Jacqueline L. Wolf, M.D., assistant professor of medicine at Harvard Medical School and co-director of the Inflammatory Bowel Disease Center at Brigham and Women's Hospital in Boston. It affects more than one million men and women across the country about equally, and although 10 to 25 percent of cases may have a genetic link, no one really knows what causes it.

The Two Faces of IBD

Dr. Wolf's theory is that IBD is caused by a three-step process. First a genetic predisposition somehow sets the stage. Then a virus or bacterium in the intestine penetrates the intestinal wall. Finally, the immune system goes on the attack, trying to rout the invader—and ends up decimating the intestine instead.

There are two types of inflammatory bowel disease, identified by where the inflammation occurs and how deeply it penetrates the intestinal wall.

When the inflammation starts along the lining of the rectum, moves upward into the large intestine, starts in pretty much the same place every time and sticks largely to the gut's surface, it's called ulcerative colitis.

This condition pops up out of nowhere, usually between the ages of 15 and 35. Sometimes a flare-up will scorch the surface of the intestine and cause seemingly endless bouts of nausea, diarrhea and pain. Surgically removing the affected area will usually eliminate the disease.

When the inflammation moves around the gut, involving the intestinal wall anywhere from the mouth to the anus, it's called Crohn's disease.

Crohn's can trigger waves of pain and diarrhea, sometimes with bleeding and, on rare occasions, nausea and vomiting. And sometimes the disease takes off on its own and sets fire to adjoining tissue. It can actually pass through the intestinal wall to other organs, triggering infection and leaving scar tissue that can lead to intestinal obstruction, fecal incontinence, infertility and perhaps even cancer. Surgery is not very helpful with Crohn's disease, because the problem will simply move to another section of the bowel.

Preventing Flare-Ups

Since inflammation is the common problem in both diseases, the strategies doctors have devised to prevent flare-ups are similar, says Dr.

Wolf: a variety of drugs to smother or suppress inflammation and a healthy regimen of diet, exercise and stress control aimed at keeping the gut cool and calm. Here's how you can do it.

EAT WELL. "People feel better if they follow a good, healthy diet," says Dr. Wolf. Although the tendency may be to eat as little as possible, a well-rounded diet of fresh fruit, steamed fish and vegetables, lean meats and lots of carbohydrates—pasta, potatoes, breads and cereals—can all help prevent the malnutrition and weight loss that can potentially undermine the health of someone with IBD.

WATCH FOR DIETARY LAND MINES. You should also monitor how various foods affect your gut, says Dr. Wolf. "Some people have a specific food that causes them to flare. Other people can eat the same food and it causes no problem." For example, some patients find that they cannot eat red meat. Unfortunately, no specific diet has been found that will get the inflammation under control.

USE FIBER CAUTIOUSLY. Check with your doctor about the amount of fiber you eat if you have Crohn's disease, cautions Dr. Wolf. Women with Crohn's disease frequently develop a narrowing somewhere along the intestine, and too much fiber—particularly in a bowel where walls are swollen—can cause obstructions.

MANAGE STRESS. You should also avoid stress where you can, says Dr. Wolf, since "there are reports that when people are under stress, the disease flares."

The best way to keep stress under wraps? Maintain a positive attitude, exercise every day and join a support group, says Dr. Wolf. There are support groups to help families cope with the stress caused by IBD.

DOUSE THE FIRE. In ulcerative colitis, daily use of the prescription drugs sulfasalazine (Azulfidine) and 5-aminosalicylic acid components (Asacol) have been shown to prevent flare-ups, says Dr. Wolf—"not 100 percent, but they're pretty good." In Crohn's disease, daily use of Asacol can prevent a relapse.

If you take sulfasalazine, you should also take a daily one-milligram supplement of folic acid, a B vitamin, says Dr. Wolf. It will compensate for the way sulfasalazine upsets your body's ability to absorb the essential nutrient, and it may also help prevent colon cancer—a disease for which women with IBD are at increased risk.

RECONSIDER BIRTH CONTROL PILLS. There is some question as to whether oral contraceptives trigger Crohn's disease in genetically susceptible women, scientists say. In a study of 303 women with IBD, for example, researchers from the University of North Carolina at

Chapel Hill found that women who used oral contraceptives had a 50 percent greater risk of developing Crohn's disease than other women.

Overcoming Sexual Difficulties

Many women with IBD take their worries to bed with them, where their sex life may be affected by fear of soiling the sheets and pain during intercourse.

In a study of 50 women with Crohn's disease at Leicester General Hospital and the University Hospital of Wales in Cardiff, researchers found that even though 45 of these women were in stable, ongoing relationships, more than a quarter were abstaining from sex. Of those who did have sex, 60 percent reported it was painful and 22 percent reported difficulty conceiving.

Luckily, there are several things you can do to prevent these problems.

MOVE YOUR BOWELS. "If there's stool in the rectum when you're going to have intercourse, have a bowel movement ahead of time," says Dr. Wolf. Then you won't have to worry about fecal material leaking out at the wrong moment.

CHECK FOR STRUCTURAL PROBLEMS. Painful intercourse may be caused by pelvic nerves that are irritated when your partner pushes on the posterior wall of the vagina, says Dr. Wolf. Or it may be caused by a fissure or fistula—a hollow tube forged between two organs by the inflammatory process. If either a fissure or fistula opens into a vagina that's being stretched during intercourse, the result can be painful intercourse.

In any case, the best way to tackle the problem of painful intercourse is to first visit your doctor, says Dr. Wolf. If there's a fissure or fistula, she can correct it.

SMOOTH THE WAY. Use lubrication before intercourse, make sure you have enough foreplay and suggest that your partner enter slowly and/or not go in quite all the way, says Dr. Wolf.

Preventing Problems in Pregnancy

Most women with IBD will not have any more difficulty getting pregnant than other women—as long as inflammation has not spread from the bowel to the ovaries and left scars that block the fallopian tubes.

What can be a problem, however, is the potential father's sperm if *he* has IBD and is being treated with sulfasalazine, says Dr. Wolf. The drug will reduce the number of sperm, slow them down and twist them into odd shapes that will have difficulty penetrating an egg. Within three months of stopping the drug, however, the sperm will resume their usual form.

"A lot of doctors tell women with IBD they shouldn't get pregnant," says Dr. Wolf. But a woman with IBD can carry a baby to term without exacerbating the disease or harming her baby.

Studies indicate that results of pregnancies among women with IBD are similar to those of women who do not have it. Among pregnant women with ulcerative colitis, 76 to 97 percent produce healthy babies, 1 to 13 percent miscarry, and up to 3 percent experience stillbirths or give birth to babies with congenital abnormalities.

Among pregnant women with Crohn's disease, studies show that 70 to 93 percent give birth to healthy babies, 1 to 4 percent miscarry, and up to 1 percent have stillbirths or give birth to babies with congenital abnormalities.

Here's how you can better the odds of a successful pregnancy.

SCHEDULE THE PREGNANCY. Get pregnant while IBD is in remission rather than during a flare-up, says Dr. Wolf. This is because when a woman is very ill—with IBD or any disease—the baby won't grow as well.

STAY ON MEDICATION. You can continue taking the drugs prescribed by your doctor to suppress the inflammation, Dr. Wolf says—they're safe during pregnancy. You should, however, discuss your IBD history with your obstetrician and get her okay to continue your medication.

AVOID DRUGS THAT SUPPRESS IMMUNITY. Experimental studies indicate that prescription drugs that inhibit your immune system in order to prevent gut inflammation can cause low fetal birthweights and double the number of birth defects. Two such drugs are azathioprine (Imuran) and 6-mercaptopurine (Purinethal).

Some scientists are so uncomfortable with 6-mercaptopurine's potential for birth defects that they recommend discontinuing the drug three months prior to conception—no matter which partner is taking it.

Similar drugs that should be avoided during pregnancy are ciprofloxacin (Cipro) and metronidazole (Flagyl), says Dr. Wolf.

If you are pregnant, go over all your medications with your obstetrician and don't take anything without her blessing.

Inhibited Sexual Desire

GETTING BACK IN THE MOOD

Movies, music videos, magazine articles and radio talk shows send out a resounding message: sex, sex, sex.

Yet some women's bodies say no, no, no.

These women have inhibited sexual desire (ISD), a common disorder in which there is a chronic disinterest in sex. Forty to fifty percent of couples who show up at sexual dysfunction clinics are said to have it, making it the most common issue for couples who seek help for sexual problems.

Men are as likely as women to have it, says Richard A. Carroll, Ph.D., director of the Sex and Marital Therapy Program at the Northwestern Medical Faculty Foundation of the Northwestern Medical Center in Chicago. But women tend to get it at a younger age than men—in their midthirties as opposed to their fifties—and they tend to experience more emotional distress with it and go for longer periods of time without seeking help, he says.

When Desire Drops

Women with ISD experience more than just an occasional ebb in desire, says Jo Kessler, a licensed nurse practitioner and certified sex therapist in San Diego. These women can go for long periods of time—maybe six months, nine months, a year or longer—without feeling the urge. They go without masturbating, thinking about sex or having it. Some say they don't miss it at all, Kessler says. If it weren't for their partners, they wouldn't really care about having sex.

The situation can be a difficult one, says Kessler. With all the information about sex and sexuality that's available, women know that some amount of sex is considered "normal." "The woman knows if she's not having sex, or if she's not interested in sex, something is wrong. She feels defective, she feels guilty and she feels helpless." And if she perceives her partner as always ready to have sex, the woman may feel that she's the one with the problem and that she's totally to blame for the unsatisfactory sex life, says Kessler.

What's Really Wrong

ISD is probably best thought of as a symptom of an underlying problem, says Dr. Carroll. The most common causes are more likely to be psychological than physical, he says. At the top of the list is depression, he says. "Depression can affect one's ability to enjoy anything. Sex is just one of those," he says.

Next in line is interpersonal conflict. Problems in a relationship often manifest themselves in sexual problems, experts say. "Sex is a metaphor for the relationship," says Susan E. Hetherington, Dr.P.H., a certified nurse-midwife and sex therapist and professor in the School of Nursing at the University of Maryland in Baltimore. "People end up fighting out in the bedroom what they should be fighting out in the living room and dining room," she says. When the couple doesn't deal with issues or problems by talking about them as they occur, the conflict comes out in other ways—often through the sexual relationship. Unexpressed anger is often part of the picture. With ISD, "in general the relationship isn't working or isn't providing the woman with what she wants or needs to be sexual," says Kessler.

The problem often develops gradually, she says. It may begin with a lack of enthusiasm for sex that causes the woman to decline sexual overtures sporadically, she says. Then, often without deliberately planning it as a sexual avoidance maneuver, the woman may get involved in activities that keep her chronically busy, unavailable or tired, so the likelihood of sex is reduced.

"Eventually a couple comes in and they haven't had sex for six months," she says. "The partner is frustrated and angry and upset. The woman is puzzled and upset and feeling pressured by her partner or by her own expectations. She's feeling overwhelmed. If she was depressed before, she's even more depressed. It can be a real downward spiral for the woman as well as for the relationship."

Physical changes, such as those occurring after pregnancy, might also trigger ISD. "It's not uncommon for a woman to be less interested in sex when there is a new baby at home. The woman is recovering physically and she's adapting to motherhood. All of the demands that having a new baby put on a woman contribute to fatigue," says Kessler. Often women will have a lower sex drive for six to nine months after having a baby, she says.

Despite common belief, women going through menopause won't automatically experience ISD. "If she's had a healthy sex drive and a healthy attitude about sex and has liked it and it's been a positive force in her life, unless there's some untoward problem with the menopause, it doesn't really affect her drive at all," says Kessler. "There used to be the notion that when women got older or went through menopause they lost interest in sex, and that's just not holding true." The sex drive of some women actually goes up after menopause, she says. "There can be such a sense of freedom that women are more interested sexually. Some report it as the best sexual time of their life."

Keeping Desire Strong

ISD can be prevented. Here's what you can do.

PAY ATTENTION TO PROBLEMS. "Have some mechanism to resolve conflict in the relationship. When couples are fighting, they don't feel particularly congenial," says Kessler, and they usually won't want to have sex. Instead of letting one issue color the whole relationship and all your interactions, set aside a specific time to address it. "For example, talk about the issue for 30 minutes, then set it aside. Agree that you'll do that every second or third day for two weeks and that at two weeks you'll have formed some resolution. That's one way to keep it from constantly being up in your face and

INHIBITED SEXUAL DESIRE

being the total focus of your relationship with each other," she says.

KEEP THE LINES OF COMMUNICATION OPEN. When you are upset, try to deal with the problems instead of pushing them under the rug, says Dr. Hetherington. Try using "I" statements and avoid using "you" statements, she says. Start with "I feel this way" or "I am frustrated," instead of "You make me mad." Another way to express and defuse feelings of anger or resentment is to write them out first, says Dr. Carroll. Then figure out how you can relay the message in an effective way, he says.

MAKE TIME FOR INTIMACY. Couples need to set aside time to be together in an intimate way, says Dr. Carroll. "Set one night aside to be together—alone—without the kids or distractions. Make a commitment to time for the relationship," he says.

VARY YOUR SEXUAL ROUTINE. Try new things with your partner to keep from getting in the same old habit. "People with ISD have fairly rigid sexual scripts. This is how sex is done—A, B, C and D," says Dr. Carroll. "A varied sexual repertoire can help prevent ISD."

THINK ABOUT SEX. "One way to keep sex drive alive is thinking about sex. Have three erotic thoughts a day, from mildly romantic to whatever any individual woman thinks of as sexually explicit," says Kessler. "If you don't ever think about sex, then it's not very likely that you're going to keep your appetite stimulated. It's important for a woman to help get herself in the mood," she says. Having some romantic or sexual thoughts during the day can serve as a kind of warm-up for sex later that night, she says.

Coping with ISD

If you have ISD or think you may be developing it, experts have some suggestions.

TAKE TIME TO TOUCH. One way to stay physically close when desire is low is to defocus from intercourse and orgasm and refocus on more generalized touching of the body, says Kessler. No breasts or genitals at first; wait until you are *both* ready before you include those parts. Set aside periods twice a week when you and your partner spend up to half an hour touching each other in affectionate, nonsexual ways. Do this in a room that's warm and relaxed, and perhaps light candles or play a tape to augment the mood. Be sure to talk to each other, too, expressing feelings.

"Use a touch with no sexual expectations or demands in the beginning," she says. "The idea is for each to get comfortable with themselves and their partner's bodies, not immediately turn each other on." The 'turn-on' will follow as you learn how to 'tune in' first, she says.

PUT YOURSELF IN THE MOOD. Try reading romantic novels or short stories that you like that have a romantic story line, says Kessler. Or rent a movie geared toward sensuality. "Find a love story you like that will create the mood," for sex for you, she says.

MAKE TIME FOR SEX. If a woman's desire is low and she's not too interested in sex, she may avoid her partner for fear that if she touches or kisses him, it will be interpreted as an overture for sex, says Kessler. If the couple sets a time when they both agree to have sex, that can take the pressure off. The woman will feel free to kiss or touch her partner affectionately at other times and know it won't have to lead to sex. And "making a date for sex can be a lot of fun," she says.

GET HELP EARLY. If you feel that you're starting to have problems, take care of it sooner rather than later, says Dr. Carroll. "If it goes on a long time, it's likely to get worse," he says. Consult a neutral third party, says Kessler. You might try calling a therapist who specializes in sexual dysfunction and asking if what you're experiencing sounds like something you should be worried about, she says. When you decide on therapy, ideally both partners should be involved, says Kessler.

●

Insomnia

FINDING YOUR WAY
TO DREAMLAND

You toss. You turn. You roll over on your stomach, twist around to your back, slide a half-turn onto your side.

Nothing feels right. Nothing feels relaxed. The sheets are too wrinkled, the blanket's too rumpled, the pillow's too soft, and your body's so wired that you just *know* you're never going to get to sleep tonight.

You're in the grips of insomnia, a problem that haunts women twice as often as it does men. It may keep us awake for a night or two as we struggle with temporary problems at work or at home. Or it may hang around for several weeks as we work our way through a family crisis or begin a corporate transition. In severe cases, it may be a constant companion due to some ongoing problem such as depression or arthritis. At some point in her life, experts say, virtually every woman will experience some degree of insomnia.

But insomnia isn't just a hard time getting to sleep at night. It can also get you up much too early in the morning. And either way, the result is a woman too exhausted to cope with the demands of life.

The Cycle of Sleeplessness

Doctors know that the quality of your slumber—how long you sleep, and how deeply—varies at different points in your menstrual cycle. For some women, insomnia is a regular, recurring problem once a month, just before they menstruate. Insomnia is also the number one complaint of women who experience premenstrual syndrome, doctors say, and a major nuisance for postmenopausal women—although hormone replacement therapy can make it go away.

Because estrogen influences the production of brain chemicals that keep you alert and progesterone makes you sleepy, doctors believe that hormonal fluctuations can cause a transient insomnia, which comes and goes with the ebb and flow of your hormones, says Suzanne Trupin, M.D., head of the Department of Obstetrics and Gynecology at the University of Illinois College of Medicine at Urbana-Champaign and an expert on the effects that hormones have on women's bodies.

But no one's sure of the hows, whens and whys of so-called cyclic insomnia because women have generally been excluded from sleep studies. One reason? Because sleep researchers were worried that women's hormones would distort the studies, says Mary Klink, M.D., medical director of the Sleep Disorders Program at Meriter Hospital in Madison, Wisconsin.

A Plan to Get Some Z-Z-Zs

Because there's little hard data on women and insomnia, doctors had to combine information from the few available studies that included women with their own observations to help their sleepless patients. Here are strategies Dr. Trupin has developed to give women who have hormone-related insomnia a good night's sleep.

KEEP A SLEEP DIARY. The first step is to see what is causing your insomnia, says Dr. Trupin. Keep a notebook beside your bed and jot down what time you went to bed, the number of times you awakened during the night, the number of times you got up, the first and last day of your period, any menstrual symptoms or difficulties, whether you were sleepy the next day and whether you experienced any particularly stressful events.

Keep the diary for three months, then go back over it and try to detect any patterns, says Dr. Trupin.

If you find that you have insomnia on the same day of your menstrual cycle every month, you can be fairly certain that it's caused by fluctuating hormones, says Dr. Trupin. And although you can't usually keep your hormones from zipping up and down, you can fight insomnia by taking the following measures.

PREPARE A MINERAL NIGHTCAP. Your mother was on the right track when she used to suggest that drinking a glass of milk would help you sleep, says Dr. Trupin. She just had the wrong beverage. Although the calcium in milk will help you nod off by slowing nervous system messages, other substances in milk may actually keep you awake.

Instead of a glass of milk, have a glass of water and a couple of Tums or any other 500-milligram tablet form of calcium carbonate, says Dr. Trupin.

KEEP THE MAGNESIUM COMING. Magnesium has a calming effect that helps prevent insomnia, says Dr. Trupin: "It tends to smooth out people who are angry and moody." You can get it throughout the day by eating such magnesium-rich foods as soybeans, almonds, black-eyed peas and lima beans. Or, if you don't have a history of kidney problems, you can take a magnesium supplement. The Daily Value for magnesium is 400 milligrams a day, although Dr. Trupin suggests you take 500 milligrams.

TAKE B$_6$. Since vitamin B$_6$ helps the brain release more serotonin, a chemical messenger that has a calming effect upon the body, adding B$_6$ to your nighttime regimen may help, says Dr. Trupin. But be sure to take it only under your doctor's supervision—too much B$_6$ can cause nerve damage. "Up to 100 milligrams of B$_6$ a day is safe for most people; 1 gram is not safe," she says.

WORK OUT. Everyone who suffers from insomnia should exercise, says Dr. Trupin. Women who do not have physically demanding jobs should exercise vigorously sometime during the day or early evening. The minimum amount of exercise to discourage insomnia? Thirty minutes, three times a week.

Altering Your Chemistry

Here are five natural ways to actually alter your hormonal chemistry to help prevent insomnia and encourage sleep.

CHECK YOUR ESTROGEN LEVELS. As estrogen levels begin to drop somewhere in the midthirties or forties, insomnia can become a problem, says Dr. Trupin.

If you're in that age range and your sleep diary hasn't revealed other possible causes of insomnia, have your doctor check your follicle-stimulating hormone (FSH) levels. They're one of the first indicators to change as your body prepares itself for menopause.

EAT PHYTOESTROGENS. If FSH levels indicate you're premenopausal, then think about adding fruits and vegetables rich in estrogen—called phytoestrogens—to your diet, says Dr. Trupin. Besides curbing your insomnia, these foods—apples, carrots, cherries, green beans, oats, peas, potatoes, soybeans and sprouts—can actually increase your estrogen levels enough to prevent insomnia.

MANAGE STRESS. Although most women are aware that everyday stress can cause insomnia, many don't realize that it does so by causing the release of various chemicals in the body that stimulate alertness, says Dr. Trupin.

Stress-management techniques may be effective for chronic insomnia (for stress-management tips, see page 000).

TRY A NATURAL RELAXER. Women who breastfeed after pregnancy actually modify their hormonal mix to encourage sleepiness, Dr. Trupin says. The effect only lasts until your child graduates to a cup, of course, but it does help alleviate the insomnia that occasionally plagues new mothers.

TREAT UNDERLYING DISEASE. Various diseases that affect the body's endocrine system—heart disease, depression or diabetes, for example—can also trigger production of "fight or flight" chemicals in the body, says Dr. Trupin. The only way to prevent insomnia is to treat the disease.

How to Chase Insomnia Away

Although many of us may experience cyclic insomnia, there's hardly a woman alive who hasn't had difficulty sleeping at one time or another. Here are three simple strategies to prevent it from happening to you.

CREATE A COMFORTABLE ENVIRONMENT. Make your bedroom quiet, cool and dark. Do not use the bedroom for anything but dressing, sleep or sex, suggests Dr. Trupin.

SCHEDULE YOUR SLEEP. Keep yourself on a sleep schedule. Go to bed at the same time every night, wake up at the same time every morning, and do not take naps, recommends Dr. Trupin.

LET THERE BE LIGHT. "Sleep onset time is highly related to light," says Dr. Klink.

The pineal gland produces a hormone called melatonin, which regulates sleep. When melatonin levels go up as it gets dark outside, you get sleepy. When melatonin levels go down as the day dawns, you become more alert.

So how can light prevent insomnia? "If you have trouble falling asleep at night, exposing yourself to light for an hour or so immediately following wake-up time in the morning may reset your biological rhythms," says Dr. Klink. "It may allow you to shift the beginning of your sleep time to earlier in the evening."

These lights are not the ones you have sitting in the living room, however, says Dr. Klink. They're called full-spectrum, high-intensity lights. The special high-intensity bulbs fit into any normal light sockets, and you can get them at most health food stores.

They may be particularly helpful in preventing insomnia among the 22 percent of employed women who work shifts, adds Dr. Klink. Several studies show that exposure to high-intensity lights, which mimic daylight, can shift women's biological rhythms and synchronize them with a work schedule within several days, she says. As a result, people who have to be up late at night, like shift workers, will be less likely to experience insomnia—and to escape the impaired judgment, slowed reflexes and all-around grouchiness that frequently result from it.

The Medical Option

While drugs are never the answer on a long-term basis, they may have a place in treating insomnia in the short term, doctors say. Here's the way doctors suggest you use them.

AVOID OVER-THE-COUNTER SLEEPING PILLS. Although OTC medications may help some people who have insomnia, the risks generally outweigh the benefits, according to a joint study by Tufts University School of Medicine in Boston and the University of New Mexico School of Medicine in Albuquerque. One problem is that the sleeping pills may cause daytime grogginess. And some people who take sleeping pills may experience forgetfulness the next day.

STAY AWAY FROM SLEEP DISRUPTERS. Don't drink caffeine within six hours or alcohol within two hours of bedtime, says Dr. Trupin. Caffeine stimulates alertness chemicals in the brain, and although alcohol might initially make you drowsy, your sleep will be so light that the slightest noise will probably disrupt it.

Irritable Bowel Syndrome

HELP FOR THE SENSITIVE GUT

The report is due on your boss's desk by 10:00 A.M., and already your insides are starting to churn.

The morning's stress has met up with last night's meat loaf and rumba-ed down your intestinal tract. Now, just when mind and body need to focus on your work with total concentration, the unholy alliance between meat loaf and stress is promising explosive results. You jump up from your desk and run for the bathroom, where, just in time, you groan, "Why me?"

Everyone has a bout of diarrhea once in a while, particularly when they're under pressure, says Douglas A. Drossman, M.D., professor of medicine and psychiatry in the Division of Digestive Diseases and Nutrition at the University of North Carolina School of Medicine at Chapel Hill. But days of painful diarrhea frequently alternating with days of painful constipation are something else entirely.

When this bouncing from one intestinal extreme to the other is uncomfortable enough that you consult a doctor, says Dr. Drossman, the diagnosis you're likely to hear is irritable bowel syndrome.

How Women Cope

Irritable bowel is the most common reason women are referred to gastroenterologists. It affects approximately 20 percent of all Americans—60 to 65 percent of them women—although no one has a clue as to its cause. Its symptoms range from an occasional bout of after-dinner cramps to chronic constipation or diarrhea with severe pain. Either constipation or diarrhea can predominate, doctors say, although women are more likely to have constipation.

Seventy percent of those who have the problem have such mild symptoms that they generally can handle it themselves with an over-the-counter drug to control diarrhea or constipation. Twenty-five percent have symptoms so severe that they interfere with their daily activities. And 1 to 5 percent will experience such pain and daily disruption that they'll do little with their lives other than visit doctors.

Why such a wide range of symptoms?

Because how you feel depends on how you cope with the condition, doctors say.

"Let's say two women have the same amount of bowel disturbance causing pain," says Dr. Drossman. "One woman has no current life stress and has good coping skills, and the other is experiencing psychological distress at work and home and has poor coping skills." The first woman talks about her feelings, is assertive and takes responsibility for her health, and the second is passive, doesn't talk about her feelings and expects her doctor to resolve her problems.

Because of the complex connection between brain and gut, the psychological distress can cause the second woman's intestines to react even more, says Dr. Drossman. That means that her intestines may move food through so quickly that she has diarrhea or so slowly that she becomes constipated. Poor coping skills may also lower her pain threshold so that it takes less of anything—stress, food or hormones—to trigger pain than it does in someone who copes well. In a sense, she becomes oversensitive to everything—even a normal stool pressing against the bowel wall.

Preventing Irritable Bowel Symptoms

There is no cure for irritable bowel syndrome. People may find short-term relief by using an over-the-counter drug such as Imodium to stop diarrhea, a laxative to relieve constipation or a prescription antispasmodic to relieve pain, says Dr. Drossman. But relying solely on medication is not enough. He advises women with irritable bowel to learn to prevent the onset of symptoms. Here's how.

LEARN TO RELAX. Stress is a killer for anyone with irritable bowel. It stimulates various neurochemicals in the brain and sends them skittering down the nervous system pipeline to the gut. There they can aggravate the gut's already overreactive tendencies and trigger a bout of misery.

"Our thinking is that stress accounts for 10 to 15 percent of flare-ups," says William E. Whitehead, Ph.D., research professor of medicine at the University of North Carolina School of Medicine in Chapel Hill. He encourages people to learn a relaxation technique to help control it.

"The simplest one for Americans seems to be progressive relaxation," he adds. It involves focusing on each group of muscles from head to toe, then consciously tensing and relaxing each group. He says it's more acceptable to Americans than meditation, a relaxation technique in which you focus your mind on a single thought or word and simply sit.

"Americans like to relax by trying harder," Dr. Whitehead says, chuckling. "And progressive relaxation meets that need."

KNOW WHAT PUSHES YOUR BUTTONS. Progressive relaxation can be particularly effective when you also learn to identify what pushes your stress button and what goes on *inside* the body when it gets stressed, adds Dr. Whitehead.

In a study of 13 women and 6 men with irritable bowel, researchers at the State University of New York at Albany found that 12 one-hour training/education sessions over an eight-week period significantly reduced symptoms.

USE THE SIDE EFFECTS OF ANTIDEPRESSANTS. Antidepressants are sometimes prescribed to alleviate abdominal pain in women with irritable bowel, says Dr. Whitehead.

This is not because people with irritable bowel are depressed but because one of the side effects of antidepressants is that they reduce the amount of a brain chemical known to stimulate contractions in the bowel. "Antidepressants also lower the sensitivity to pain, which is caused by distention of the bowel with gas or food residue," Dr. Whitehead says.

GET UP AND GO. "We also recommend exercise," says Dr. Whitehead, because it can prevent the constipation associated with irritable bowel, probably the most difficult symptom to overcome.

In a study of ten men and women who jogged, Dr. Whitehead and his colleagues found that even a single hour of this intense exercise stimulated the bowel so that it literally doubled the number of contractions it normally generated to push food residue through the intestine.

LIFT WEIGHTS. Strength training three days a week cut the amount of time it took for food to pass through the bowel by about 56 percent, according to a 13-week joint study conducted by Dr. Whitehead and researchers at Johns Hopkins University and the University of Maryland, both in Baltimore.

Study participants warmed up on a stationary bike for three minutes, did stretching exercises for another ten minutes, then performed 15 repetitions on each of a variety of weight machines to exercise upper- and lower-body muscles. Weights were initially set close to each participant's maximum strength, then made progressively lighter to allow them to complete all 15 repetitions.

ADD FIBER. Dietary fiber also fights constipation, says Dr. Whitehead. The best type is insoluble fiber, which helps form a larger, softer stool that is passed easily and quickly. Bran, whole grains and fruits and vegetables are good sources of insoluble fiber. (For a list of high-fiber foods, see page 122.)

The Food Relationship

Although avoiding stress and constipation will help keep a cranky gut calm, food is the one irritable bowel trigger that's impossible to avoid.

Food normally initiates contractions and stimulates a bowel movement 30 to 60 minutes after a full meal, doctors explain. But with the super-sensitivity of an irritable bowel, instead of contractions and a bowel movement, food can lead to cramps and diarrhea. And it does so in about 75 percent of those with irritable bowel.

The key to preventing an irritable bowel from throwing a tantrum after meals is directly related to what you eat and how many calories you consume at once, doctors agree. Here's what to do.

THINK LEAN. Since any form of fat is the strongest food stimulus of intestinal contractions, keep your diet as lean as possible, doctors suggest. Trim fat from meat, switch to low-fat cheeses and avoid fried foods.

THINK SMALL. Large meals have been found to trigger both cramping and diarrhea. So try eating smaller meals, more often.

BLOCK IT WITH MEDICATIONS. If eating lean and small doesn't do the trick, says Dr. Whitehead, ask your doctor to prescribe an antispasmodic drug such as atropine, propantheline (Pro-Banthine) or dicyclomine (Antispas). Taking the drug before you eat will block the nerve signals that trigger bowel spasms.

BE A PICKY EATER. A particular food may irritate some people and not others. So if certain foods or certain ingredients seem to bother you, either decrease the amount you consume or avoid them altogether, doctors say.

Common irritants include dairy products, caffeine, alcohol, the artificial sweetener Sorbitol, beans, spicy foods, concentrated fruit juices and raw fruits or vegetables.

Understand the Problem

Many women have symptoms of irritable bowel syndrome but don't seek health care. Others continually seek a cure that doesn't exist at this time, says Margaret M. Heitkemper, Ph.D., professor of physiological nursing at the University of Washington in Seattle.

This can be particularly frustrating when irritable bowel symptoms are regularly exacerbated by menstruation. "Many women with irritable bowel will very likely have variations in symptom severity based on menstrual cycle phase," says Dr. Heitkemper. For most women, she adds, the symptoms will be worse a day or two before their periods or when they're actually menstruating.

What can you do about it? Here are two things.

ACCEPT YOUR BODY. Just keep the bowel as calm as you can with diet, exercise and stress reduction and try to understand that menstruation is a natural, common occurrence, says Dr. Heitkemper.

AVOID SURGERY. Do not try to push your doctor into unnecessary surgery to find a cure for irritable bowel, cautions Dr. Whitehead. "Our data suggest that at least some women seek out hysterectomy or other surgical procedures" in an attempt to find a cure, he says. "Hysterectomy is *not* a treatment for irritable bowel," he emphasizes. "But if a patient keeps insisting on finding a cause for irritable bowel, the likelihood of a decision being made to do an operation like a hysterectomy—or an appendectomy—is high."

Dr. Whitehead can't explain why. "It isn't rational," he adds. "But if a patient really presses for surgery, she's likely to get it."

Lactose Intolerance

Making Peace
with the Dairy Family

During your twenties you barely gave milk a second thought. But now that you're over 30, you're making a concerted effort to get enough calcium, and milk is a major part of your plan. So are cheese and yogurt—in their low-fat forms, of course. Finally, they're all becoming a regular part of your daily diet.

Only your body doesn't seem too happy about it.

Drink some milk before bedtime and you get a lot of gas. Have a bowl of ice cream and diarrhea sets in. With dairy foods, sometimes you get bloating, other times an upset stomach.

So what's all the gastrointestinal fuss about?

It's related to lactose, a type of sugar found in milk and milk products. Sometimes the body has a hard time digesting it, a condition doctors refer to as lactose intolerance. The problem affects an estimated 50 million Americans and is most prominent in people of African American, Asian and Indian descent. Researchers don't know how many women are affected.

Milk-Induced Mayhem

Lactose intolerance develops when your body makes insufficient amounts of lactase, the digestive enzyme responsible for breaking down milk sugar into a form the body can easily absorb. Without lactase, the milk sugar remains in the digestive tract, where it attracts water, causing bloating and diarrhea. And when the enzyme is lacking or absent, bacteria in the intestines try to pick up the slack and go to work on the milk sugar in an effort to digest it. Their activity produces gas, and flatulence and cramping result.

Some women are born with lactose intolerance and have to stick to a lactose-free diet for their entire lives. Others develop a temporary form of the condition that appears during gastroenteritis, an inflammation of the stomach and intestines caused by infection or food poisoning, or after surgery. This type generally lasts for several weeks.

And some women develop lactose intolerance as adults, says Daryl Altman, M.D., an allergist and immunologist and director of Allergy Information Services, an allergy consulting service in Lynbrook, New York. Women who have consumed milk for years may develop the problem in their twenties, thirties, forties or fifties. "It's really just part of the aging process," she says. "The enzymes that we used to have in our gut, the lactase enzyme that breaks down milk sugar, just gradually decreases."

How a woman feels when she has lactose intolerance varies from person to person, says Chesley Hines, M.D., a staff physician at the Center for Digestive Diseases at Southern Baptist Hospital and clinical associate professor of medicine at Louisiana State University Medical School, both in New Orleans. Some women lack quite a bit of the enzyme, so very little lactose gets broken down and their symptoms are more severe. Others have a little bit more lactase, so some lactose is digested and their symptoms are milder.

How you feel also depends on how much milk sugar you ingest: While a little might be okay, larger quantities may cause problems, says Dr. Hines.

There are other sources of lactose aside from milk and dairy products. Some medications contain lactose as filler, says Dr. Altman. And it is an ingredient in some other foods, namely breads and salad dressings.

But What about Calcium?

Women don't necessarily have lactose intolerance more than men do. And their symptoms aren't really any different, either. Yet lactose intolerance can pose some special challenges for them.

A particular concern for women is maintaining bone strength. One out of every four women develops osteoporosis, a disease in which the strength of the bone, particularly in the wrists and hips, declines. And each year, an estimated 1.5 million Americans suffer osteoporosis-related fractures.

Milk and milk products are often a primary source of calcium and a major weapon, along with exercise, in the war against osteoporosis. So if you have trouble with milk products, getting the right amount of calcium can become more complicated.

But there are ways you can do it.

That's because the good news about lactose intolerance is that there's a pretty easy, straightforward solution: Replace the enzyme that's missing from the gut. You can do this by drinking Lactaid, a milk product that contains lactase. Or you can replace the lactase your body lacks by taking lactase caplets or adding lactase drops to milk.

Yogurt with live and active cultures—bacteria, that is—can also be substituted for milk. While yogurt does contain lactose, actually more per gram than whole milk does, the bacteria in yogurt release the lactase necessary to break down milk sugar.

You can also turn to nondairy sources of calcium, such as broccoli, kidney beans, tofu with calcium salts and dark green leafy vegetables such as kale, says Rosemarie Bria, Ph.D., director of nutrition at Allerex, a Greenwich, Connecticut, company that advises food companies about adverse reactions to food. Calcium is also found in sesame seeds, sardines, nuts and dried figs, she says.

Finally, an easy way to get calcium is to take calcium carbonate, such as Tums or Mylanta, says Dr. Altman. While ideally food sources are best, it can be difficult to get the recommended 1,000 milligrams or more of calcium that way, so taking calcium carbonate is a quick and simple way to make sure women get the calcium they need, she says.

Pregnant women and nursing moms who have lactose intolerance need to be extra careful about getting adequate calcium, says Dr. Altman. "In order for your body to make milk, it needs calcium," she says.

If it can't find it in the bloodstream, it will draw it from your bones, she says. Women can take calcium carbonate or go for calcium supplements. But avoid dolomite-derived calcium substitutes, Dr. Altman says, since they may contain lead.

Know the Difference

Sometimes lactose intolerance is confused with milk allergy, and it's important to distinguish between the two, experts say. While lactose intolerance is a digestive problem, milk allergy, the number one food allergy, involves a change in the immune system. If you're lactose-intolerant, you'll have discomfort, but it's not life-threatening, and you can solve the problem by ingesting lactase. But with milk allergy, it's possible to have a severe, life-threatening reaction called anaphylaxis, in which the throat swells, breathing is blocked, blood pressure drops and the body goes into shock.

Milk allergy may go away, but you have to avoid milk as long as you have it. And if you do stay off milk as long as you have the allergy, it's likely to go away faster.

Regain the Calm

Lactose intolerance can cause a lot of misery for the people who have it, says Dr. Hines. But it is a manageable condition. Here's what you can do for relief.

TEST YOURSELF. If your symptoms are limited to gastrointestinal problems, there's a simple test you can give yourself to see if you're lactose-intolerant. Try eliminating milk and dairy products from your diet for one week, says Dr. Hines. If your symptoms go away or decline, it may be lactose intolerance. Try slowly reintroducing dairy products into your diet and see if your symptoms return.

SEE YOUR DOCTOR. The best way to know for sure whether your discomfort is from lactose intolerance is to see your doctor. She can perform tests, including a lactose intolerance test and a breath hydrogen test. The lactose intolerance test is a blood test that measures your glucose level after a lactose challenge. Doctors often use other tests after this one because it has a low rate of accuracy. The breath hydrogen test measures the amount of hydrogen you expel after ingesting lactose. Hydrogen is produced by the bacteria that try to break down lactose when lactase is missing, so the higher your rate of hydrogen, the more severe your condition.

DRINK LACTAID. Once your doctor has diagnosed lactose intolerance, you can replace the milk you usually drink with Lactaid, milk that's been fortified with lactase. It's available in most supermarkets in the dairy case.

GO FOR YOGURT. Yogurt with live and active cultures is generally okay for those with lactose intolerance, says Dr. Altman. Check the label; it should specify "live and active cultures."

POP SOME DROPS OR PILLS. You can also replace missing lactase with enzymes that come in drop, caplet or capsule form. Supermarkets and drugstores carry a variety of brands. You can add the drops to dairy products 24 hours before you plan to consume them. The foods may be slightly sweeter than normal, but the lactose content will be reduced by nearly 100 percent. You can also take lactase as a caplet or capsule before or within 30 minutes of consuming milk products. Generally, two caplets are recommended to tackle the lactose in an eight-ounce glass of whole milk, but follow directions on the label.

READ FOOD LABELS. If you've got lactose intolerance and it's on the severe side, check the labels of the food and medicine products you use. Some medicines, as well as some breads, cereals and salad dressings, contain lactose, says Dr. Altman.

GET YOUR CALCIUM. If you cut back on dairy products, be sure to turn to other sources for calcium. The National Institutes of Health recommend that premenopausal women get at least 1,000 milligrams of calcium a day, though many doctors recommend increasing that to 1,200 milligrams. Menopausal and postmenopausal women need more—about 1,500 milligrams.

In addition to Lactaid, you can get calcium from a number of possible food sources, says Dr. Bria. Tofu made with calcium salts has about 154 milligrams in four ounces, a cup of broccoli has about 178 milligrams, a half-cup of kidney beans contains about 110 milligrams, and a cup of collard greens has about 350 milligrams, she says. You can also take calcium supplements.

Laryngitis

BREAKING THE SILENCE

There are 20 people gathered around the conference table. Each is looking at you expectantly. Each is waiting for the words of wisdom that will bring new insight to their work and maybe their lives.

You're humbled by all this attention. You stand, arrange the papers in front of you, clear your throat and open your mouth to speak.

And . . . nothing comes out. Nothing except a hoarse whisper that can't be heard past the woman sitting directly to your left.

This is not a nightmare—at least not the kind you have when you're asleep. It's the kind you get when you have laryngitis, that peculiar hoarseness and altered pitch that can make you sound like a cross between Lauren Bacall and Flipper. Sometimes your words come out in a low, breathy contralto, sometimes they come out with a high-pitched squeak. Sometimes they simply don't come out.

In any case, hormonal changes, bulimia, viruses, allergies, smoke-filled rooms and alcohol are frequent causes of laryngitis in women, says Michael Benninger, M.D., chief of otolaryngology at Henry Ford Hospital in Detroit. They trigger the inflammation, irritation or swelling in and around the vocal cords that physically alter the normal voice.

What's more, overuse, misuse or frank abuse can also cause laryngitis, says Dr. Benninger. Lecturing for a couple of hours when you're not used to it, carrying on a loud conversation on the subway or screaming for the home team at your annual alumni football game are all likely to send you into a day or so of silence.

The Hormone Connection

Most women experience some changes in their vocal cords a day or two before menstruation. In most cases the changes will be minor—a slightly lower pitch or a momentary hoarseness that generally goes unnoticed—but in others the change will be so significant that they may have difficulty carrying on prolonged conversations. They may even develop mild laryngitis.

"Just as there are certain women who have terrible premenstrual syndromes and others who have mild syndromes, we expect that same variation to occur," says Dr. Benninger. Other common premenstrual symptoms like bloating, cramping and headaches can also contribute to vocal changes.

How do hormones actually affect the vocal cords? Changing levels of estrogen and progesterone can cause body tissues to swell with fluid, says Dr. Benninger. The cords become heavier than normal, and your voice can sound low and hoarse. The hormonal changes at menopause have a similar effect.

For most of us these changes are not a problem. But for any woman for whom the nuances of voice are an important part of how she makes a living, here are Dr. Benninger's suggestions for dealing with premenstrual voice changes.

UNDERSTAND THAT IT'S NATURAL. "Number one is be aware that it's a normal process," he says. "It can be a normal component of the natural menstrual cycle. Don't worry about it—you don't have cancer and you're not going to have a permanent change in your voice—particularly not if the laryngitis happens at the same time every month and then goes away."

SEE A SPEECH PATHOLOGIST. "If voice changes or laryngitis affect your livelihood, voice therapy may be helpful," says Dr.

Benninger. "Voice therapy is actually teaching you to use your voice in a way that helps you overcome the deficiencies that are occurring." A speech/language pathologist may help you offset some of the vocal problems caused by hormonal changes by teaching you certain posture or breathing techniques.

CHANGE YOUR REPERTOIRE. "If you're a speaker, you may want to do less—schedule fewer appointments around that time and do more paperwork instead," says Dr. Benninger. If you're a singer, you may not want to try to reach high "C"—you may want to change your repertoire a little so that you only reach high "A."

At the turn of the century, there were a substantial number of European opera houses that excused women from singing just before their periods. It was part of their contract. And there's some speculation that some of the most famous opera singers of all time—Maria Callas and Joan Sutherland—had premenstrual changes in their voices and therefore chose not to perform just before their periods.

CONSIDER HORMONE THERAPY. "In women who have really severe problems, hormone therapy may be necessary," says Dr. Benninger. If laryngitis is really sabotaging your life and your career every month, discuss the idea of taking hormones with your gynecologist.

When the Problem Isn't Hormonal

If you are prone to laryngitis as a result of overusing your vocal cords, here's what you can do to prevent it.

STAY AWAY FROM SMOKE. "Smoking has a direct effect on the vocal cords," says Dr. Benninger. Don't smoke yourself and don't hang out in places where others will blow smoke in your face.

STAY AWAY FROM ALCOHOL. "Alcohol has an indirect effect on the vocal cords," says Dr. Benninger. "It's a diuretic, so it dries the mucous membrane." In addition, alcohol loosens people up, often leading them to talk more loudly and for a longer period of time. The vocal cords then become irritated, with voice changes and laryngitis a natural result.

MOISTEN YOUR THROAT. Rev up the humidifier when you turn on the heat every winter, says Dr. Benninger. That can make a big difference in whether you get laryngitis.

KEEP YOUR MOUTH SHUT. Avoid talking, yelling or even whispering when you have laryngitis, says Dr. Benninger. It will only irritate your throat further.

Lung Cancer

A WOMAN'S RISK IS RISING

If you still smoke, here's your best reason to stop: The American Cancer Society (ACS) estimates that 59,000 American women were killed by lung cancer in 1994, representing a whopping 500 percent increase in deaths from this disease among women over the past 30 years. That's four times the increase experienced by men. And it's not expected to peak until well into the next century.

The reason?

"Lung cancer in women is mostly caused by smoking," says researcher Ellen R. Gritz, Ph.D., chairman of the Department of Behavioral Sciences at the University of Texas M. D. Anderson Cancer Center in Houston and former director of the Division of Cancer Control at the Jonsson Comprehensive Cancer Center at the University of California at Los Angeles.

"There are other factors such as radon and occupational ex-posures," she adds. "But they pale in magnitude compared to deaths attributed to smoking."

"You've Come a Long Way, Baby!"

The facts of smoking bear evidence: As the rate of smoking rises in women, so do the rates of lung cancer. In 1935, about 18 percent of all American women were smokers, and by 1965 the percentage rose to a peak of 33 percent, says Dr. Gritz. About 1977, the proportion of women smokers began to decline until, by 1992, less than 25 percent of American women were smokers.

The number of deaths due to lung cancer also increased—approximately 20 to 40 years after the increase in smoking. Now that smoking rates have dropped among women, lung cancer rates will eventually begin to drop as well, says researcher Linda Sarna, D.N.Sc., professor of oncology nursing at the University of California at Los Angeles. But the decline won't begin until about 2020 because of the time lag between when a woman starts to smoke and when she develops cancer.

In addition to not smoking, you need to avoid other people's smoke. Several thousand U.S. nonsmokers develop lung cancer annually because smoking friends, lovers, spouses, co-workers and even complete strangers give it to them.

A study of 1,800 nonsmoking women from five urban areas across the United States indicates that nonsmoking women increase their lung cancer risk by 24 percent when they live with a smoker. Their risk is increased 39 percent when they work with people who smoke and an astounding 50 percent when they hang out with smokers in social settings such as bars and restaurants.

"The findings indicate that there is an increased risk in each setting," says Elizabeth Fontham, Dr.Ph., the Louisiana State University researcher who led the study.

The March of Cancer

Once tobacco smoke or some other carcinogen has damaged the DNA in lung cells or activated oncogenes that trigger growth of a tumor, most lung cancer evolves into one of two forms, either small-cell cancer, which is treated primarily with chemotherapy, or non-small-cell cancer, which is generally treated with surgery and radiation.

Women seem more likely to develop adenocarcinoma, a type of non-small-cell cancer, says Robert Ginsberg, M.D., head of thoracic surgery at Memorial Sloan-Kettering Cancer Center in New York City. No one knows why. But because there are rarely symptoms of cough, bloody sputum or chest pain until the disease's later stages, 60 percent of those who have any type of lung cancer don't get to a doctor until the disease has advanced too far to be cured by treatment. As a result, most people with lung cancer die within a year of diagnosis.

A study at the University of Texas at Houston indicates, however, that shrinking even an advanced tumor with chemotherapy before and after surgery will increase average survival time from one to five years. But the best way to make sure you won't die of the disease is to prevent it, says Dr. Sarna. Here's what experts suggest.

STAY SMOKE-FREE. Any woman who smokes should quit, experts agree.

That's easier said than done, of course. Statistics show that most people average around seven tries before they actually quit forever. So don't be discouraged if you've tried and failed. (For tips on the best ways to stop, see page 492.)

AVOID EXPOSURE. You may not smoke yourself, but you can be in a whole lot of danger from those around you who do, says Dr. Sarna. Ask friends and significant others not to smoke in your presence, she suggests. Avoid restaurants that don't have—or don't enforce—smoke-free areas. And find out what local and state laws govern smoking in your workplace.

GORGE ON VEGGIES AND FRUIT. A study of approximately 3,000 women at the University of Minnesota in Minneapolis found that women who ate 31 or more servings a week of vegetables had a 50 percent lower risk of lung cancer, while women who ate 18 or more servings of fruit each week had a 25 percent lower risk.

"The most striking finding was that the more vegetables women ate, the less likely they were to get lung cancer," says nutritional epidemiologist Kristi Steinmetz, Ph.D., the researcher who led the study.

That's why you should integrate as many fruits and vegetables as possible into your diet, she adds, a suggestion that Demetrius Albanes, M.D., a researcher at the National Cancer Institute in Bethesda, Maryland, supports.

EAT INTERNATIONALLY. One way to increase the fruits and vegetables in your diet may be to move away from the All-American, hamburger-and-french-fry diet toward a more international cuisine, suggests Dr. Steinmetz.

Other cultures tend to use more vegetables more often and in frequently innovative ways. Try vegetarian tacos or ratatouille as a start, then experiment as you find time.

You might want to schedule an occasional vegetarian meal, says Dr. Steinmetz. And whenever you serve a nonvegetarian meal, double your veggies and cut back on the meat on your plate.

DITCH THE BURGERS AND CHEESE. At least one study suggests that there may be a link between saturated fat and lung cancer. In a study of 1,400 nonsmoking women in Missouri, researchers at the National Cancer Institute found that the women who ate the most saturated fat—more than 15 percent of their total calories—had a sixfold increase in the risk of lung cancer. What's more, women who ate the most saturated fat were 11 times more likely to develop adenocarcinomas—the most common type of lung cancer among women.

Among the foods that can contribute a lot of saturated fat are hamburgers, cheeseburgers and meat loaf, followed by cheese, cheese spreads, hot dogs, ice cream and sausage. According to Michael Alavanja, Ph.D., the researcher who led the Missouri study, decreasing your fat intake to less than 30 percent of total calories and saturated fat to less than 10 to 12 percent of total calories can reduce your risk of cancer and heart disease.

INCREASE VENTILATION. If you live in a house that has high levels of radon, you could be putting yourself at increased risk for lung cancer. A radioactive gas emitted as the earth's rock formations age and decay, radon is prevalent in various areas throughout the United States. A study of more than 4,000 men and women at the Karolinska Institute in Stockholm found that lung cancer nearly doubled in those who lived in homes with elevated levels of radon emissions for 32.5 years.

Have your home tested for radon, recommends Clark Heath, M.D., vice-president for epidemiology of the ACS. Current government guidelines suggest that you increase ventilation in your home through special ventilating systems whenever your house air exceeds specific emission levels. You can call 1-800-SOS-RADON to find out where to get test kits and brochures on how to reduce radon in your home.

Lupus

WHEN THE IMMUNE SYSTEM GOES AWRY

You wouldn't know that Mary Pat Whiteley has a chronic disease. In her early thirties, she works full-time photographing crime scenes and collecting evidence for the police department in Baltimore.

But Whiteley has lupus, a disease in which the immune system doesn't function the way it should. It makes her tired a lot, and it makes pregnancy a high risk. She had four miscarriages before her doctors were able to get the lupus under control. She adopted a child, then delivered a baby under the careful guidance of her doctor, and now she's expecting another. To help decrease the risk, she took early maternity leave.

She has the most common form of lupus, called systemic lupus erythematosus; 90 percent of those who have it are women of child-bearing age. While the total number who have lupus is unknown,

343

researchers estimate that the disease strikes 1 in 400 Caucasian women and 1 in 250 African American women.

An Attack from Within

With lupus, there's a glitch in the immune system. Instead of performing its normal duty of fighting off infections, the immune system demolishes normal tissue, says Michelle Petri, M.D., associate professor of medicine and co-director of the Lupus Pregnancy Center at Johns Hopkins University in Baltimore. It does this by producing more antibodies than normal and by producing antibodies that are excessively destructive. The skin, joints, kidneys, lungs and nervous system can be affected. Some patients have a limited form of lupus called discoid lupus, which involves only the skin.

A butterfly rash on the face, extending from one cheek over the bridge of the nose to the other cheek, which many consider to be a classic sign of lupus, actually appears in only about 50 percent of patients.

Common symptoms include fatigue, arthritis pain, fever, hair loss, muscle weakness and tenderness. Women with lupus are also prone to Raynaud's disease, a circulatory ailment that affects the hands and feet, and are often sensitive to light. Some can develop life-threatening complications such as kidney disease and problems with their lungs and heart.

How Do You Know It's Lupus?

Diagnosis is based on having 4 of 11 symptoms established by the American College of Rheumatology. One of these is a positive blood test for a group of antibodies called antinuclear antibodies (ANA). Other signs may include arthritis, the butterfly rash, mouth sores, seizures or psychosis, pleuritis (inflammation of the lining of the lungs), pericarditis (inflammation of the lining of the heart) or skin lesions.

Women who test negative for ANA may have a condition in which subtle signs of lupus are present. Usually this condition doesn't develop into lupus, but women should still seek medical advice.

A woman may test positive for ANA but have no symptoms, says Philip Mease, M.D., clinical associate professor of rheumatology at the University of Washington School of Medicine in Seattle. These women often ask whether they will eventually develop full-blown lupus, but that's hard for doctors to predict, says Dr. Mease.

In a few cases the disease can be fatal, says Dr. Petri, but most women with lupus can have a normal life expectancy. And the chances of living a full life are greater now than ever, she says.

Dr. Petri says good medical care and following the doctor's advice should help anyone with lupus "do quite well." Women with lupus can lead full lives, says Dr. Petri. Marriage, children and career are more than possible, she says.

A Complex Puzzle

Researchers don't know what causes lupus, but they have identified several factors that may predispose women to it or trigger its onset.

Genetics is first on the list. There appear to be at least four genes involved in lupus, says Peter H. Schur, M.D., professor of medicine at Harvard Medical School. The probability of inheriting the disease is fairly low. There's about a 5 percent chance that if a parent or sibling has lupus, you'll develop it, too, says Dr. Schur. (Some researchers believe the chances of inheriting lupus may be as low as 2 percent.) But women can get lupus even when it doesn't run in the family.

If a woman does carry lupus, a wide variety of factors may spur a flare-up of symptoms. Among the possible culprits are certain medications like sulfa drugs and penicillin, viral infections, exposure to the sun and possibly even stressful events, says Dr. Schur.

Because lupus occurs more often in women than in men during the years that women menstruate, researchers suspect that female hormones play a role—though they don't know what that role might be. Ten women for every one man get lupus during their childbearing years. Before and after that time, the rate of diagnosis is equal for both genders.

Further support for the role of hormones comes from laboratory studies. The introduction of male hormones in mice has been shown to suppress development of the disease, whereas female hormones accelerate it. Studies have also determined that lupus symptoms get worse during the hormonal fluctuations of pregnancy and the postpartum period.

And, through questionnaires answered by 104 women who had lupus, Dr. Petri found that two symptoms—joint pain and the facial rash—were worse in the two weeks prior to menstruation, when hormone levels change.

A Strategy for Pregnancy

Pregnancy can be tricky for women with lupus. Besides the possibility of a worsening of symptoms, they're at risk for complications of pregnancy. About 15 percent of these pregnancies end in miscarriage, and women with lupus are three times more likely to deliver prematurely than women who do not have it.

Pregnancy risk varies from woman to woman, however. Those who have certain types of antibodies that interfere with the circulation of blood to the placenta and fetus are said by experts to be at greater risk for miscarriage in midpregnancy. It's best to get pregnant when the disease has been inactive for at least three to six months, researchers say.

Living with Lupus

Lupus has no cure and can't be prevented. But it can be managed with medication, and there are ways to keep your symptoms under control. Here are some suggestions.

SEE A SPECIALIST. Lupus is a complex disease that's best managed by a specialist. A rheumatologist or internist with a specialization in lupus should coordinate your care, says Dr. Schur.

Once you're in the care of a specialist, you're likely to be put on a program that includes medication and careful observation. Different women require different medications, says Dr. Schur. Most are treated with nonsteroidal anti-inflammatory drugs, antimalarial drugs, corticosteroids or drugs that suppress the immune system. Lupus can be monitored through kidney function tests, x-rays, MRIs, ultrasound and EKGs. Specialists can also observe lupus through exercise tolerance tests.

GET A SECOND OPINION. If you have any doubts about your diagnosis or treatment, get a second opinion, says Dr. Schur. And if the two opinions conflict, get a third, he says.

JOIN A SUPPORT GROUP. Some women find such groups helpful, says Dr. Petri. The Lupus Foundation of America and the American Lupus Society have groups all over the country, she says. If a group is not your style, the Lupus Foundation can also put you in contact with another woman with lupus whom you can call to talk with about your disease. Sometimes doctors can put you in touch with other lupus patients, too, says Dr. Mease, so don't be afraid to ask.

DON'T FEEL GUILTY. Some people feel they did something wrong that led to the disease, says Dr. Petri. "Because we don't know what causes it, you don't have to feel guilty about it," she says.

CONSIDER A COURSE. A series of self-help courses has been designed and tested by Carrie Jo Braden, Ph.D., professor of nursing at the University of Arizona School of Nursing in Tucson. They help women gain coping skills, improve communication, boost self-esteem and deal with depression that can accompany chronic disease. Contact your local chapter of the Arthritis Foundation for information.

TAKE IT EASIER. Lupus causes fatigue, so it's important

for women to get the rest they need, experts say. If you work full-time, explore options for flex-time. Ask family members or friends to run errands, help clean the house, take care of the yard and help with the shopping and other chores— or hire outside help if you can afford it.

GO WALKING. "We are very big believers in exercise, even though lupus is a disease that causes fatigue," says Dr. Petri. If you can keep up with a walking program, she says, you may be less fatigued. Or pick another activity that you like that has some aerobic benefit, adds Dr. Schur. Try to do some activity every day, for as long as you can.

PROTECT YOURSELF. Exposure to sunlight can trigger a lupus flare-up, so be careful not to get too much. Women don't have to avoid outdoor activity altogether, says Dr. Petri, but they do need to wear sunscreen with a sun protection factor (SPF) of 15 and a brimmed hat. Be especially careful around sand and water, because they reflect sun.

DEVELOP AN EMERGENCY PLAN. Having a plan for what should happen if you go into the hospital with a flare-up can help make things a little less stressful, says Dr. Braden. Write out a list of who has keys to the house, who can take care of the kids and who will feed the pets, she says. Update the plan every six months.

THINK OF ALTERNATIVES. Unexpected lupus flare-ups can require you to change plans—from simple things like maintaining your work schedule to something more unusual like going camping— at the last minute. It helps to practice coming up with different options so when a flare-up occurs, making plans is easier, says Dr. Braden. Practice brainstorming, either alone or with others, she says.

REVIEW YOUR CONTRACEPTIVE CHOICE. Talk to your doctor before you choose a contraceptive. Women with lupus used to be advised against using oral contraceptives for fear that the Pill's high estrogen content would stimulate the disease. Some newer products, however, contain less estrogen and may be considered if you choose not to use barrier contraception. However, women with lupus and at risk for blood clots should not take estrogen-containing oral contraceptives, says Dr. Petri. Other hormonal options for women with positive ANA tests are Norplant and Depo-Provera, two contraceptives that contain progesterone but no estrogen, she adds.

CONSIDER HRT AFTER MENOPAUSE. Some medications for lupus, particularly prednisone, increase a woman's risk for osteoporosis and heart disease, experts say. Talk to your doctor about hormone replacement therapy (HRT), which can lower your risk for both of these diseases, says Dr. Petri.

Menopausal Changes
SIGNS OF A NEW BEGINNING

You protect your skin by staying out of the sun, control your cholesterol by sticking to a low-fat diet and keep your bones strong by exercising regularly and getting enough calcium.

But among the physical changes life can bring, there's one you can't prevent. And that's menopause.

Okay, so you don't want to hear about it. You don't even want to think about it. You figure you're too young for menopause. And besides, you've heard about its discomforts—hot flashes, mood swings and vaginal dryness, to name a few.

But menopause doesn't have to be terrible. In fact, when women share their experiences they often find that some of the myths about it just don't hold water. They find that it doesn't have to be the beginning of old age. Instead, it can mark the start of a new phase in life, one that is vital, productive and fulfilling.

What May Happen

An estimated 40 to 50 million women—more than ever before—will enter menopause in the next two decades. Most American women hit menopause around age 51. Some women go through it earlier, and an estimated 1 percent do so before age 40.

Menopause begins after a woman's last period. A woman is considered to be in menopause after she hasn't menstruated for a full year. But before that happens, women go through a phase known as the climacteric, or perimenopause. At this time, the ovaries get smaller and produce less estrogen. This drop is what causes the hot flashes, night sweats, vaginal dryness, skin changes, sleep difficulties, mood swings, depression and weight gain experienced by some women. The drop in estrogen often alters a woman's period, which may become heavier or lighter, longer or shorter or irregular. And symptoms of premenstrual syndrome (PMS) can worsen.

It's often difficult for women to tell whether menopause has started because the onset of physical changes can be gradual. Doctors can do a follicle-stimulating hormone (FSH) test to see if menopause has started. This test measures the amount of FSH a woman is producing; at menopause the amount increases because more FSH is necessary to stimulate the ovaries to release an egg. An FSH level of about 40 indicates that you may be in menopause.

Menopause can bring physical and emotional changes, which may be both uncomfortable and troublesome. Because of hormonal shifts, women sometimes can feel out of control. "It can be a real up-and-down time," says Joan Borton, a licensed mental health counselor in Rockport, Massachusetts, who runs workshops for menopausal women and is the author of *Drawing from the Women's Well: Reflections on the Life Passage of Menopause*. "That is very disconcerting for women, particularly those who have been able to feel like they are on top of things."

But the changes women fear do not always occur, experts say. Studies indicate that between 16 and 38 percent of menopausal women are symptom-free—no hot flashes, no dryness, no nothing.

And even if women do have symptoms, they don't happen overnight, and they don't turn women into wrinkled old ladies. On the contrary, women often feel sexy, productive, bright and relieved that they no longer need to worry about getting pregnant, says Ellen Klutznick, Psy.D., a psychotherapist in San Francisco who counsels menopausal women.

At this time, some women truly branch out. "A lot of women are starting new businesses or new careers," says Dr. Klutznick. During menopause many women evaluate what they have done, what they are doing and where they are going, says Borton. "There is a sense of excitement among many women at this time, as well as a real sense of urgency," she says. Women commonly tell her, "For this last third of my life I really want to be giving my energy to things that are real core concerns to me. I am not going to give my energy to peripheral stuff anymore," she says.

How the Body Responds

But even if a woman approaches menopause with positive feelings, there are changes going on inside her body that put her at risk for certain diseases.

When estrogen drops, for instance, a woman's risk of heart disease increases: Before age 65, one in nine women develops heart disease, compared to one in three after age 65. Estrogen exerts a protective effect on the heart by keeping levels of "good" cholesterol, or HDL, high, and levels of "bad" cholesterol, or LDL, low.

Declining levels of estrogen also place women at increased risk for osteoporosis and the debilitating fractures that can result from it. This is because estrogen plays a key role in stimulating bone growth and promoting the absorption of calcium. When estrogen levels drop, these effects do, too. After menopause, between 25 and 44 percent of women experience hip fractures due to osteoporosis. And women are nearly twice as likely to fracture their hips as men when they reach their nineties.

Hormone Replacement: Yes or No?

These disease risks and the physical changes that some women go through are why some women consider hormone replacement therapy (HRT)—formulations designed to replenish a woman's diminishing hormones.

While there are different types of HRT, most doctors recommend ones that include estrogen and a synthetic form of progesterone called progestin. Estrogen is used for its beneficial effect on the heart and bones, among other things. But when given alone, estrogen can stimulate cancer growth in the uterus and breast. Progestin cuts that risk.

Whether to take HRT is one of the biggest questions women confront about menopause, says Borton. It is a difficult personal decision, she says, because there are pros and cons.

Among the benefits of HRT is relief from hot flashes and vaginal dryness—the two symptoms that drive most women to ask about the therapy, says Brian Walsh, M.D., director of the Menopause Clinic at Brigham and Women's Hospital in Boston.

Between 75 and 85 percent of menopausal women who have symptoms get hot flashes. Of those who do, 80 percent have them for more than a year, while 25 to 50 percent have them for more than five years. Frequency and intensity vary, Dr. Walsh says. For some women they can be mild and last a couple of minutes, while for others they can be more intense, cause flushing and sweating and last as long as 12 minutes. When hot flashes come at night—what's commonly called night sweats—they can disrupt sleep, leaving women exhausted and irritable the next day.

Without estrogen, the vagina can become dry and less elastic. HRT replenishes estrogen, so moisture is restored.

Regarding the Risks

From a health standpoint, a big plus for HRT is the protection from heart disease it provides, experts say. In studies of women who took just estrogen, doctors found that it appeared to lower women's risk of heart disease by 50 percent compared to women who didn't take it. Thorough studies on HRT—which provides both estrogen and progestin—have yet to be done, but initial research shows that HRT may also offer substantial protection against heart disease.

Hormone replacement therapy can also prevent women from developing osteoporosis. Research suggests that women who take HRT reduce their risk of osteoporosis-related fractures by 50 percent.

And women who have the disease may be able to increase their bone density by 5 percent through HRT.

But HRT is not without its risks, cautions Dr. Walsh. The greatest concern is whether taking HRT will increase the risk of uterine or breast cancer.

Of postmenopausal women not taking HRT, 1 in 1,000 will develop uterine cancer, according to studies. For women who take estrogen alone, that risk increases between two and ten times, depending on how much estrogen is in the formulation they take and how long they take it.

Studies indicate, however, that when progestin is taken with estrogen, the risk of uterine cancer is lower than when estrogen is taken by itself. In a ten-year study of 398 women taking both hormones, none of the women who took progestin for at least 10 days out of 25 developed uterine cancer. Whether women who take HRT are at lower risk for uterine cancer than women who don't take any hormones has not been conclusively proven, but based on preliminary studies, doctors suspect that the risk may be lower by an estimated 30 to 40 percent.

If a woman decides to take only estrogen, she can be monitored for uterine cancer by her doctor.

Breast cancer is a concern for women on HRT. Estrogen promotes cancer growth in lab animals, so there's reason to suspect that giving women estrogen might stimulate breast cancer. While research on breast cancer risk from HRT has yielded no definite conclusion, a study con-

THE DIFFERENT FACES OF HRT

If you decide to go on hormone replacement therapy, there are some things you need to know, says Brian Walsh, M.D., director of the Menopause Clinic at Brigham and Women's Hospital in Boston.

First of all, not all HRT prescriptions are the same. There are different timetables for taking the formulations, which can come as a cream, patch or pill.

One type of HRT is what doctors call sequential therapy. Estrogen is taken every day for two weeks. Then, on the 15th day, progestin is taken as well. Both estrogen and progestin are continued from day 15 through day 25, and then both are withdrawn. It's at this time that menstruation-like bleeding begins. The dose of each hormone used varies from physician to physician, but the standard dose is 0.625 milligrams of estrogen (Premarin) and 10 milligrams of progestin (Provera).

Another method is continuous combined therapy. Just as implied by the name, both estrogen and progestin are taken every day. This method was developed as a means to eliminate the bleeding that occurs with sequential therapy, and it's currently the most common regimen used. Initially, women on continuous therapy do experience irregular bleeding. In time, the bleeding will cease, but that can take up to six months. This therapy usually involves 0.625 milligrams of estrogen (Premarin) and 2.5 milligrams of progestin (Provera).

ducted at the Centers for Disease Control and Prevention in Atlanta determined that a woman's risk may be relative to how long she's on the therapy. Women in the study who took hormones the longest—for more than 15 years—had the greatest risk, and it was 30 percent higher than for women who did not take HRT or took it for less than 5 years.

Women who take HRT are also at risk for gallstones, particularly during the first year of therapy, says Dr. Walsh.

If you've had cancer of the breast or uterus, have active liver disease or have had major problems with blood clots, HRT is not usually recommended.

Estrogen creams are often used by women who are having trouble with vaginal dryness. The cream is inserted with an applicator directly into the vagina, where it works to replenish vaginal tissue. Two types of estrogen cream are Dienestrol and Premarin. In the beginning, vaginal estrogen cream is used three to four times a week, until vaginal symptoms improve. Then it's used less frequently.

Estrogen patches are often the choice of women who want to take HRT but can't take estrogen orally because of gallbladder disease. The patch, called Estraderm, is the size of a small bandage and is worn on the lower abdomen. The estrogen is absorbed through the skin and then released directly into the bloodstream in timed sequences.

Estrogen pills are taken by mouth, according to the regimen set by your doctor. Premarin, the most commonly used pill, is a natural form of estrogen—mare's estrogen—whereas some other estrogen pills are synthetic.

How effective HRT is in fighting heart disease depends on which type of estrogen you use, according to Dr. Walsh. Estrogen creams and the patch are not as effective as pills. With the pill, estrogen passes through the digestive tract and liver, where it exerts its impact on cholesterol. With the patch and cream, however, estrogen goes directly into the bloodstream, and the effect on cholesterol is diminished.

Looking Ahead to Menopause

Menopause may bring some physical changes, but there are some steps you can take now to help you get through it. Here are some suggestions.

GET IN THE EXERCISE HABIT. Do some form of weight-bearing, aerobic exercise for 30 minutes at least three times a week, and more if possible. Weight-bearing activities—such as walking or running—help increase or maintain bone density. Aerobic exercise, the kind that gets your heart rate up continuously for at least 20 to 30 minutes, will also help keep your cholesterol levels down and boost your feelings of well-being, Dr. Walsh says.

WATCH YOUR FAT INTAKE. Each day, 25 percent or less of the calories you eat should come from fat, experts say. Eating a diet low in saturated fats will help bring your cholesterol level down.

GIVE UP THOSE CIGARETTES. Smoking can worsen any menopausal symptoms you have, Dr. Walsh says. Smoking not only brings on menopause sooner, it also reduces the small amount of estrogen women do have after menopause. In addition to making you feel better at menopause, giving up smoking will also be better for your bone health—you'll have more estrogen available to maintain bone strength.

BONE UP NOW. Get enough calcium to keep your bones strong and healthy. After age 35, women begin to lose about 1 percent of their bone mass per year. The Daily Value for calcium for premenopausal women is 1,000 milligrams, but some doctors recommend getting between 1,000 and 1,200 milligrams. An eight-ounce glass of 1 percent low-fat milk and one cup of low-fat yogurt with fruit contain about 300 milligrams each. Three ounces of canned sockeye salmon, with bones, contains about 203 milligrams, and a half-cup of tofu contains about 258 milligrams.

Calcium supplements are another option. When deciding how many supplements to take, read the label to see how much "elemental" or "bioavailable" calcium each tablet contains; that's the number of milligrams your body will actually absorb. Take the supplements with food and a glass of water to help your body absorb them easily and efficiently, says Kendra Kaye, M.D., clinical assistant professor of medicine at the University of Pennsylvania School of Medicine and attending physician at Graduate Hospital, both in Philadelphia.

HAVE YOUR CHOLESTEROL CHECKED. Ask your doctor to check your cholesterol levels to make sure you are in the healthy range, says Dr. Walsh. She should measure the ratio of your total cholesterol to your good cholesterol, or HDL. A total cholesterol/HDL cholesterol below 3.5 indicates that you are at low risk for a heart attack. A ratio between 3.5 and 6.9 means you are at moderate risk, and a ratio over 7.0 means you are at high risk. Menopause can cause your ratio to go up, because levels of LDL (bad cholesterol) go up and levels of HDL go down.

SEE YOUR DOCTOR ABOUT PMS. If you've got PMS and your symptoms are getting worse, see your doctor; you may have begun menopause, says Dr. Klutznick. Your doctor can perform an FSH test to determine whether that is the case.

ASK MOM. If the uncertainty of menopause weighs on your mind, talk to your mother about it. It's not uncommon for women to follow the same pattern as their mothers, says Dr. Walsh, especially if they have a similar health history.

BRING YOUR HUSBAND INTO THE PICTURE. Share information you learn about menopause with your husband, says Dr. Klutznick. One way to do that is to ask him to read a book or two on menopause, she says. Some books have chapters just for men.

SAVOR THE MOMENT. It can make the menopausal transition easier if you appreciate where you are in your life and enjoy it, says Borton.

When Menopause Arrives

Don't just sit back and worry, or try to ignore it. Here are tips to help you cope.

TALK ABOUT IT. "Talk to other women," says Dr. Klutznick. Find out what symptoms they're having, what causes them difficulty and what they do to cope. A lot of women are doing their own research and information-gathering, and they can be a tremendous resource for you, she says.

FIND SOMEONE TO LOOK UP TO. Some older women who have been through menopause can serve as wonderful mentors, says Borton. Find a woman 10 to 15 years older who's living a lifestyle you admire and respect and talk to her about what has meaning in her life. Make her a role model.

CONSIDER HRT. Talk to your doctor about your symptoms and options for dealing with them. Deciding to take hormones is a very individual decision, experts say. Talk to several doctors if you need to, Dr. Klutznick says, until you find one you are comfortable with and who is willing to respect what you want to do to manage your menopause.

CREATE A SENSE OF COMMUNITY. "Women need to have a community of other women," says Dr. Klutznick. This can help you feel connected and productive during this transitional time, she says. So join a book club or take art lessons or a course that stimulates your intellect, she says.

EXPECT SEXUAL CHANGES. For some, sex will change during menopause, says Dr. Klutznick. Some women find that sex is not as passionate but becomes more affectionate. And this can be fine, since their mate's testosterone levels may be dropping as well, lowering his sex drive. Some women also find that certain places on the body that used to be highly sensitive are less so, and that other places that were not sensitive now are, she says.

STAY SEXUALLY ACTIVE. Sex may feel different, but try to stay active, doctors say. Women who do so undergo fewer vaginal changes than those who slow down, studies show. Not having sex can cause your vagina to change in size and elasticity, which can make sex painful. Communicate to your partner the changes you are feeling and explore new and different ways to have sex that may be more comfortable. You may take longer to lubricate than you used to—it may take one to three minutes for your vaginal area to become aroused, compared to the 6 to 20 seconds it used to take.

Besides allowing yourself more time, you can also use water-based vaginal lubricants. Try K-Y Lubricating Jelly or Replens, which are available in drugstores.

If you do not have a partner, masturbation helps promote circulation and moistness in the vagina, helping it to maintain its size and elasticity, says Dr. Klutznick.

TRY HERBS. Black cohosh, blue cohosh, sarsaparilla, wild yam root and dong quai are among some of the herbs doctors often recommend to alleviate menopausal symptoms. These herbs contain phytoestrogens, plant sources of estrogen similar to that produced in the body.

The levels of phytoestrogens found in these herbs are lower than the doses of estrogen in HRT and are believed by some doctors to relieve menopausal symptoms without causing harmful side effects. Consult with your doctor before using these remedies.

Menstrual Problems

GET BACK IN SYNC WITH YOUR CYCLE

Cramps. Heavy bleeding. Light bleeding. Being a few days late.

At some point, most women have experienced one or all of these menstrual problems. In fact, in one survey, about 400 working women between the ages of 18 and 72 were asked what health problems doctors had told them they had. Almost one-quarter of the women reported having menstrual problems. "Menstrual problems are very common," says Christine Wells, Ph.D., professor of exercise science and physical education at Arizona State University in Tempe and a researcher on the study.

Many times menstrual problems are nothing to worry about. A change in menstrual flow or cycle length, for instance, happens now and then and is perfectly normal. In fact, perfect regularity is rare, experts say.

Other times, lifestyle changes or new events, whether positive or negative, can trigger a variation in your cycle. Maybe you've started a new exercise program, or maybe you've had an accident or undergone surgery.

But sometimes changes can be a sign that something is not right physically. Uterine fibroids, pelvic inflammatory disease (PID), endometrial polyps, cancer and early menopause all can lead to changes in cycle length or flow.

Monitoring Your Menstrual Health

There are some basic steps you can take to detect menstrual problems early and make managing them easier. Here are some suggestions.

GET CHECKED REGULARLY. Having an annual gynecological exam won't necessarily prevent all menstrual problems, but it can help detect them early and make treatment easier and more successful. "We certainly recommend that everyone have an annual exam," says Natalie Blagowidow, M.D., an obstetrician-gynecologist at Crozer-Chester Medical Center in Upland, Pennsylvania. Women who have a family history of ovarian cancer or who have had benign ovarian tumors in the past should be seen twice a year, she says.

KEEP AN EYE ON CHANGES. Know what is normal for you and pay attention to any irregularities. There's probably no need to get too upset over small variations. "If one month it's a little different and then it's back to what is normal for you, that's probably not a reason to worry," says Dr. Blagowidow. "But if you notice a change that is consistent and that's more severe than what you experienced before, you should certainly be examined and evaluated."

KEEP A MENSTRUAL RECORD. Recording when your period starts and stops and whether you bleed heavily or lightly will help you keep track of whatever changes develop. "I tell everyone to keep a menstrual history," says Annamarie G. Hellebusch, R.N., a certified nurse-practitioner in the obstetrics-gynecology department at the University of Pennsylvania Medical Center in Philadelphia. It's often hard for women to remember over a span of several months exactly when their periods started and stopped, she says.

CONSULT YOUR DOCTOR. If you notice what you believe is a change, tell your doctor what's going on. Whether you'll need an appointment depends on what the change is, says Margaret M. Polaneczky, M.D., medical director of women's health and assistant professor of obstetrics and gynecology at the New York Hospital–

Cornell Medical Center in New York City. If there is unusual discharge or pain or you miss a period, go right away, she says. If, over two or three cycles, your cycle is lengthening or you have spotting or a different flow, your doctor may perform blood tests or other tests to rule out physical or hormonal causes, she says.

Here are some common menstrual problems and what you should do about them.

Heavy Bleeding and Spotting: Fighting the Flow

There are many things that can cause heavy bleeding in women whose flows are generally light to moderate.

The two most common causes are benign uterine growths known as fibroids and cycles in which a woman doesn't ovulate, says Dr. Polaneczky.

Whether fibroids require surgical removal "depends on the size, growth rate and degree of pain and bleeding," says Dr. Polaneczky. Smaller fibroids may be left alone. For larger ones, some women opt to have a surgical procedure called a myomectomy, in which fibroids are removed. For women who have completed childbearing, a hysterectomy that removes the uterus but preserves the ovaries is also an option.

Endometriosis, a disease in which the uterine lining proliferates beyond normal bounds, can also cause heavy bleeding. So can PID, benign endometrial polyps, thyroid problems and diabetes. Rarely, for older women or those with a long history of irregular periods, heavy bleeding may indicate a precancerous condition.

Sometimes aging can cause heavier bleeding. The uterus continues to grow in small increments until women are about 35 years old, says Dr. Blagowidow. So after 35 they may bleed a little more heavily than they did when they were younger because the uterus is slightly larger and there is more uterine tissue to bleed.

Spotting is normal for some women, says Dr. Blagowidow. Some women spot around the time of ovulation, and they do it every month in a regular pattern, she says. Other women spot for up to a week prior to the start of their menstrual flow. In these cases, the cause is often a hormonal imbalance called luteal phase defect, in which women don't have enough of the hormone progesterone. This is a common cause of spotting in women who are 30 to 45 years old, she says.

When spotting occurs at different times of the cycle, Dr. Blago-widow says, something other than a hormonal imbalance is usually causing it. Possibilities include pregnancy, polyps, fibroids and cancer, she says. For some women, spotting may signal the onset of menopause. And it's been observed in women on the Pill who've contracted a sexually transmitted disease (STD) called chlamydia.

If you're having heavy bleeding or spotting, here is some advice from the experts.

MONITOR YOUR FLOW. If you start bleeding more heavily than usual, keep track of how much. This will help your doctor. You can monitor the increase by writing down how many times you have to change your pads or tampons in one or two hours and what size products you are using, says Dr. Blagowidow.

KEEP A RECORD. In addition to noting your flow, make a record of the activities and events surrounding the episode, says Dr. Blagowidow. Did you have sex the day before? Are you suffering

TAKE CONTROL OF YOUR CYCLE

Planning a vacation? Don't want to hassle with your period? Preliminary research indicates that women may be able to prolong the time between their periods and to essentially delay them. They may also be able to decrease the pain of menstrual cramps.

It's done with a program of mental imagery, says Maureen Groër, R.N., Ph.D., program director and professor in the Graduate Program in Nursing at Massachusetts General Hospital Institute of Health Professions in Boston.

Over a three-month period, women listened to an audiotape of guided mental imagery. The tape included 7 minutes of progressive muscle relaxation instruction followed by 5 minutes of guided imagery. During the imagery portion, a voice on the tape advised the women with statements about controlling their cycles. Phrases such as "I am in control" and "I can alter the length of my cycle" were repeated over and over. Meanwhile, in the background, a clock was ticking; the beat of the ticking slowed down progressively as the 12-minute tape continued.

By listening to the tape one to several times a week for three months, women were able to lengthen their cycles from an from any illnesses? Have you had an unusual amount of exercise? These details will also assist your physician.

CONSIDER THE PILL. If you normally have heavy menstrual flow or have endometriosis, the Pill is an option. It usually decreases flow. Consult with your doctor on whether the Pill is right for you.

GET CHECKED FOR STDs. If you have spotting, ask your doctor to test you for sexually transmitted diseases. Spotting may be an indicator for chlamydia in women who are taking the Pill and have had regular periods while on it.

Cramps: Acing the Ache

Who among us hasn't had cramps? Some of us get them occasionally, others every month. It's estimated that 50 percent of all women get cramps and that 5 to 10 percent have pain that's bad enough to incapac-

---

average of almost 30 days to an average of 31 days. Playing the tape more often seemed to have a greater effect, says Dr. Groër. One woman lengthened her cycle to 56 days, which meant she went for over two months without having a period (it eventually returned to normal). Of all the women in the study, she listened to the tape the most frequently.

Some women also experienced a decrease in the pain that accompanied their periods.

The technique appears to work only temporarily, Dr. Groër says. Eventually the body's regulatory mechanism kicks in and women's cycles return to their usual pattern.

The process is similar to those of biofeedback and meditation, in which regulation of the mind is used to control bodily functions such as heart rate and skin temperature.

Women can make a tape of their own and try it, says Dr. Groër, using a metronome to simulate the ticking clock.

Dr. Groër tried it. She didn't want to have her period while on vacation in Greece, and it was due to arrive. After using the technique, she was able to delay the start of her period for about a week—until the plane trip home.

itate them every month for anywhere from one hour to three days.

The culprits behind cramps are substances called prostaglandins. Prostaglandins are produced by cells in the lining of the uterus and are released when the lining begins to slough off during menstruation. That release triggers contractions of the uterus that we feel as cramps.

Cramps tend to start 2 to 24 hours before menstrual bleeding begins and last about 24 to 35 hours. Studies indicate that the severity of cramps declines after ages 25 to 30. And many women report that their cramps lessen in severity after they have had a baby.

While you can have your period even if you haven't ovulated—known as an anovulatory cycle—you usually get cramps only when you ovulate, says Dr. Polaneczky. So if nothing is physically wrong and you have cramps, that's a signal that an egg was released from your ovary at midcycle.

While cramps can be normal, they can also result from something more serious, such as endometriosis, PID or fibroids.

If your cramps are not caused by a disease or fibroids, you can take steps to make them milder. Here's how.

WATCH YOUR DIET. "I often counsel women to cut back on caffeine and heavy meals," says Hellebusch. Though it's not clear why this may help lessen cramps, it has worked for many women, she says. Avoid heavy meals and spicy foods that may cause gastrointestinal upset, and increase your intake of fluids, especially water, seven to ten days before your period starts, she advises.

REACH FOR THE MEDICINE CABINET. Several over-the-counter medications are effective for relieving cramps. Acetaminophen works, but at the top of the list are the nonsteroidal anti-inflammatory drugs (NSAIDs) ibuprofen and naproxyen sodium (Aleve), which block prostaglandin activity and thereby help eliminate cramps. If you're regular and can anticipate when you will start bleeding, you can take an NSAID the day before, says Hellebusch. That way it will already be in your system, she says. If you can't forecast the date of your period's arrival, it's not essential to start the medication ahead of time. You can start it with the onset of bleeding or pain, says Dr. Polaneczky.

SWITCH MEDICATIONS. Research indicates that 80 to 85 percent of women respond to antiprostaglandin medications. But if you try one and it doesn't work, don't give up. Try another. Also, if you use one medication for months and then it stops working as well, switch; you may have developed a resistance to the first type. Finally, if the over-the-counter antiprostaglandin medications don't provide enough relief for you, talk to your doctor, who may prescribe higher doses or other NSAIDs. Prescription forms are also available.

TRY BIRTH CONTROL ACTION. For women with severe cramping, oral contraceptives are an option. The Pill decreases the amount of menstrual tissue—the source of the chemicals that cause cramping. So less tissue, less prostaglandins, less pain.

MOVE IT. Regular exercise may help keep cramps to a minimum, experts say. "Women who regularly exercise will tell you that when they do exercise, their cramps are less severe," says Dr. Polaneczky.

Although it's not clear exactly how exercise helps, experts point to brain chemicals called endorphins, which are released when you work out. These chemicals are thought to mediate the perception of pain, and it's possible that they interfere with the pain mechanism responsible for menstrual cramps.

Coping with the Unexpected

In women over 30, changes in the cycle appear to be the biggest concern among patients, doctors say. "The most common thing is that the timing of bleeding is different," says Dr. Blagowidow. "The cycle is a week earlier or a week later. Their concern is 'This is not the way I usually am. I'm usually regular,' " she says.

Many things can cause the timing of your period to change. The many sources of stress—travel, a job change, moving—and the beginning of menopause can cause cycle changes.

Women who have sporadic sexual activity or who are celibate tend to have cycles that are unusually long or short. And women who spend more time with men—sexually or otherwise—tend to have more regular cycles.

Some women always have irregular cycles, and some have cycles that are much longer than the usual 28 days. A small study of ten women at the University of California at San Diego shed some light—literally—on the problem of longer cycles. Researchers there observed that the length of women's cycles was shortened when they were exposed to a light source while sleeping.

For two months, women were exposed to light while they slept. The light source was a table lamp or a light mask (a Hollywood-style sleep mask with a built-in light source) timed to come on about a half-hour after the women went to sleep. The women were exposed to white light for the first month and to red light for the second month. Before the study, the average length of the women's cycles was about

40 days. After the study, the cycles of the women exposed to white light shortened to an average of about 33 days. Women exposed to red light had average cycles of about 37 days.

While they can't guarantee that light exposure will work for all women, researchers say it's worth a try. Simply turn on your bedside lamp before you go to sleep or set it on a timer so it turns on after you've fallen asleep.

While doctors say there's little you can do to control irregular cycles or cycle changes, there are some things you can do to make living with them a little easier.

PAY ATTENTION TO THE SIGNS. Your body often gives signals that your period is on the way. You may feel breast tenderness, bloating and cramping, experts say. Listen to your body.

PLAN AHEAD. Have tampons or pads handy for those times when your period arrives unexpectedly. Stash them everywhere—in your car, in your briefcase, in your office, in your pocketbook. "Just be prepared," says Dr. Blagowidow. If you don't want to be bothered with a pocketbook, try a hip pack. They're big enough to hold tampons or the thinner pads. Wear blazers with big outside pockets or inside breast pockets and stash a tampon or pad there for emergencies during the workday.

CHANGE PANTY LINERS OFTEN. Wearing panty liners is one way to be prepared for unexpected bleeding. Just be sure to change them often. Their plastic bottom traps moisture, which can trigger yeast infections, says Hellebusch.

FIND OUT YOUR FAMILY HISTORY. If you find yourself in early menopause, check out your Mom's history. You may be following the same pattern she did. "Women who go through premature menopause may be more likely to have family members that did, too," says Dr. Polaneczky.

ACCEPT CHANGE. If you've seen your doctor and any physical cause for your problem—such as pregnancy, fibroids, endometriosis or PID—has been ruled out, understand that your cycle may change as you age. "Women think their body will stay the same forever and ever. It takes a lot of reassurance that nothing's wrong," says Dr. Polaneczky. "It's normal for periods to change in women over 30," she says.

Breast Tenderness: Soothing the Pain

Breast tenderness preceding menstrual periods is a frequent complaint, and in most cases it is normal.

"Breast tenderness is very common," says Kathleen Mayzel, M.D., director of the Faulkner Breast Centre and assistant clinical professor of surgery at Tufts University School of Medicine in Boston. "Most is hormonally related. As estrogen levels go up right before your period, the breasts get more tender. Then as they go down after your period, the breasts get less tender. And there's no need to do anything about it."

But if you're really uncomfortable, there are a few things that you can try.

CUT OUT CAFFEINE. "One thing that is effective is to stop caffeine intake," says Dr. Blagowidow. Cut it out as much as you can, she says. Sources of caffeine to keep an eye out for are coffee, sodas, tea and chocolate. If you feel that quitting caffeine altogether is impossible, at least try to cut back the week before your period is due, says Hellebusch.

TAKE VITAMIN E. The use of vitamin E for breast tenderness is controversial, but some women find it works, says Hellebusch. Women start taking 400 international units a day ten days before their period starts and continue until they stop menstruating for the month, she says.

SEE YOUR DOCTOR. If none of these measures helps, talk to your doctor. She may want to check you out for cysts—tiny fluid-filled sacs—and costochondritis, an inflammation of the ribs that can cause pain in the breast.

Doctors don't know what causes either of these conditions, says Dr. Mayzel, although cysts may have something to do with fluctuating hormone levels. Postmenopausal women do not get these cysts, she says.

Fortunately, either of these types of breast tenderness can be relieved. "Cysts can be aspirated—drained—in a physician's office with a needle and syringe," says Dr. Mayzel, "and costochondritis can be relieved with anti-inflammatory medication from your doctor."

Motion Sickness
SMOOTHING A ROUGH RIDE

When motion makes you miserable, travel is torture. The fishing boat is pitching and rolling on choppy seas. The jumbo jet hits turbulence and shudders. The car is hot, the radio's too loud, and the road to the beach is a maze of hairpin turns.

And you? You've broken out in a cold sweat. You're green around the gills. Your stomach lurches. How soon, you wonder, will you lose your lunch?

Whether you're carsick or airsick, seasick or even trainsick, take comfort in the fact that motion sickness strikes 90 percent of Americans at some point in their lives. Women and men seem equally disposed to this nightmare, but a woman may suffer the effects more if she's pregnant or premenstrual—times when hormone levels can make her feel nause-ated anyway. Studies at Pennsylvania State University in University Park also suggest that people of Asian descent are more prone to motion sickness than those of European or African descent.

It's All in Your Head

Why does a bumpy trip make some people ill? Because their brains are receiving contradictory signals from motion sensors in their eyes, inner ears, joints and tendons. Say you're on a ferry boat: Your eyes follow the moving waves, but your ears and body sense the rocking of the ship. Somehow, this "sensory mismatch" activates nausea and vomiting centers in the brain.

Researchers aren't sure how this happens, but one theory suggests that the brain misinterprets the mixed signals as food poisoning and—thus fooled—tries to eject toxins it thinks must be in the stomach. But all that really comes up is your breakfast.

So far, motion sickness has no cure. But there's plenty you can do to steady yourself and your stomach.

TAKE MEDICATIONS EARLY. Dramamine, Bonine, Marezine and other over-the-counter motion sickness drugs are most effective when taken at least an hour before your journey. The scopolamine patch, which releases a prescription drug through your skin into your bloodstream for up to three days, must be applied behind the ear several hours in advance.

But beware—all of these medications can make you drowsy, and blurred vision and dry mouth are additional side effects of the patch. If drowsiness is a worry for you, says gastroenterologist Kenneth L. Koch, M.D., a researcher in the Division of Gastroenterology at the Pennsylvania State University/Milton S. Hershey Medical Center in Hershey, try Marezine. He says it makes you less groggy than Dramamine does, and "it lasts up to six hours." Pregnant women should check with their doctors before using the patch or any motion sickness drugs.

TRY GINGER. Some medical studies show ginger is better than Dramamine or other drugs at keeping motion sickness at bay. Start with two 900-milligram capsules of ground ginger root 15 to 20 minutes before a trip, says researcher Daniel Mowrey, Ph.D., director of the American Phytotherapy Research Laboratory in Salt Lake City. Take more whenever feelings of nausea arise. How much at one time is the right dose? "You know you've had enough when you can taste ginger at the back of your throat," Dr. Mowrey says. He says it works for up to 60 percent of people with motion sickness. "It's worth a try; ginger cannot hurt you," he adds.

But ginger didn't do as well as the patch in studies at the Louisiana State University Medical Center in New Orleans, where 28 people were tested. When they sat on a rotating chair to stimulate motion sickness, ginger did not avert or lessen their distress, but the patch did.

FACE FORWARD. Always ride so your eyes see the same motion your body and inner ears feel. Sit in the front seat of the car and watch the road ahead, choose a forward-facing seat on the train and observe the scenery, sit by the window on an airplane and look outside or stand on the deck of the ship and keep your eyes on the horizon ahead. "You want to match the swerves, bumps, starts and stops that your inner ear is sensing, so the same signals go from your eyes and ears to the brain," says Robert M. Stern, Ph.D., professor of psychology at Pennsylvania State University.

DON'T READ. Reading in a moving vehicle sends your brain the very mixed signals that cause nausea: Your eyes track across the printed words, while your inner ear detects every swerve of the car. Look out the window and let someone else read the map.

BREATHE FREELY. Avoid food odors and smoke-filled spaces. "Get cool air," says Dr. Koch. "Nobody knows quite why, but it seems to help."

EAT, BUT LIGHTLY. Steer clear of spicy or greasy foods before a trip, but don't go hungry. A small, easily digestible meal—try bread, crackers, cereal or granola bars—will keep your stomach occupied with normal digestion without burdening it with foods that may irritate or, like fatty items, take longer to digest. "And take some crackers with you," Dr. Stern says. "Try to eat something very small every two hours or so."

SQUEEZE YOUR WRIST. According to the ancient Chinese practice of acupressure, stimulating the "Neiguan point" relieves nausea. You can find it between the tendons on the underside of your wrist, three finger-widths below the crease of skin where your wrist joins your hand.

Muscle Cramps
PUT THEM AT EASE—FOR GOOD

They seem to come out of nowhere. One minute you're lying in bed reading quietly. The next, you're sitting up, clutching your leg, rocking back and forth and swearing at an intense muscle cramp shooting through your calf.

You know the feeling. That's because muscle cramps, which are involuntary muscle contractions that can occur anywhere in the body, are very common. A whopping 95 percent of college students questioned in a survey said they had experienced muscle cramps. And a survey of patients at a health clinic found that 50 percent had suffered at least one leg cramp in the previous month.

An Unsolved Mystery
The most common type of muscle cramp occurs at night in the legs, says Baltimore physical therapist Z. Annette Iglarsh, Ph.D., vice-

president of Theraphysics, a rehabilitation managed-care corporation, and president of the Orthopedic Section of the American Physical Therapy Association. These cramps can be extremely painful and can even rouse you from a deep sleep. Daytime cramps are also possible in muscles throughout the body, including the thighs, back, hands and arms.

Doctors suspect that muscle cramps are often related to mineral deficiencies, says Dr. Iglarsh. Magnesium and calcium in particular are believed to play central roles in muscle contraction and relaxation, so a lack of them may bring about cramps. So might shortages of potassium and sodium, which also trigger the contraction and relaxation of muscles.

Exercise can reduce the body's mineral reserves because potassium and sodium are lost in sweat. Dehydration is also thought to cause cramps.

People who are out of shape run an increased risk of getting cramps because poorly conditioned muscles get fatigued more easily, says Paul Davidson, M.D., associate clinical professor of medicine at the University of California in Greenbrae and medical director of the Fibromyalgia Clinic at Kentfield Rehabilitation Hospital in Kentfield, California.

Changes in circulation—such as swelling in the feet and ankles, which many pregnant women experience—can lead to cramps, says Dr. Iglarsh. That's because swelling deprives the calf muscles of the nutrients they need. Also during pregnancy, the fetus draws on the mother's mineral stores, which may lead to depletion, she says.

Your sleeping position may also be the culprit. When blankets press down on your foot, forcing it into a pointed position, your calf and foot muscles are shortened and a cramp can result.

Medications can trigger muscle cramps. Diuretics, for example, which are used to treat kidney disease and high blood pressure, cause frequent urination. Because you lose minerals when you urinate, mineral balances in the body are altered.

Muscle cramps can also be due to diseases, including hypothyroidism, in which the thyroid gland produces too little hormone. Peripheral vascular disease, in which the small blood vessels in the extremities deteriorate, and atherosclerosis, in which the walls of small blood vessels thicken, both cause circulatory problems and possibly cramps.

Don't Cramp Your Style

Lots of people get muscle cramps, and usually they are not a sign of anything serious, says Dr. Davidson. There are some things you can do to lower your chances of getting one, however, and to get relief when one strikes.

STAY ACTIVE. Do your best to participate in an exercise program on a regular basis, says Dr. Iglarsh. This may help prevent leg cramps by keeping your muscles in shape. Any kind of aerobic exercise, such as walking, running or biking for at least 20 minutes three times a week, is generally sufficient to maintain muscle fitness.

QUIT SMOKING. Smoking decreases the size of the arteries that supply blood to your muscles, says Dr. Davidson. This improper blood flow can cause cramps, so do your best to cut back or quit.

PREPARE FOR SLEEP TIME. Slowly unwind at least one hour before you go to sleep, says Dr. Iglarsh. Too often we rush around all day, exercise after work, race home to prepare dinner and do some chores, then jump right into bed without a relaxation period, she says. Taking time to calm down may reduce the likelihood of cramps because you won't be placing great demands on your muscles and then stopping suddenly.

STRETCH IT OUT. To deter leg cramps, do calf stretches before you go to bed or when you wake up, says Dr. Iglarsh.

Stretching can also help if you get a cramp, she says. The aim is to stretch the cramping muscle, whether it's in your calf, foot, thigh or hand, in the opposite direction. For example, if you have a cramp in your calf, sit on the floor with the cramped leg extended straight in front of you. Pull your toes back toward your kneecap. You may want to pull back gently on your toes with your hand to assist the stretch.

STAND UP. If you're in too much pain to sit down and do a calf stretch, standing will also provide a prolonged, moderate stretch, says Dr. Iglarsh. In fact, one of the best things for foot and calf cramps is weight-bearing, she says. So if you get a cramp, stand on the affected leg. Be careful not to lose your balance, warns Dr. Iglarsh.

DRINK UP. Muscle cramps that occur during exercise are often from dehydration, so drink water. Drink six eight-ounce glasses each day, and drink as much as you can in the hour after you exercise. A recommendation is to drink 8 to 12 ounces of water for every 20 to 30 minutes that you exercise, says Margot Putukian, M.D., team physician at Pennsylvania State University in University Park and assistant professor of orthopedic surgery and internal medicine at Pennsylvania State University/Milton S. Hershey Medical Center in Hershey.

GET ENOUGH POTASSIUM. Since muscle cramps may be due to insufficient potassium, give your body what it needs. The

Daily Value (DV) for potassium is 3,500 milligrams. Foods high in it include bananas, orange juice, oranges, prune juice, broccoli, baked potato with the skin and red snapper.

LOAD UP ON OTHER MINERALS. Calcium, magnesium and sodium are also important. The DV for calcium is 1,000 milligrams; good food sources include milk, yogurt, canned pink salmon, Swiss cheese and broccoli.

The DV for magnesium is 400 milligrams. Halibut, long-grain brown rice and spinach are magnesium-rich.

Most Americans get enough sodium, but if you use very little salt and exercise a lot, add a dash to your food.

GET IT CHECKED. If your cramps persist or are painful and frequent enough to disrupt your lifestyle, talk to your doctor about them, says Dr. Iglarsh.

ASK ABOUT QUININE. People who regularly have nocturnal leg cramps may find relief with the nonprescription drug quinine, says Dr. Davidson. A study of 27 male veterans conducted at the Veterans Affairs Medical Center in White River Junction, Vermont, found that 13 of the patients had a 50 percent reduction in the number of nocturnal cramps while taking quinine sulfate. Other studies, however, have found quinine to be no more effective than a placebo. Ask your doctor about it; quinine's side effects can include dizziness, nausea and ringing in the ears.

Neck and Shoulder Pain
EASY TO KEEP AT BAY

You sit in front of a computer for hours every day, barely moving your head. You sleep in a bed for hours every night, barely moving anything.

Oh, sure, you moved around at work and even a little afterward. You talked to your colleagues, went for a soda, leaned over some files.

But much of the past 24 hours was spent with your neck and shoulders in a single position. And now—surprise—you've got a royal pain in the neck and a shoulder that's as stiff as an old piece of leather.

We've all known someone who has complained of neck and shoulder pain, and most of us have gone a round or two with it ourselves.

It's not known whether this type of pain is more common in men or women. But doctors do know what causes it. So, starting with the neck, let's take a look at these two troublesome body parts and see if we can figure out how to keep them from being such a pain.

A Delicate Balancing Act

Poor posture, tight muscles, muscle tension and back and other injuries can cause neck pain. In fact, about 50 percent of people with back pain—and that's 80 percent of the population—also have neck pain. Diseases including rheumatoid arthritis, fibromyalgia, which causes muscle pain throughout the body, and degenerated or herniated disks can also lead to neck pain.

What to do about it? Practice good posture, for one thing, says Baltimore physical therapist Z. Annette Iglarsh, Ph.D., vice president of Theraphysics, a rehabilitation managed-care corporation, and president of the Orthopedic Section of the American Physical Therapy Association. That's because poor posture takes the spine and neck out of alignment.

A common problem is sitting or standing with your head too far forward, which makes the small muscles at the back of your neck work twice as hard as they normally would, says Dr. Iglarsh. With your head in the wrong place, the neck muscles lose the support of the spine and end up having to do all the work of holding up your head by themselves. The muscles are overworked and pain is the result.

Driving, sitting for long periods, working at a computer and lifting objects are tough on posture. So is tension, since overwrought muscles get tired and don't perform the way they should.

Physical changes that come with aging can also cause neck pain. As time passes, the disks between the spinal vertebrae start to dry up, which causes them to shrink and the vertebrae above and below them to shift.

When this happens, nerves passing from the spinal cord through holes in the vertebrae can become pinched. This is called degenerative disk disease and can lead not only to pain but to a decrease in the range of neck motion. While everyone gets degenerative disk disease to some extent as they age, good posture and limber neck muscles can reduce the chances of a pinched nerve.

The disks between the bones of the spinal column can also crack, or herniate. When this happens, the jellylike substance inside the disk leaks out and presses on the nerves leading to the neck, causing pain.

Every year there are roughly one million cases of whiplash, a well-known cause of pain in which the ligaments are strained when the neck is "whipped" forward and back—or slammed backward, then forward—during an automobile accident. Women are twice as likely as men to have pain after a whiplash, possibly because a woman's neck is smaller and usually weaker than a man's.

Being Nice to Your Neck

Although necks are vulnerable to disease and injury, preventing pain is frequently simply a matter of common sense. Here's how to apply it.

KEEP IT IN NEUTRAL. Having your neck in a neutral position can prevent excessive strain, says Dr. Iglarsh. To see if your neck is in the right position, place two fingers on your upper lip and push your head back until your ears are in line with your shoulders.

USE A GOOD PILLOW. Your head should be in the neutral position when you sleep, says Dr. Iglarsh. That is, when you lie on your back, your pillow should be low enough so that your chin is not on your chest. And it should be fat enough so that when you roll onto your side, the pillow fills the space between your shoulder and the bed, she says.

MAKE YOUR OWN. An orthopedic pillow can keep your neck in neutral, and while there are lots of these pillows on the market, it's easy to make your own, says Dr. Iglarsh. To increase neck support, fold a thick bath towel lengthwise into quarters. Using safety pins, fasten the folded towel to the lower long edge of your pillow and slip your pillowcase over it. Sleep with the folded-towel portion of the pillow under your neck.

For a pillow shaped like a bow-tie, fold the towel in quarters again, says Dr. Iglarsh, and pin the towel tightly around the center of the pillow, pinching the pillow into the "bow-tie" shape. Then slip the pillowcase over it. This shape can support your neck in neutral when you're lying on your side. Give these pillows a try before spending money on a commercial model, and use these pillow-making techniques when you travel, says Dr. Iglarsh.

TRY A NECK ROLL. If you prefer to sleep without a pillow, try a neck roll instead, says Dr. Iglarsh. Just fashion a towel into a small roll that fits into the curve of your neck.

TAKE CARE ON THE ROAD. Sleeping with your neck in awkward positions while you travel in a plane, bus, car or train can lead to neck pain, says Edward Hanley, M.D., chairman of orthopedic surgery at the Carolinas Medical Center in Charlotte, North Carolina. Try one of the cervical pillows designed for travel.

STRETCH YOUR NECK MUSCLES. Preventing muscles from getting too tight can forestall pain and relieve aches caused by tension and fatigue, says Dr. Iglarsh. Stretches that involve trying to touch one ear to the shoulder beneath it and alternately turning your chin toward each shoulder are effective.

DON'T CRACK YOUR NECK. Cracking the neck to relieve pain isn't good, says Dr. Iglarsh. It can loosen up the neck joints, which will make them less stable and more prone to injury, she says.

LIGHTEN YOUR LOAD. Carrying a heavy handbag, briefcase, gym bag or other bag on one shoulder is dangerous, says Dr. Iglarsh. Must you really carry all that stuff around? For must-haves, like lipsticks or hairbrushes, keep one in your office, one in the car or gym and one at home, she says. Also, put travel bags on wheels, she says.

USE THE HEADREST. Sixty-two percent of people in car accidents report to the emergency room complaining of neck pain. To avoid this problem—and the whiplash that generally causes it— adjust the headrest on your seat so that the top of the headrest is in line with the top of your ear.

Strain, Then Pain

Shoulder pain in women is frequently caused by muscle strain, tendinitis, arthritis or a condition called frozen shoulder, where the shoulder gets stiff and can't move freely. Fibromyagia, which occurs more often in women than men, can also cause pain.

The shoulder is a ball-and-socket joint that is held together by muscles, tendons and ligaments that allow the shoulder a wide range of motion but also keep it stable. The central stabilizing force in the shoulder are the four muscles of the rotator cuff. Lifting too heavy an object or overdoing it with exercise can strain the muscles and cause pain.

The fact that most women have less shoulder power than men doesn't make them more prone to shoulder injuries, says John M. Fenlin, Jr., M.D., clinical professor of orthopedic surgery at Thomas Jefferson University in Philadelphia. He says most women's shoulders are actually strong relative to their body size.

What can make women more susceptible to shoulder pain and injury, however, is that their shoulders are naturally more lax, or loose, than men's. This can make women candidates for dislocation and impingement, in which tendons in the shoulder become pinched against a bone. According to Dr. Fenlin, some people are more predisposed to this because the bone at the top of their shoulder has a little beak on it that is more likely to rub on the tendon. Others can develop it when tired muscles don't function as they should and the tendon gets pinched as a result.

Women who play tennis, work as baggers in grocery stores or work at a computer keyboard are most likely to get shoulder pain, says Dr. Fenlin.

Another common problem for women is frozen shoulder. For some reason, the ligaments that go around the ball-and-socket joint become inflamed, says Dr. Fenlin. The pain causes a reduction in use of the shoulder. As a result, the ligaments don't get stretched and the shoulder starts to tighten up.

Saving Your Shoulders

You may be able to carry the world on your shoulders, but only if you keep them in good shape. Here's how to do it.

STRETCH OUT. Before engaging in exercise or strenuous chores, warm up and stretch your shoulders to get them ready for exertion, says Dr. Fenlin. Simple forward and backward arm circles can help limber them up.

TAKE BREAKS. When you use your muscles for a sustained period of time to do things like clip the hedge, paint a room or turn over the garden, muscle fatigue and pain can result, says Dr. Iglarsh. "Take breaks," she says. And divide the task into segments instead of trying to do it all at once. Work for half an hour or so, do something else that does not use the same muscles for a while, then come back to your original task for another short period of time. Do this until the task is done.

WATCH YOUR WORK SURFACE. Whether you're working in the office or in the kitchen, make sure your work surface is at a height that's comfortable for you, says Dr. Iglarsh. A surface that's too low will cause you to hunch your shoulders and upper back, and one that's too high will cause you to arch your back too much.

LIFT IT RIGHT. When you lift something, pay attention to the position of your head, says Dr. Iglarsh. Bend at the knees to pick something up, and hold the item close to your body. (If your head moves forward, the weight is too heavy: don't lift it at all.) If you're lifting a child, have her climb onto a chair so you can pick her up from there, says, Dr. Iglarsh.

STRENGTHEN YOURSELF. The stronger the muscles in your shoulder, the more stable—and less prone to injury—it will be. Ask a physical therapist to put you on a shoulder-strengthening program. But make sure your therapist helps you adjust any weight machines to your particular size. Since weight machines designed for men are too big for a woman's frame, you may need to customize the machine by adding extra seat cushions and back pads.

SEE A DOCTOR. If you develop shoulder pain, check with a physician if it lasts longer than a month, says Dr. Fenlin.

Oral Cancer

OPEN WIDE AND CHECK FOR CHANGES

You do all the right things to support an active, healthy life: You eat right, get plenty of sleep, exercise regularly and do a monthly breast self-exam, plus have an annual pelvic exam and Pap test. But did you ever think that your health might also depend on whether you pull out a hand mirror, open your mouth and look around?

Who would've thought?

Yet oral cancer, which is frequently preceded by an easily detectable precancerous red or white patch that can appear anywhere in the mouth, is expected to hit nearly 10,000 women this year alone—continuing an upward trend that has increased the number of oral cancer deaths among women by 9 percent over the past three decades.

What puts women at risk? "Cigarette smoking, smokeless tobacco, alcohol, alcohol-based mouthwash and—especially among young women—the human papillomavirus," says Waun Ki Hong, M.D., chairman of thoracic/head and neck medical oncology at the University of Texas M. D. Anderson Cancer Center in Houston.

Alcohol and tobacco are the most common causes of oral cancer, particularly when they're used in combination, says Dr. Hong. No one knows exactly how long you need to smoke or drink before cancer appears, but scientists estimate that the risk is just about doubled in someone who smokes one to two packs of cigarettes a day or drinks one or two drinks a day.

The risk is quadrupled when someone does both at that level, while smoking and drinking heavily—with heavily defined by experts as more than two packs and four drinks a day—increases the risk nearly 40 times.

It's difficult to calculate a woman's risk of oral cancer from the human papillomavirus, says Dr. Hong. The virus, which causes genital warts and is a first cousin to the virus associated with cervical cancer, has no symptoms and no known cause. It cannot be prevented or treated and is usually identified only under a microscope—when it's already set the stage for cancer.

Prevention: The Best Defense

Oral cancer is a formidable disease. Once the cancer has invaded the oral cavity, the survival rate after five years is only 52 percent even with today's technically advanced surgery, radiation and chemotherapy.

The problem is that the carcinogens causing the cancer have been bathing the entire oral cavity for years, says Dr. Hong. As a result, the proliferation of cancer cells is probably under way in several areas by the time any changes are detected. And that means that the premalignant or malignant changes that first appear in the mouth may be only the first of many.

In contrast to its gloomy prognosis, however, oral cancer is a highly preventable disease. Here's how experts suggest we do it.

AVOID THE DEADLY DUO. The most effective way to reduce your risk of oral cancer is to avoid alcohol and tobacco, says Dr. Hong. As men have modified their lifestyles over the past couple of decades, their rate of oral cancer has dropped a whopping 22 percent.

USE LOW-ALCOHOL MOUTHWASHES. A study by the National Cancer Institute (NCI) in Bethesda, Maryland, revealed that women who regularly used mouthwash with an alcohol content of 25 percent or higher were nearly twice as likely to develop oral cancer as those who didn't. That's why women should check the ingredient label on any mouthwash they use to make sure that it contains less than this amount of alcohol, says Dr. Hong.

STUFF SNUFF. Several years ago doctors from Memorial Sloan-Kettering Cancer Center in New York City estimated that 1.3 percent of all women in the United States were using smokeless tobacco.

Dipping snuff, as the habit is called, is just as harmful as smoking a cigarette or chewing tobacco, says Dr. Hong. A study of more than 600 North Carolina women found that long-term users—many of whom had started to use smokeless tobacco by the age of ten—increased their risk of cancer nearly 50 times.

FIT FRUIT INTO YOUR LIFE. A federal study of nearly 2,000 men and women from across the country found that those who regularly ate a variety of fresh fruits and vegetables containing a naturally occurring cancer-fighter called glutathione reduced their risk of oral and throat cancer.

"Consumption of raw fruits and vegetables looks protective, but we don't know if this effect was due to glutathione or to some other constituent in raw vegetables and fruit," says Gloria Gridley, one of the NCI researchers who conducted the study.

Researchers aren't sure whether the glutathione may have helped repair cells injured by cancer-causing agents, enhanced immune system function or simply grabbed cancer-causing free radicals and escorted them out of the body.

Top fruit sources of glutathione in the study were grapefruit, orange juice, cantaloupe, watermelon and oranges.

ADOPT A SOYBEAN DIET. A series of laboratory and animal studies at the University of Pennsylvania in Philadelphia may show that soybeans contain Bowman-Birk inhibitor (BBI), a substance that may help prevent cancer.

"BBI prevents the transformation of precancerous cells into cancer," explains Ann Kennedy, D.Sc., professor of research oncology at the university. And it may be the single biggest reason that the Japanese, who eat a diet rich in soybeans, have such a low rate of many different kinds of cancer.

Dr. Kennedy and her associates are studying whether a soybean-based mouthwash will prevent the transformation of precancerous patches into cancer in the mouths of 24 people. The mouthwash, which is swallowed after it's swirled around the mouth, contains the equivalent of less than an ounce of a soybean preparation.

Preliminary indications are that the mouthwash is likely to prevent oral cancer. But until it's commercially available, why not borrow a book on Japanese cooking from the library and figure out how to work more soy into your diet?

THINK ABOUT VITAMIN E. In a study at the NCI, women who took vitamin E supplements in any amount had half the risk of oral cancer of those who didn't, says Gridley, the researcher who led the study. Although researchers are not yet recommending vitamin E, they note that studies indicate that vitamin E neutralizes cancer-causing free radicals, protects cell walls against carcinogenic changes and may even enhance the immune system's work.

MONITOR YOUR MOUTH. Get into the habit of checking your mouth for red or white patches whenever you brush your teeth, says Dr Hong. It only takes a second, and constant vigilance pays off.

PUT YOUR DENTIST ON THE ALERT. Also ask your dentist or hygienist to keep an eye out for precancerous patches and to give you an oral cancer check during your six-month checkup.

"Cancer of the oral cavity is a multistep process," says Dr. Hong. "So if we can catch a precancerous lesion, there's a possibility we can prevent the cancer."

Osteoporosis

THE TIME TO THINK ABOUT IT IS NOW

For Debbie, life isn't what it used to be.

She can't go biking and hiking with her husband anymore, and her ability to travel is severely limited. She can't even take a car ride for longer than an hour and a half, because when she does, she's so stiff and sore afterward she can barely walk.

When she goes grocery shopping, she can't lift any packages weighing more than five pounds. Somebody has to take the bags from her car to her house.

Debbie says her days are very routine. She does her exercises at the same time every day, has a list of certain foods she must eat and follows a strict medication regimen. She's too afraid to veer from her set schedule for fear that any changes might send her disease into a tailspin.

Debbie has severe osteoporosis. She's 40 years old.

A Disease for the Young, Too

If you expected Debbie to be 78 or 85, you're probably not alone. Osteoporosis, the steady, progressive loss of bone density, is typically associated with elderly women because the results of the disease don't become apparent until those later decades, when we can see the loss of height and the dowager's hump that can be a precursor of fractures.

But osteoporosis has its roots much earlier. It starts slowly and silently and progressively gets worse if not attended to. It can begin at menopause, when estrogen levels start to drop. Sometimes the foundation is laid in the thirties or forties when, for a number of reasons, a woman doesn't achieve peak bone mass. And it may come even earlier, as it did for Debbie. Doctors don't know why she has the disease, but they think she probably started developing it in her late twenties, about ten years before she was diagnosed at the age of 37.

Debbie's case is unusual in that few women have severe osteoporosis at her age. But it's a reminder that while you may not have the disease yet, as a woman you are at risk for it. And now—not later—is the time to do what you can to prevent it.

Osteoporosis is much harder to treat than it is to prevent, says Harold Rosen, M.D., instructor of medicine at Harvard Medical School. Once there's a loss in bone density, it's very hard, and sometimes impossible, to regain what's already lost, he says.

"We're trying to get the message out to younger women that there are things they can do to help prevent osteoporosis," explains Kendra Kaye, M.D., clinical assistant professor of medicine at the University of Pennsylvania School of Medicine and attending physician at Graduate Hospital, both in Philadelphia. "We don't want women to wait until they already have the disease to start paying attention to it," she says.

The Risk for Women

While men can get osteoporosis, women are at much greater risk. An estimated 25 million Americans have the disease, and four-fifths of them are women. Hip fractures are a particular problem. The rate of hip fractures is two or three times higher in women than in men, and osteoporosis is the underlying cause of many of these injuries.

Bones tend to get stronger and build up through the teen years and into the twenties and thirties, says Dr. Kaye. In other words, the osteoblasts, or bone-building cells, outpace the osteoclasts, or bone-destroying cells, and bone continues to get stronger. When you're between 25 and 40, the bone reaches its maximum strength, she says.

Afterward, the process that leads to bone buildup slows down. That is, the osteoclasts take the lead, and bone loss is greater than bone buildup. "At that point, you start to lose bone strength as the bones become thinner and thinner," Dr. Kaye says.

So bones can lose density just through aging. But there are two reasons women are at greater risk for osteoporosis, says Dr. Kaye. The first is that for whatever reason, women tend to achieve lower bone mass than men do. So whatever decline takes place after 40 affects their bones faster. The second is that women's bone loss accelerates at menopause. Estrogen helps stimulate bone growth; in addition, "estrogen improves the intestinal absorption of calcium," says Lorraine A. Fitzpatrick, M.D., associate professor of medicine at the Mayo Clinic and Mayo Foundation in Rochester, Minnesota. So when estrogen levels decline, there's not enough to protect bone, and that's when density drops.

Postmenopausal women lose about 2 to 3 percent of their bone density per year, and the loss continues at that rate for the first five to ten years after menopause. While that may not seem like much, if bone loss continues at that rate for a number of years, the total bone loss can be substantial. If a woman loses 3 percent per year over ten years, that's a 30 percent decrease in bone strength.

This substantial drop in bone density at menopause and during the first ten years after is the reason doctors often recommend that women take hormone replacement therapy (HRT), a formulation of hormones that replenishes a woman's declining level of estrogen. Research indicates that the use of HRT can decrease the risk of osteoporosis-related hip fractures by 50 percent. If you already have osteoporosis, HRT may increase bone density by as much as 5 percent.

How long women need to take HRT for it to be effective is a matter of debate. The Framingham Osteoporosis Study, which analyzed the bone density of 670 white women from the Framingham Study—which began in 1948 and followed women through their lives to evaluate risks for heart disease—indicates that HRT was most effective in women who took it for at least seven years. The study also found that women who took HRT for seven to ten years and then stopped were protected against declining bone strength only until the age of 75.

How the Risks Go On

Just the fact that you're a woman places you at risk for osteoporosis, but a slew of other risk factors are involved, ranging from things you can control, like your diet, to things you can't, like your family history.

If you're Caucasian or Asian, you're more likely to be affected by osteoporosis than if you're African American, says Dr. Kaye. And if someone in your family, say your mother or grandmother, has had the disease, that places you at increased risk as well, she says.

Although researchers aren't clear how the disease gets passed through the generations, there's some indication that a "vitamin D" gene may have something to do with it. Research from Australia indicates that there are different types of vitamin D receptors and that some are associated with good bone density, while others are associated with bad bone density, says Dr. Fitzpatrick. Women who inherit a certain type of vitamin D receptor may be more at risk for osteoporosis. The ultimate hope is to develop a screening test that could tell which women are at greater risk and that such a test could motivate high-risk women to take preventive measures early on, says Dr. Fitzpatrick.

Women whose diets are low in calcium are also at greater risk, says Dr. Kaye. Calcium is one of the central building blocks for bone, so if you're not getting enough, new bone can't form to replenish old. The National Institutes of Health recommend that premenopausal women get at least 1,000 milligrams of calcium a day, though many doctors recommend increasing that to 1,200 milligrams. Menopausal and postmenopausal women need more—about 1,500 milligrams.

Leading a sedentary lifestyle also places you at risk. Exercise such as walking or running, which places weight-bearing stress on bones, stimulates the bone tissue and triggers bone growth.

Women who smoke have also been found to be at increased risk. The reason is unclear, but experts suspect that smoking enhances the metabolism of estrogen, making less available to feed bone growth.

Overweight women appear to have somewhat less risk of bone fractures than women with low body weight. Possibly this is because extra weight stimulates additional bone formation. In addition, heavy women have more fat stores, which convert androgen hormones to estrogen, so they may have more estrogen available to spur bone growth.

But women who have been on and off diets, a phenomenon called yo-yo dieting, and women who have or have had an eating disorder, may be at increased risk because their bodies have been deprived of proper nutrition. And women who have amenorrhea (lack of menstrual periods), either because of an eating disorder or through exercise, may also be at increased risk. Since the absence of periods indicates a decline in estrogen, these women may be lacking the levels of estrogen necessary to stimulate bone growth.

Certain diseases and medications can be responsible for osteoporosis, experts say. Women with certain thyroid diseases, cancer, liver disease and rheumatoid arthritis are at greater risk for osteoporosis, says Dr. Fitzpatrick. And medications, particularly steroid hormones and anti-seizure medications, can contribute to the development of osteoporosis.

No Time like the Present

The stronger your bones are when you hit menopause, the better. If you're between 30 and 50 and haven't hit menopause yet, there's a lot you can do now to build up and maintain your bone strength.

GET YOUR CALCIUM. The typical American diet includes only about 300 milligrams of calcium, so most women need to add a lot more. Each serving of dairy food—an eight-ounce glass of low-fat milk, a cup of low-fat yogurt, a hunk of cheese—is worth about 300 milligrams. So aim to eat three additional servings of dairy foods a day.

DON'T FEAR THE FAT. Don't shy away from dairy products because of their fat content. Practically every dairy product out there is available in a low-fat version, says Laurie Gibson Lindberg, director of patient education and information at the National Osteoporosis Foundation in Washington, D.C. Milk, yogurt, cheese and cottage cheese all come in low-fat and nonfat forms, she says.

SUPPLEMENT YOUR DIET. Another quick, easy, fat-free way to add calcium to your diet is to take calcium supplements. "The most economical is calcium carbonate," says Dr. Rosen. Take supplements with a meal to aid absorbtion of the calcium from the stomach.

Read the label on your bottle of calcium supplements carefully. "Look at the fine print," says Dr. Kaye. Look to see how many grams of your tablet are considered "elemental" or "bioavailable"—that's the form of calcium that your body will absorb. If you're taking a 750-milligram supplement, probably only 300 milligrams will be elemental. So check to see that you are really getting the amount you think you are.

LOOK AGAIN AT THE LABEL. Check the label to see if the tablets will dissolve in time to be absorbed by the body. (If they don't dissolve within 30 minutes, they will be excreted, and the calcium won't be absorbed.) Some pills don't dissolve in the stomach in a half-hour, says Dr. Kaye. Look for something like "this calcium supplement has passed the rigorous 30-minute dissolution test," she says. This will confirm that the pill has been tested for dissolvability.

CHECK THE PILLS YOURSELF. Test whether your calcium supplements will dissolve in your stomach in time through a simple home test. Put some vinegar in a glass, then put a supplement in it and let it sit for half an hour, says Dr. Kaye. Vinegar has roughly the same pH as the acid in your stomach, so if you come back after a half-hour and the supplement is dissolved, you can rest assured that your supplements will be absorbed by your body. If the pills you purchased don't dissolve, don't take them; try another brand. You might consider chewable calcium carbonate tablets (Tums) so dissolvability isn't a problem.

SET A TIME TO TAKE IT. Plan to take your calcium at a specific time each day to make taking it a habit, says Lindberg.

GET A MOVE ON. Weight-bearing and impact-loading exercise have been shown to stimulate bone growth, so do your best to get enough. Generally, three sessions a week of about 20 to 30 minutes each are sufficient, says Dr. Kaye. But "if you can do more, that's wonderful," she adds. Things like walking, running, aerobics, or climbing stairs are best, whereas non–weight-bearing exercise like swimming is of little help. "Walking is one exercise that almost anyone can do that's good," says Dr. Kaye. Pick an exercise you like, adds Dr. Rosen.

STAY STRONG. "Work on strengthening your lower extremities," says Dr. Rosen. Fractures tend to happen when people fall, and people often fall because they're weak, he says. So strengthening your leg, hip, thigh and back muscles through weight training will help you build and maintain your strength and may help prevent a fall.

GIVE UP THE CIGS. Quit smoking or cut back as much as you can. Smoking increases your risk for osteoporosis. Researchers suspect it's because smoking accelerates the metabolism of estrogen, making less available to stimulate bone growth.

CUT OUT CAFFEINE. Reduce your caffeine intake as much as you can. While the results are contradictory, some studies indicate there may be a link between high caffeine intake and osteoporosis. The thinking is that caffeine may draw calcium from the bone and also cause it to be excreted rather than absorbed, since caffeine increases urination. If you're drinking about two cups a day, you probably don't have to worry, says Dr. Kaye. It's women who are drinking five cups or more a day who should try to cut back. Try weaning yourself off caffeine by mixing your caffeinated coffee with decaf a little at a time, she says.

GET YOUR D. Vitamin D plays a key role in helping your body absorb calcium, so do your best to get enough. The current Daily Value is 400 international units. A cheap and easy way to get an adequate amount of vitamin D is to take a multivitamin, says Dr. Rosen. Because it is toxic in high doses, doctors do not advise taking vitamin D supplements with more than 800 international units.

Getting your vitamin D from milk is another possibility, but the amount of D in milk is not closely regulated, says Dr. Rosen. Many foods, including cereals, are fortified with vitamin D.

SCHEDULE A FAMILY VISIT. If it's an option, take your mother and daughters with you to the doctor for a joint visit, says Dr. Fitzpatrick. That way the doctor can get a full family history and recommend some preventive measures for all the women in the family.

What to Do at Menopause

If you're in menopause, you're at higher risk for osteoporosis because your estrogen levels are declining. Here are some things to consider.

CONSIDER HRT. Weigh the pros and cons of hormone replacement therapy with your doctor. By replacing diminishing levels of estrogen, HRT helps prevent the dramatic bone loss that occurs during menopause.

If your main objective for taking HRT is to prevent osteoporosis, you probably should continue taking it for at least seven years, research indicates. The therapy will prevent bone loss while you are taking it, but once you stop, bone density starts to decline again, experts say.

SEE YOUR DOCTOR. Even if you have decided that you don't want to take HRT, it's a good idea to be evaluated by a doctor to see if you have any other medical conditions that might increase your risk for osteoporosis, says Dr. Fitzpatrick. Contact the National Osteoporosis Foundation at 1150 17th Street NW, Suite 500, Washington, DC 20036 for a list of doctors who have a special interest in osteoporosis.

GET SCREENED. If you're not going to take HRT, you should probably undergo a screening test to assess your bone mineral density. Different tests are available.

KEEP EXERCISING. Stay as active as you can through menopause; any weight-bearing activity or weight-lifting exercise you can do will stimulate your bone and help you maintain the bone mass you already have. It's best to consult a doctor and have a physical before embarking on any exercise program.

BOOST THAT CALCIUM. Increase the amount of calcium you take in to about 1,500 milligrams a day, experts say. Women in menopause require more calcium because as they get older, the absorption of calcium from the intestines drops, says Dr. Fitzpatrick.

Ovarian Cancer

FRIGHTENING BUT
FREQUENTLY PREVENTABLE

One year after she was diagnosed with ovarian cancer, Christine Peloghitis, director of student services at Allentown College in Pennsylvania, embarked on a 2,935-mile foot race from Huntington Beach, California, to New York City.

Peloghitis entered the race not knowing if the surgery she'd had to remove one ovary and part of another had cured her cancer. But Peloghitis, who managed to finish 1,000 miles in nearly 22 days of running, did know this: At age 27 she wanted to be the toughest woman this disease had ever attacked. So far, she's succeeding in her fight against it.

"Ovarian cancer is the fifth leading cause of cancer deaths in the United States," says Michael Muto, M.D., co-director of the Familial Ovarian Cancer Center at Brigham and Women's Hospital in Boston and assistant professor of obstetrics and gynecology and reproductive biology at Harvard Medical School. Its only symptoms are the common complaints of bloating, constipation and a swollen waistline. It attacks 24,000 women every year—5 out of every 100,000 women over age 30, 8 of every 100,000 women over age 35 and 12 of every 100,000 women over age 40. A woman's risk of getting the disease over her entire life span is 1 in 80.

While the chances that Peloghitis would develop ovarian cancer were low, the chances that she'll survive it are high.

Younger women like Peloghitis who are of childbearing age are more likely to get a lazy, slow-growing tumor with what doctors call low malignant potential, meaning it takes a long time to invade other parts of the body. Older women, particularly postmenopausal women in their fifties, are more likely to develop invasive epithelial cancer, that is, cancer that grows rapidly and literally strangles organs, like the bowels, then rapidly spreads to other parts of the abdomen. Any woman of any age, however, can develop either type of ovarian cancer.

When tumors with low malignant potential are confined to the ovary, surgical removal results in a cure rate of 90 percent, Dr. Muto says. Even if the tumor spreads to other parts of the abdomen, the survival rate is better than that for epithelial cancer, which spreads more aggressively.

"Our track record in treating advanced disease is quite poor," says Dr. Muto. "Take a look at the survival rates in 1969 and then again in 1994. Just pull an old book out of the library, look up the survival rates over the last 30 years and you won't find a bit of difference."

Who's at Risk?

One of the difficulties in finding better ways to treat ovarian cancer is that its cause is still a mystery.

Some scientists feel it's caused by a gene that has been preprogrammed by heredity to cause trouble. Women who have a mother, sister or daughter with ovarian cancer have a 1-in-20 chance of getting the disease themselves, says Dr. Muto. Women who have two or more close relatives with the disease have a 3-in-10 chance of getting it. And the rare woman who has a defect in the gene that has been identified as a cause of ovarian and breast cancer has an 8-in-10 chance of getting one or both diseases.

Still, scientists point out that heredity accounts for only 5 to 7 percent of all ovarian cancer. What causes the rest?

Some scientists feel that it's triggered by a virus or a chemical carcinogen that travels from outside the body through the vagina and cervix, into the uterus and out through the fallopian tubes into the abdominal cavity, where the rich hormonal mix from a woman's reproductive system promotes malignant growth.

But others suspect the cause is more direct. "It may have something to do with the trauma and wound healing experienced by the ovary," says Alice Whittemore, Ph.D., professor of epidemiology and biostatistics at Stanford University Medical School, who has conducted epidemiological research on ovarian cancer.

"Every month an egg literally bursts through the outer layer of this walnut-size ovary. It's then caught by the fallopian tube and sent on its way to the uterus. The trauma of ovulation, followed by the repeated wound healing, may set off the cancer."

The Best Protection

The data suggests, says Dr. Whittemore, that "the more you ovulate, the higher your risk."

That's why the common denominator of most strategies that researchers suggest to reduce risk involves reducing the number of times you ovulate over your life span. Here's what they have in mind.

TAKE THE PILL. "Data suggest as much as half of ovarian cancer can be prevented if we use the Pill for four years sometime before menopause," says Dr. Whittemore. "Since 24,000 women get the disease every year, that means we could save 12,000 women every year."

GET PREGNANT. Women who don't have children have twice the risk of ovarian cancer of women who have two or three, says Dr. Whittemore.

BREASTFEED. "Breastfeeding also reduces risk," says Dr. Whittemore. In fact, breastfeeding for a total of 12 to 24 months can reduce your risk of ovarian cancer by about one-third.

POWDER YOUR NOSE, NOT YOUR BOTTOM. A study of more than 400 women at Harvard Medical School found that women who used talc on their genitals on a daily basis for many years were three times more likely to get ovarian cancer than women who did not.

"The female genital tract is wide open," says Dr. Muto. "Anything you put on your external genitals will get into your abdomen. It goes into your vagina, into your uterus, into your tubes and right on out to your ovaries. So the talcum powder can get right up there."

Since few talc fibers have actually been found within an ovarian tumor, however, Dr. Muto is not so sure that the talc causes cancer.

Nevertheless, he adds, until more research has been done, it's probably a good idea to forgo the powder.

EAT GREEN AND ORANGE VEGETABLES. A study of 213 women at Ohio State University found that loading up on foods rich in beta-carotene, such as dark leafy greens, carrots and sweet potatoes, reduces the risk of ovarian cancer. Even eating as few as three medium carrots every five days was associated with fewer cases of cancer.

JUMP UP AND DOWN. A collaborative study between the National Cancer Institute in Bethesda, Maryland, and the Shanghai Cancer Institute in China indicated that women who hold jobs requiring lots of physical activity may have a reduced incidence of ovarian cancer. Women in the study who sat for long periods of time on the job had an increased incidence of the disease; women who were more active had less.

TIE YOUR TUBES. Having your fallopian tubes tied when you're finished with childbearing also reduces your risk, says Dr. Whittemore. A study of more than 120,000 nurses at Harvard Medical School revealed that women who got their tubes tied reduced their risk of ovarian cancer by 67 percent.

Researchers don't know why tying the tubes cuts your risk, adds Dr. Whittemore, but some researchers suspect that it prevents various contaminants from reaching the ovaries.

"My own bias is that it impedes blood flow to the ovaries," says Dr. Whittemore, "but so far surgeons won't admit the possibility."

THINK TWICE ABOUT OVARY REMOVAL. Only women with two or more close family members who have ovarian cancer should even consider having their ovaries removed as a preventive tactic, concluded a panel of experts at a National Institutes of Health conference on ovarian cancer. And they should consider it only after childbearing is complete.

Although getting rid of your ovaries sounds like a good way to prevent ovarian cancer, in women with a strong family history of the disease, it does not reduce the risk of ovarian-like cancers growing somewhere else in the abdominal cavity, says Dr. Muto.

Overweight
TAKE AIM AT A SLIMMER SHAPE

Judging from the tidal waves of low-fat foods washing up on supermarket shelves and the multitude of health clubs popping up in cities, you'd think that America had become the land of the lean and the home of the fit.

Not by a long shot. In fact, one in three Americans—the highest number ever—is now seriously overweight, the National Center for Health Statistics in Bethesda, Maryland, has reported. Experts call obesity an epidemic—and it's one that's spawning major health problems in women. Heart disease, endometrial cancer and possibly breast cancer, high blood pressure, high cholesterol, immune problems, gallstones, gout, diabetes, osteoarthritis, stroke and sleep apnea are all associated with overweight.

But do we really know what our healthiest weight is? How many of us are on target? And what are those who *are* on target doing differently from those who *aren't*?

To answer these questions, *Prevention* Magazine surveyed women readers and got more than 10,000 responses. Here's an overview of the survey results.

Frustrations of Fat-Fighting

Frustration fairly leaped off the pages of the responses. Ninety percent of the respondents confessed they needed to lose weight (on average, 27 pounds). Only 14 percent described themselves as "well-toned," and just 7 percent said they were "very satisfied" with their bodies. More than half admitted they were "not very" or "not at all" satisfied.

But are so many female fat-fighters really overweight, or do we just want to look slimmer?

In the opinion of top medical researchers and experts on obesity, many of the respondents had valid reasons for being concerned about their weight.

"Slimmer is definitely healthier," observes William P. Castelli, M.D., medical director of the famed Framingham Heart Study, which followed 5,000 Massachusetts residents for 40 years to assess their risk for heart disease.

Fortunately, researchers are exploring ways to evaluate optimal body weight based on the latest research on weight-related health risks. Two approaches, used together, are emerging as the new "gold standard" for such evaluations: body mass index and waist/hip ratio.

An Index of Your Risk

Body mass index (BMI) is a ratio of height to weight. It's determined by a mathematical formula: First you divide your weight (in pounds) by your height (in inches) squared, then multiply the resulting number by 705. You should get a BMI that's somewhere between 19 and 30. But you don't have to do the calculations: just see "Calculating Your BMI" on page 396.

Several large medical studies, involving thousands of people, have suggested that 21 to 22 is the optimal BMI. At this level, there are no weight-related health risks, according to Dr. Castelli.

One large-scale study that points to a BMI below 22 as ideal for preventing heart disease in women is the Nurses' Health Study, based at Harvard University and Brigham and Women's Hospital in Boston. In it, researchers followed 115,886 initially healthy American women ages 30 to 55 for eight years. During that time, 605 of the women experienced coronary artery disease, leading to 83 deaths.

There was no elevated risk of heart disease among women whose BMIs were under 21 (the lean group). For women whose BMI was between 21 and 25, the risk of heart disease was 30 percent higher. It was 80 percent higher for women with a BMI between 25 and 29. And women whose BMI was greater than 29 had more than twice the risk of heart disease (230 percent) of those with a BMI under 21.

"Obesity is a strong risk factor for coronary heart disease in middle-aged women," the researchers concluded. "Even mild-to-moderate overweight is associated with a substantial elevation in coronary risk." Other large-scale studies have reached similar conclusions.

Safety Measures

Beyond heart disease, there seems to be a broader safety range. A BMI between 23 and 25 isn't ideal, some experts insist, but the excess risk for cancer and other weight-related diseases seems to be small at that level. Around a BMI of roughly 26, these health risks appear to rise, although scientists don't agree on exactly where to draw the line.

Most scientists do agree that a BMI over 27 increases risk for many people. But risk also depends on other factors, including waist/hip ratio, notes Jean Pierre Despres, Ph.D., associate director of the Lipid Research Center at Laval University in St. Foy, Quebec.

Researchers have determined that the fat most associated with health risks is on the upper body—the abdomen and above—rather than on the thighs and hips. (A pattern of upper-body fat is often called central obesity.)

Some Hip Calculations

One way to judge whether you have too much upper-body fat is by measuring your waist (at the midpoint between your bottom rib and your hipbone) and your hips (at their widest point). Then divide the waist measurement by the hip measurement. The resulting number is your waist/hip ratio (WHR).

If your waist is 30 inches and your hips are 37 inches, for example, you would divide 30 by 37 to get a WHR of 0.81.

What's an ideal WHR? While scientists quibble over hundredths of a percent, most target 0.80 or less as desirable for both women and men.

This technique isn't very reliable for women who are very thin or very overweight. But in most cases, it can prove very predictive of cardiovascular disease risk.

"Central obesity is turning out to be the most lethal risk factor associated with excess body weight," says Dr. Castelli. That's because upper-body fat is strongly correlated with visceral fat, which is fat that's packed around our internal organs.

While more of the research on the health risks of upper-body fat has been done with men, more research with women is beginning. Researchers at the University of Miami School of Medicine and the

CALCULATING YOUR BMI

To find your body mass index, or BMI, locate your height in the left column. (If you've lost inches over the years, use your peak adult height.) Move across the chart to the right until

HEIGHT	BODY WEIGHT IN POUNDS					
4'10"	91	96	100	105	110	115
4'11"	94	99	104	109	114	119
5'0"	97	102	107	112	118	123
5'1"	100	106	111	116	122	127
5'2"	104	109	115	120	126	131
5'3"	107	113	118	124	130	135
5'4"	110	116	122	128	134	140
5'5"	114	120	126	132	138	144
5'6"	118	124	130	136	142	148
5'7"	121	127	134	140	146	153
5'8"	125	131	138	144	151	158
5'9"	128	135	142	149	155	162
5'10"	132	139	146	153	160	167
5'11"	136	143	150	157	165	172
6'0"	140	147	154	162	169	177
BMI	19	20	21	22	23	24

University of Minnesota School of Public Health, for example, examined data on 32,898 healthy women ages 55 to 69. In a four-year period, there were nearly three times as many heart disease deaths among women with the highest WHR (over 0.86) as among women with the lowest.

A high WHR has also been associated with diabetes, hypertension, breast and endometrial cancers and high cholesterol.

Dr. Castelli is one of several scientists who believe that WHR is even more important than BMI in predicting risk. "If someone has a

you find your approximate weight. Then follow that column down to the corresponding BMI number at the bottom of the chart. For optimal health, your BMI should be in the 21 or 22 range.

119	124	129	134	138	143	148	153
124	128	133	138	143	148	153	158
128	133	138	143	148	153	158	163
132	137	143	148	153	158	164	169
136	142	147	153	158	164	169	174
141	146	152	158	163	169	175	180
145	151	157	163	169	174	180	186
150	156	162	168	174	180	186	192
155	161	167	173	179	186	192	198
159	166	172	178	185	191	197	204
164	171	177	184	190	197	203	210
169	176	182	189	196	203	209	216
174	181	188	195	202	207	215	222
179	186	193	200	208	215	222	229
184	191	199	206	213	221	228	235
25	26	27	28	29	30	31	32

healthy body mass index but a high WHR, it is important to try to bring that WHR down," he explains. "Someone with a higher BMI but a low WHR might not be quite as bad off."

Overweight or Overfat?

According to weight-control experts, some women may be confusing overweight with overfat. If you're in the "optimal" range, you may not need to lose pounds. But even so, you may need to lose fat and improve muscle tone.

Along with BMI and WHR, muscle tone does have relevance to health risks and weight. After all, scientists agree that the danger of overweight generally is not from heavy bones or muscles; it's from excess fat.

Exact standards don't exist for how much body fat a person can carry without increasing risk, but at the Cooper Aerobics Center in Dallas, they aim for 18 to 22 percent of total weight as optimal for women, slightly higher than for men.

Unfortunately, it's not easy to determine percentage of body fat. There are several ways to go about it, from pinching skin folds with calipers to bioelectric impedance (running a mild current through the body to measure resistance) to underwater weighing. These methods are not widely available outside health clubs or specialists' offices and are not always reliable.

But you can often eyeball it, according to Joan Marie Conway, Ph.D., research chemist at the U.S. Department of Agriculture (USDA) Human Nutrition Research Center in Beltsville, Maryland. An easy way to judge whether you're overfat is by looking in a mirror, she explains. If, despite good BMI and WHR numbers, you look flabby, you probably are. And you'd do well to embark on an exercise regimen that burns fat and tones muscle.

Through all the weighing and measuring, it's important not to get too hung up on the scale or measuring tape, she adds. "You could never use one number to tell someone their risk for disease," says Dr. Conway.

Other doctors agree. "There are other factors, like family history, good and bad health habits like smoking and exercising or personal health risks like high cholesterol, low HDL cholesterol (the good kind) or high blood pressure to consider, too," says Dr. Despres. "People with more risk factors must be more careful of their weight."

Clearly, finding your perfect weight for health is not yet a precise science. But it's safer to err on the side of slender, says Dr. Castelli. "You may be on the borderline today, but where are you going to be five years from now? Get in the habit of controlling your weight before you have a problem, not after."

Flexing Your Way to Success

Many of the women who responded to the *Prevention* survey found that weight loss wasn't so hard. The toughest challenge, many said, was keeping the weight off. For them, exercise was an important factor. Forty-eight percent of the women with optimal weight were in the habit of exercising four or more times weekly.

Based on the experience of these women, here are some exercise tips that will help you go the extra mile.

STRETCH YOUR EXERCISE TIME. "It's known that the only way to maintain weight loss forever is to increase the amount of physical activity you do," says Miriam Nelson, Ph.D., research scientist at the USDA Human Nutrition Research Center on Aging at Tufts University in Boston.

"People with desk jobs think, `I walk up and down stairs a lot and I run around doing household chores in the evening—I get plenty of exercise'; even if that adds up to 90 minutes of physical activity, it's not enough," says Dr. Conway. "You need intentional exercise like fitness walking or cycling to call yourself anything but sedentary."

Indeed, though women of optimal weight were no more active in their daily lives than overweight respondents, they did participate in more intentional exercise. In the optimal weight group, most women said their workout sessions lasted between a half-hour and an hour. Severely overweight women most commonly report the shortest exercise sessions—less than 20 minutes.

GO FOR PLEASURE. To exercise consistently, of course, you must find a form of exercise (or a combination of exercises) that you actually enjoy. "It needs to be something people like and feel they can continue doing indefinitely," says James O. Hill, Ph.D., associate director of the Center for Human Nutrition at the University of Colorado Health Sciences Center in Denver.

For people at risk from overweight, Dr. Despres recommends walking, walking, walking. The risk of injury is lower than for many other exercises. "We have shown that this is an excellent form of exercise to decrease excess abdominal fat and the complications associated with it," he explains.

"Even if you don't lose a lot of weight, your risk profile will improve with a brisk 45-minute walk four or five days a week," he continues. "If you don't exercise that much, you won't burn enough fat to get the substantial improvement in your risk profile that you'd see with that program."

WEIGHT UP. The *Prevention* survey also revealed that women who have optimal body weight do more strength training. Thirty-five percent of those in the optimal group were hefting small weights or using resistance machines to strengthen muscle, compared with 14 percent or fewer of those in heavier groups.

Why is strength training so important to maintaining healthy body weight? "Large muscle mass helps burn calories," Dr. Nelson explains. "More muscle means a faster metabolism." That's because muscle requires more oxygen and more calories to sustain itself than fat does. And strength training is more effective than aerobic exercise at building and maintaining muscle.

Some Food Advice

Of course, low-fat eating goes hand-in-hand with exercise. "When you combine strength training and aerobic exercise with sensible eating, you'll look trimmer, feel more fit and be able to eat more," observes Wayne Westcott, Ph.D., strength consultant to the YMCA of USA, IDEA: International Association of Fitness Professionals and the American Council on Exercise.

But how do you find comfortable limits without going on a diet? Here are the strategies recommended by experts.

LEARN YOUR BODY SIGNALS. Have you lost the ability to distinguish between emotional and physiological hunger and just plain boredom? If you have, your best bet to dump those unnecessary pounds and maintain a stable weight is to tap into what your body wants and doesn't want, says Steven C. Strauss, M.D., an internist in New York City specializing in nutrition and weight control and author of *The Body Signal Secret.*

As you eat, become aware of how you feel when you're satisfied, when you're full and when you're stuffed, Dr. Strauss advises. Then decide to stop eating whenever you hit the full mark. "If you eat only when you're hungry and stop when you're satisfied, your body will reach its optimal weight," says Dr. Strauss.

MULTIPLY MEALS, SHRINK PORTIONS. If you're a devotee of three meals a day, you may be consuming more calories than you need at those meals and storing the rest as fat. That's because "your body can only use a certain amount of calories at a time to function," says Debra Waterhouse, R.D., author of *Outsmarting the Female Fat Cell.* Eating four or five mini-meals a day will prevent the problem.

BREAK THE MORNING FAST. "Never, ever eliminate breakfast," says Dr. Strauss. "Try to eat grains, fresh fruits and vegetables."

If "just a cup of coffee," is your basic M.O. for starting the day, your metabolism is probably sluggish, burning fewer calories than it should from subsequent meals. Since our bodies burn calories at a slower rate while we sleep, breakfast acts as reveille for our metabolism. In fact, a study at George Washington University in Washington, D.C., showed a metabolic increase of 3 to 4 percent above average in morning eaters.

FILL UP ON FIBER. "High-fiber foods promote a feeling of fullness more readily than low-fiber meals," says Dr. Strauss. So "you feel more satisfied with less food."

Try hot oatmeal for breakfast, vegetarian chili for lunch and five-bean casserole for dinner. Aim for 35 grams of fiber a day. (For good sources of fiber, see page 122.)

FORGO EXCESS FAT. Fat calories are much harder to burn than calories from carbohydrates and proteins. They're also easily converted to body fat. "When you eat fat calories your body doesn't need, only a tiny fraction are used to digest and metabolize the fat; the rest store themselves in your fat cells," says Dr. Strauss. That's why you should keep fat calories to 25 percent or less of your daily diet.

How? First, avoid deep-fried or breaded and fried foods. Instead, go for broiled, grilled or baked fish and skinless chicken. Use a nonstick pan or oil sprays or chicken broth for sautéing. Try evaporated skim milk as a substitute for whole milk or cream.

Also, be sure to trim the fat off all meats before cooking. And for sweet treats, reach for fruit and nonfat products. Just be sure to read labels and check how much fat is in each product. "If the percentage of fat is greater than 15 percent, you may want to replace that item on the shelf," says Dr. Strauss.

Painful Intercourse
Bringing Back the Pleasure

You and your partner begin making love one night. You're in the mood and plenty excited, but when you start having intercourse, it hurts so much you can't continue. So you stop, leaving the two of you frustrated, unsatisfied, disappointed and concerned.

If this scenario sounds familiar, you're not alone. Many women experience painful intercourse. Doctors call it dyspareunia, and it's estimated that 10 to 50 percent of all sexually active women will have it at some time, says Richard A. Carroll, Ph.D., director of the Sex and Marital Therapy Program at the Northwestern Medical Faculty Foundation of the Northwestern University Medical Center in Chicago.

The problem—how it feels and what causes it—varies widely from woman to woman. Some women have pain during thrusting because of fibroids, chronic constipation, pelvic infections, endometriosis, hemorrhoids, pelvic inflammatory disease or surgical scar tissue. Others have pain with penetration because of insufficient lubrication, yeast infections, sexually transmitted diseases (STDs), allergic reactions to contraceptive products or an improperly healed episiotomy—the surgical incision that's made during vaginal childbirth. And some women can't even begin intercourse: They have vaginismus, a condition in which the opening of the vagina closes, making penetration painful or even impossible.

In all its different forms, painful intercourse is something women need to pay attention to. Yet not all do. Even today, a lot of women assume that discomfort during sex is kind of normal, says Jo Kessler, a licensed nurse-practitioner and certified sex therapist in San Diego. But women need to realize that intercourse is not supposed to hurt and that if it does, it's the body's signal that something is wrong.

When You're a Little Too Dry

A major cause of painful intercourse in women over 30 is insufficient lubrication, experts say. Hormone levels often have a lot to do with it. Estrogen plays a role in stimulating vaginal secretions, so when it's low, you may be drier. This can happen right after your period, while you're breastfeeding and during menopause, when the ovaries produce less estrogen. Medications can also be responsible. Cold formulas are one example; they contain antihistamines, which dry up mucous membranes throughout the body, including the vagina.

You also may have trouble lubricating properly if you don't become sufficiently aroused; this can happen if your partner isn't stimulating you enough or in ways that you need. "Sometimes a woman is not ready for intercourse and is not able to tell her partner what she's feeling," says Dr. Carroll. If she has sex, there can be friction and pain.

You need to be aware that it's possible for a vicious cycle to develop between physical pain and anxiety, says Dr. Carroll. "A woman may experience a little bit of friction or painful intercourse and that makes her more hesitant the next time," he says. So when she and her partner try to have sex again, she's more anxious and even less likely to become lubricated, and sex is bound to be more painful. This cycle can go on and on, often leading to a complete avoidance of sex, he says.

Insufficient lubrication can also be connected to feelings about your partner and the relationship, experts say. If you have repressed anger toward your lover or resent him, or you're just turned off that day, you may have trouble getting aroused and sufficiently lubricated, making sex painful.

When Your Body Says No

The connection between your emotions and the way your body responds to sex is even more apparent in the case of vaginismus. Here, a woman's anxiety about sex triggers a dramatic physical reaction: The muscles of her pelvic floor spasm and her vaginal opening closes, making sex difficult and often impossible.

Vaginismus is not usually caused by medical problems, says Dr. Carroll. "It's a learned physical response caused by anxiety about impending intercourse," he says. Women who've had traumatic sexual experiences, such as rape or sexual abuse, or who've been raised in households with very conservative, negative attitudes about sex, often develop it, says Dr. Carroll.

If Something's in the Way

While emotions can play a role in painful sex, sometimes the cause is strictly physical. Chronic constipation is one example. During sex, the wall of the vagina gets pinched between two hard objects, the man's thrusting penis and the stool sitting in the colon, says Kessler. Because the wall of the vagina is sensitive to this compression, it hurts, she says. Fibroids or endometriosis can cause similar problems. If there are growths in the uterus or endometrial tissue outside it, during sexual intercourse it can feel as if the penis is bumping against a bruised area.

Sometimes sex is painful because a woman's uterus is tipped backward or because her vagina is short, either congenitally or due to surgery or other medical treatments.

Another physical factor that can cause painful sex is childbirth. Some women find sex painful after they've had a baby, particularly if they've had a vaginal delivery that required an episiotomy. If sensitive scar tissue results, it can make penetration painful.

Vaginal infections, STDs such as trichomoniasis and genital warts, and allergies to contraceptive products can also cause irritation of the vaginal opening and make sex painful.

What You Can Do

There are things you can do to prevent painful intercourse or cope with it if you're already experiencing it. Here are some suggestions.

STAY HEALTHY. Since painful intercourse can be caused by medical problems, including endometriosis and fibroids, it's important to have a gynecological exam annually, experts say. Yeast infections and STDs can cause pain as well, so protect yourself. Keep the vaginal area clean, use condoms to prevent sexually transmitted diseases and get immediate treatment for vaginal irritations and infections.

NURTURE YOUR RELATIONSHIP. Negative feelings about your relationship or your partner can affect your sex life, experts say. Deal with problems as they come along, instead of letting them accumulate. Talk to your partner using "I" statements such as "I'm having a problem with . . . " instead of "you" phrases like "You always . . . ," which can place blame and cause bigger rifts. Try writing about your anger as a way to express and defuse it, says Kessler.

DON'T FORCE IT. "I talk to women about how not to have intercourse when they don't want to," says Kessler. There are other ways to be sexual. You can still have sex without putting the penis in the vagina. Talk about various options with your partner before you get in a romantic situation.

STAY LUBRICATED. If you are not sufficiently lubricated, take steps to become so. Either extend foreplay until you are naturally lubricated or use artificial lubricants. Go with a water-soluble lubricant, like Astroglide, that's best absorbed by the body, says Dr. Carroll. And be aware that your ability to lubricate may vary from day to day, he says. If you are on medications like antihistamines that make you drier, use water-soluble vaginal lubricants while you're taking them, says Kessler.

DRINK FLUIDS AND EAT BRAN. If you are constipated a lot and it causes painful sex, try increasing the amount of fluids you drink, says Kessler. And add bulk to your diet with fresh fruits, whole grains, vegetables or some form of bran. "When you clear up the constipation problem, then you don't have firm stool in the colon for the penis to thrust against," she says.

With fluids, aim for six to eight glasses a day. If you're having trouble getting to the water fountain, try a sports fluid bottle, says Kessler. Many of them hold 16 ounces, and you can fill it up three or four times a day. "Have one at breakfast, one at midmorning, one at lunch, one at dinner and one at bedtime," she says.

TRY DIFFERENT POSITIONS AND TECHNIQUES. Painful sex might be "something as simple as a position not being compatible with a woman's anatomy," says Kessler. If you're feeling discomfort with one position, try another. Having sex side by side or with the woman on top allows the woman to "control how fast and at what angle and how deep the penis is inserted into the vagina," she says.

TAKE IT SLOW AFTER PREGNANCY. Scar tissue left

behind after an episiotomy can cause discomfort, so use lots of lubrication, says Susan E. Hetherington, Dr.P.H., a certified nurse-midwife and sex therapist and professor in the School of Nursing at the University of Maryland in Baltimore. She suggests that your partner put a dab of water-soluble lubricant on his finger, then, with your assistance, gently place that finger in the vagina. You should bear down, as if going to the bathroom, and that will release the muscle that stimulates the vaginal opening. This allows his finger to slip in more. Gentle touching will relax the vagina. Then, with proper lubrication, the penis will slide in. It should be a slow process with no deep thrusting initially, she says.

KEEP A DIARY. If you are experiencing pain with sex, keep a record of what kind of pain you have and when, says Kessler.

Keep track for two to three months and look to see whether the discomfort occurs on entry or with deep thrusting, whether it only occurs while intercourse is going on or if it continues after the penis is withdrawn, whether the pain always occurs at the same time of the month and whether it happens with every position or only with one. And if a woman has multiple partners, she needs to pay attention to whether she has the pain with all partners or just one, says Kessler.

FIND THE RIGHT DOCTOR. "The main thing is to know that if it hurts, that's a signal that you need to do something about it. I always want them to get a medical exam as soon as possible," says Kessler. It's important to find a doctor who understands the problem, too. Some will do a pelvic exam and say they don't see anything, leaving the woman with the impression that it's all in her head, Kessler says. "Women need to keep seeking an answer. If one doctor says, 'I don't see anything,' and offers no other options, be persistent and get a second opinion," she says.

GET HELP FOR VAGINISMUS. Doctors do have a technique—called vaginal dilation—for helping women with vaginismus. With supervision, women first learn techniques to help them relax. Then, starting with a dilator about the size of the small finger, they learn to penetrate the vagina. Slowly, at a pace at which they are comfortable, they work their way up to a dilator that has a circumference equal to that of their partner's penis.

When women start the process, they're often anxious and scared, says Kessler. "Once they realize they won't have to jam something into the vagina and won't have to progress any faster than they are ready to, they relax, and that brings relief and results," she says.

Panic Attacks
GETTING A GRIP ON FEAR

Driving across a bridge, a young woman suddenly feels she's going to lose control. She worries she may suddenly drive off the bridge. Frantic, she stops in the middle of the road—terrified and unable to get out of the car.

Another woman begins graduate school in New York City. While riding the subway to class one day, her heart starts racing. Suddenly her palms are sweating, her breathing is rapid and she feels like she's got to get out. She gets off at the next stop and rushes home.

Finally, a woman who once dreamed of a career in acting now has a fear of leaving home. Even though she lives near the school her children attend, she cannot bring herself to go to any school events.

Each of these women has panic disorder, which affects from 3 to 5 percent of Americans. The third woman has panic disorder and also has agoraphobia, a condition in which individuals develop such an intense fear of going out that they can't leave their homes.

Twice as many women as men develop panic disorder, and as many as 5 percent of women will experience it sometime in their lives, says R. Bruce Lydiard, M.D., Ph.D., professor of psychiatry at the Institute of Psychiatry at the Medical University of South Carolina in Charleston.

Understanding the Disorder

Panic disorder usually begins between the ages of 20 and 40, says Dr. Lydiard. But women tend to develop it later than men, according to the National Comorbidity Survey conducted by the Institute for Social Research at the University of Michigan in Ann Arbor.

The disorder begins with an initial panic attack, which includes the typical symptoms of the fight-or-flight response: a racing heartbeat, hyperventilation and hot and cold flushes. An attack may also include chest pains, dizziness, trembling, shaking, sweating, choking and numbness. "These come on for some individuals as if a thunderbolt has hit," says Dr. Lydiard. With no apparent stimulus to make their bodies react this way, their internal alarm system goes off, he says.

While for some a panic attack consists of just physical symptoms, others may think they've lost control of their minds, he says. In addition to feeling like they are going crazy, some people experience an overwhelming fear of dying.

Not everyone who experiences one panic attack—and an estimated 10 percent of Americans report doing so—has panic disorder. For it to be diagnosed, according to Dr. Lydiard, there must be recurrent, unexpected panic attacks with the persistent fear of having another—or the fear of a medical or mental problem. Either the incidence of panic attacks or the fear of having an attack must persist for at least one month.

Panic disorder can be traumatic. "Most people who come in complaining of it are truly devastated by the experience," says David Katerndahl, M.D., director of research and education in the Department of Family Practice at the University of Texas Health Sciences Center in San Antonio.

"It's an extremely disabling disorder. If people develop any phobic avoidance, they tend to limit their life and their activities. They become afraid to drive, or at least drive alone. They may become afraid to leave their house and become progressively housebound. They may have to quit jobs because they feel they can't function with their panic attacks or because they can't even go to work because of their panic attacks."

Panic attacks can last from a few minutes to an hour, says Dr. Katerndahl. The most common time to have one is in the middle of the night, between 1:00 and 3:00 A.M., he says.

What's behind It

Researchers don't know exactly what causes panic disorder, but they do know there are factors that can place you at greater risk for it.

For one thing, if someone in your immediate family—a parent or sibling—has panic disorder, you may be at greater risk for developing it. In a study of 2,163 female twins conducted at the Medical College of Virginia in Richmond, researchers found that women with a family history of panic disorder had a 30 to 40 percent chance of experiencing it.

Researchers also believe there is a biochemical basis to the disorder. When the fight-or-flight response is activated, usually when the brain perceives that the body is under attack or being threatened, adrenaline is released. With panic disorder, this response is triggered spontaneously, without outside stimuli.

But what causes panic disorder to develop? That's the question that stumps researchers. In some individuals a traumatic event, such as an accident, a death in the family, a divorce or some other serious event, precedes it. Eighty percent of panic disorder patients recall experiencing a critical incident prior to their first attack.

Some women develop panic disorder around the time of a hormonal fluctuation, says Dr. Katerndahl. About one-third of women who report the problem say their attacks started during pregnancy or immediately after delivery, he says. During the two to three weeks after menstruation, many women with panic disorder tend to experience relative well-being. Then, during the week prior to the start of their next period, their panic worsens, says Dr. Lydiard.

Researchers aren't sure how hormonal changes trigger panic, but they suspect it may have something to do with fluctuations of progesterone levels and the relationship of those changes to carbon dioxide levels in the body, says Dr. Lydiard. People who have panic disorder are more sensitive to carbon dioxide than those who do not have it, he says. Experts hypothesize that in these individuals, carbon dioxide triggers a "false suffocation alarm," and the body responds with a panic attack. Progesterone is a potent respiratory stimulus. After pregnancy and prior to menstruation, progesterone drops, and as it does, carbon dioxide levels rise, says Dr. Lydiard.

The Treatment Decision

Panic disorder can be treated with cognitive behavioral therapy or with medication. "Each has advantages and disadvantages," says Dr. Lydiard. It's often a matter of patient preference, he says.

With cognitive behavioral therapy, psychologists teach patients behavioral techniques that help them overcome the panic. If a woman doesn't want to take medication, cognitive behavioral therapy can be an excellent place to start, says Dr. Lydiard.

Cognitive behavioral therapy can be a potent and long-lasting form of treatment, says Dr. Lydiard. When it works, you may not need another form of treatment, ever. The downside, he says, is that it can be expensive, and it can be hard to find health professionals who know

THE AGONY OF AGORAPHOBIA

Some individuals with panic disorder also develop a condition known as agoraphobia—an intense fear of going places or being in situations where they might not be able to get help if they have a panic attack.

From one-third to two-thirds of those who experience panic attacks have agoraphobia, says David Katerndahl, M.D., director of research and education in the Department of Family Practice at the University of Texas Health Sciences Center in San Antonio. Most are women, he says.

Agoraphobia can be terribly disabling, says Dr. Katerndahl. One woman he knew missed her daughter's wedding because she was too afraid to leave home, while another was housebound for 20 years. Many people with agoraphobia work out of their homes and depend on drugstores and grocery stores that deliver.

There's some question about what causes agoraphobia, but Dr. Katerndahl says an individual will experience a panic attack first. Agoraphobia can follow if the person associates the attack with the location where it occurred and gets anxious about returning. "Some work suggests that all you need is a single panic attack," he says. People who have no explanation for their panic attack are most at risk for agoraphobia.

how to do it well. Individuals who are trying cognitive behavioral therapy should begin to see results within three months of starting treatment. If you are not seeing any results within that period, says Dr. Lydiard, consider a new therapist or some other form of treatment.

There are a number of drugs that can be used to treat panic disorder, but the most effective are benzodiazepines, including the drug alprazolam (Xanax), says Dr. Lydiard. Among its side effects are sedation and problems with coordination and memory. Physiological dependence is a very real possibility as well, says Dr. Lydiard, but withdrawal symptoms can be eased if individuals taper off the drug properly, he says.

Another drawback to benzodiazepines for the treatment of panic disorders is that they don't work for treating depression, which often

---

So how can women who've had a panic attack prevent themselves from developing agoraphobia? "The most important thing to do is to not avoid those situations you fear. As soon as you give in to the fear, you are on the road to agoraphobia," says Dr. Katerndahl.

Most therapists suggest exposure therapy, in which a woman goes to the place she associates with her panic attack. If she had a panic attack in the mall, for instance, she would visit the mall on a schedule to reduce the fear.

Exposure therapy is also used for those who've developed agoraphobia, says Dr. Katerndahl. There is no medication to treat the problem, he says.

Some women with agoraphobia have trouble only when they are alone. They can go places and do things as long as they have company. For these women, exposure therapy would emphasize going places by themselves, says Dr. Katerndahl.

When you're practicing exposure therapy, it helps to enlist the aid of a family member or friend, says Dr. Katerndahl. He or she can help you keep records of your activities and encourage you to keep it up.

appears along with panic disorder, says Dr. Lydiard. For that reason, many physicians use antidepressants such as fluoxetine (Prozac) as the first line of treatment.

An important issue for women to consider when making their treatment choice is pregnancy. While benzodiazepines and antidepressants have not been shown to be harmful during pregnancy, says Dr. Lydiard, one never knows. Women should plan to stop taking any medication before getting pregnant.

Getting Help

You don't have to be a prisoner of panic disorder. Here's some advice to help you cope.

FIND THE RIGHT DOCTOR. If you think you may have panic disorder, find a doctor and begin treatment. The treatment recommended depends on the type of doctor you see, says Dr. Katerndahl. Psychologists are more likely to recommend cognitive behavior therapy, whereas family doctors and psychiatrists may lean more in the direction of medication.

Some health professionals don't recognize panic disorder, says Dr. Katerndahl. If you don't get a satisfactory explanation of your symptoms or don't get your questions answered, find another doctor.

DON'T BE ASHAMED. Panic disorder is not a psychological problem or an inherent personality flaw, says Dr. Lydiard. People around you may not understand what you are going through, but "this should be considered a medical condition just like migraine headaches or peptic ulcer or any other treatable medical condition," he says.

Should you require treatment over the long term, you should not view that as an inherent weakness, he says. The fact that doctors may use psychological techniques to treat panic disorder does not mean it's a purely psychological problem, he says.

CONSIDER A SUPPORT GROUP. Support groups can be effective, says Diane Sholomskas, M.D., professor in the Department of Psychiatry at Yale University School of Medicine. The Anxiety Disorders Association of America has an Anxiety Disorders Self-Help Group Network; you can contact them at 6000 Executive Boulevard, Suite 513, Rockville, MD 20852.

Pelvic Inflammatory Disease

WHAT IT IS—AND ISN'T

For a long time Sarah didn't know she had pelvic inflammatory disease (PID). She had suffered bouts of pelvic pain and fever, but she lacked some classic signs of the disease, so doctors didn't detect it right away.

More than three years later, they did.

Sarah had PID caused by sexually transmitted diseases (STDs) that had gone undiscovered. She was married and doctors didn't think STDs could be an issue. But two infections, mycoplasma and chlamydia, had been bouncing back and forth between Sarah and her husband for who knows how long. In Sarah, the STDs invaded her upper reproductive tract, causing PID.

The disease had moved into her fallopian tubes, causing tremendous pain. Doctors wanted to perform a hysterectomy, but Sarah hadn't had children yet, and she was determined to find someone to help her. Eventually she found a doctor in New York who could. With surgery and antibiotics, he treated her successfully, and she went on to have two healthy children.

Sarah is one of the lucky ones. Others aren't so fortunate. In many cases, PID goes undetected for so long that it robs women of their fertility and reproductive health.

Understanding PID

PID is an upper genital tract infection that's diagnosed in an estimated one million American women every year. The disease often (but not always) develops when an STD in a woman's lower genital tract goes unchecked. The infection moves into the upper genital tract and PID develops. The disease can cause discomfort and pain—or show no signs at all, making it difficult for doctors to diagnose. One in four women who get PID experiences complications, including ectopic (tubal) pregnancy, infertility, recurrent pain and recurrent PID. Infertility occurs in 12 percent of women with PID after they've had it once, 25 percent after two occurrences and 50 percent after three or more episodes.

There are several theories on how organisms move up from the vagina into the uterus. Some experts say it is possible that organisms initially attach to the cervix. Then, during menstruation, hormonal and cervical changes occur that make it easier for the organisms to pass through the cervical opening into the uterus: A mucus plug that seals off the uterus during the other phases of the cycle is expelled at menstruation, and the cervix is open for organisms to pass through. Others believe that the organisms attach to sperm and essentially hitch a ride up.

The uterus is normally a sterile environment, so when bacteria or sexually transmitted organisms that don't belong there enter, trouble may develop. The organisms can penetrate the endometrium, or lining of the uterus, causing an inflammatory condition known as endometritis, which may be painful. They can also attack the fallopian tube, infecting and damaging its lining. This inflammation, called salpingitis, is painful and can hamper a woman's ability to become pregnant.

Infections in these areas, as well as the ovaries and lining of the pelvic area, make up PID.

Who's at Risk

Because PID is usually caused by STDs, having multiple partners and having unprotected sex are the major risk factors, says Joseph

Apuzzio, M.D., professor of obstetrics and gynecology and director of the Division of Prenatal Diagnosis and Infectious Diseases at the New Jersey School of Medicine in Newark. But other factors may play a role, too.

Frequent douching may put women at increased risk for PID. One study showed that the risk for women who douched was twice that of women who never douched, and the risk of PID increased as frequency of douching increased.

Smoking may even play a role in PID. One study showed that women who smoked were at greater risk for PID than those who never smoked, and women who smoked ten or more cigarettes per day were at greater risk than those who smoked less.

The intrauterine device (IUD) has also been implicated in placing women at increased risk for PID. Researchers say women are most at risk during the first four months after they've had an IUD inserted. "The initial risk is really from the insertion," says Dr. Apuzzio. If certain bacteria normally present in a woman's vagina get onto the IUD during insertion and get up into the uterus, they can cause infection of the uterus and fallopian tubes, he says. So after an IUD is inserted, women need to tell their doctors of any discomfort, discharge or pain.

Whether oral contraceptives increase the risk for PID is unclear. The consensus among researchers is that oral contraceptives increase the risk of contracting chlamydia if you are exposed to it, says Nancy S. Padian, Ph.D., associate adjunct professor in the Department of Obstetrics, Gynecology and Reproductive Sciences at the University of San Francisco, San Francisco General Hospital. But some researchers believe that being on the Pill will lower the chance that chlamydia will develop into PID, she says. "Somehow, even though it may increase your susceptibility to lower genital tract infections, it may decrease the likelihood that it ascends," says Dr. Padian, who adds that it is not known why.

The STD Connection

The two most common STDs responsible for PID are gonorrhea and chlamydia. Between 20 and 40 percent of women with a history of PID have shown evidence of a chlamydia infection. Chlamydia can cause silent PID—that is, there are no signs of the disease.

Gonorrhea organisms have been found in the cervixes of up to 80 percent of women with PID and in the fallopian tubes of 13 to 18 percent of women with the disease. Women whose PID is caused by gonorrhea generally have noticeable symptoms, including abdominal pain, fever, fatigue, painful intercourse and pain during pelvic exams.

Bacterial vaginosis, a vaginal infection characterized by an overgrowth of harmful bacteria in the vagina, is also believed to be a risk factor for PID. Researchers don't know why, but in some cases the bacteria overgrowth ascends into the upper genital tract, causing PID.

When discovered early, STDs can be treated with antibiotics. But if undetected and left untreated long enough, infection in the uterine lining can leave behind scar tissue that can block the fallopian tube partially or completely and threaten fertility, says Dr. Apuzzio.

Preventive Measures

The first step in preventing PID is to prevent STDs. If you already have one, the next step is to prevent a lower genital tract infection from spreading to your upper genital tract. Here are some tips.

USE CONDOMS. When used properly, condoms are effective protection against STDs. Laboratory studies show that latex condoms are impermeable to just about all STDs.

"If you really want to talk about prevention, it's the same message as it is for HIV, and that's to use condoms," says Dr. Padian. "There isn't any question about that." Latex condoms offer more protection than the more porous lambskin ones, says Dr. Apuzzio. Condoms with the spermicide nonoxynol-9, which has been shown to be effective in killing many infectious organisms, are particularly helpful in preventing some STDs.

"Even in some of our patients who want to use oral contraceptives, we still recommend that they use condoms for the prevention of sexually transmitted disease and some of the organisms that would cause pelvic inflammatory disease," says Dr. Apuzzio.

OR PUT UP OTHER BARRIERS. If your partner won't wear a condom, use a barrier method such as a diaphragm. "Using a barrier is certainly better than nothing. But first choice would be getting your partner to use a condom," says Dr. Padian.

KNOW YOUR PARTNER. Find out your partner's sexual history before you sleep together. Has he had multiple partners? Does he use condoms? Has he ever had an STD? Was he treated? Has he ever been tested for STDs? "The best thing is to try to eliminate the risk factors, and the risk factors would be having [other] sexual partners or having a partner who has a sexually transmitted disease—gonorrhea or chlamydia. Often individuals don't know they have it and pass it on," says Dr. Apuzzio.

ASK HIM TO GET TESTED. If your partner hasn't been tested for gonorrhea or chlamydia, ask him to have a test. He could have the infection, not know it, and pass it on to you. And then you may not even know it, says Dr. Padian.

CONSIDER REGULAR TESTING. Dr. Apuzzio says he provides STD testing for women who come to him for their yearly exams.

KNOW YOUR BODY. Realize what is normal for you; if you notice any changes, see your doctor. "If you think you have any kind of symptoms, any kind of discharge, dripping, irritation or whatever, get in and see your physician," says Dr. Padian. Pay particular attention when these signs appear right after your period. Women often have their first signs of PID at this time, says Dr. Padian.

"It's really pretty common to have your first symptoms of upper genital tract infection at the time of menstruation—not because you've acquired the infection then but because that's when the infection has had an opportunity to ascend into the upper genital tract," says Dr. Padian.

GET TREATMENT. If you think you may have an infection, see your doctor. Treatment for PID can vary, depending on the severity of your symptoms or the extent of the disease. Your doctor will prescribe antibiotics, which will be given intravenously in the hospital or orally at home.

"This is an infection where we really want to start with the so-called big guns right from the beginning," says Dr. Apuzzio. Treating the disease early and aggressively will decrease the pain and discomfort as well as preserve fertility, he says.

FOLLOW YOUR DOCTOR'S DIRECTIONS. Delaying or failing to complete treatment only gives the infection time to spread and cause more damage.

DON'T DOUCHE. "I don't know that women need to douche unless they are directed to do so by a health professional," says Dr. Apuzzio.

Phlebitis

WOMEN ARE MOST AT RISK

The late Richard Nixon may have been best known for the Watergate scandal, but during his presidency he also brought global attention to a disease called deep-vein thrombosis, the severe form of phlebitis, which periodically laid him low.

Nixon's form of phlebitis was indeed quite serious. More often, though, phlebitis attacks a relatively small vein close to the skin. This is called superficial phlebitis, and it is much more painful than it is life-threatening. The symptoms usually include inflammation, swelling and tenderness. You can actually feel the clot, a painful, tender lump right under the skin, and the skin surrounding the clot often feels hot and looks pink or red.

Treatment of this most common and benign form of the disease is surprisingly simple. Even if you don't do anything, most superficial vein clots will dissolve within about two to four weeks. In the meantime, your doctor will recommend applying cold packs and prescribe anti-inflammatory drugs to ease discomfort.

Frequently less painful but far more dangerous is the formation of a blood clot in a large vein deep in the muscles, called deep-vein thrombosis. Two things can happen to these clots: They can adhere to the vein wall or break off and go into a lung. In the first scenario, scar tissue may damage vulnerable valves, causing swelling and an accumulation of fluid, known as edema.

But the real threat is the latter possibility. If the clot detaches and travels to a lung, it can cause sudden death from a blockage of the lung, or pulmonary embolism. Such an occurrence is extremely rare, but it's frightening. "With horrors in mind, people often panic" when they receive a diagnosis of phlebitis, says Brian McDonagh, M.D., a phlebologist and founder of the Vein Clinics of America in Schaumburg, Illinois.

Their fears are almost always groundless, he says. In most cases when superficial veins are involved, there's no need to worry about dire consequences, he explains. But if you have any doubts, or if a fever accompanies a bout with phlebitis, see a doctor immediately. A physical examination can determine just what veins are affected. New diagnostic techniques, such as ultrasound scanning to detect blood flow patterns, can precisely and painlessly locate a clot and help doctors determine treatment.

The Female Phlebitis Factor

Although Nixon may have been the most famous person to have phlebitis, he was not really typical. The vast majority of people who experience this painful circulatory problem are women—up to 80 or 90 percent, according to Dr. McDonagh.

Doctors don't understand exactly how or why women get phlebitis so much more often than men do, but studies suggest that female hormones make the difference. Pregnant women face a particularly high risk for phlebitis—about 1 in 100 newly delivered moms develops it—because pregnancy releases "a tide of hormones that may affect the walls of the veins," says Eugene Strandness, M.D., professor of surgery at the University of Washington School of Medicine in Seattle.

Pregnancy is also the time when many women first notice varicose veins, and people with varicose veins, whether they're pregnant or not, are far and away the most likely to get phlebitis. Dr. McDonagh estimates that 80 percent of the phlebitis patients he sees are women who started out with varicose veins.

Varicose veins are most vulnerable to the kind of minor trauma that can cause a blood clot to form, according to Dr. McDonagh. "Even a slap on the knee or bumping into a coffee table can cause a clot in a superficial vein," he says.

While anybody with varicose veins is at increased risk for phlebitis, the risk rises gradually with age. Older people who are physically inactive for long periods of time are prime candidates. And prolonged bed rest slows down circulation, causing blood to pool in the veins. "One of the most common situations in which phlebitis develops is during hospitalization, particularly after major surgery," says Dr. Strandness.

Effects of the Pill

Until recently, researchers believed that women who took birth control pills were four to six times more likely to get phlebitis. But these figures are now being re-evaluated, since the oral contraceptives currently in use contain much less estrogen than the pills women took only a decade ago.

What about menopausal women on hormone replacement therapy (HRT)? "In most cases, the advantages far outweigh the disadvantages," says Dr. Strandness. There's no conclusive evidence that HRT significantly increases the dangers of developing phlebitis, he says, and the body of evidence that HRT reduces postmenopausal women's risks for heart disease and osteoporosis is growing.

The best advice is to consult your own physician if you have a problem or believe you're at risk because of your medical history or that of your family.

What You Can Do

Phlebitis doesn't have to happen. Here's how to prevent it.

STAY ON YOUR TOES. People who have varicose veins can help prevent blood clots from forming by keeping active. A regular exercise program—a brisk 20-minute walk three or four times a week, for instance—does nicely, says Dr. McDonagh.

RELAX WITH YOUR LEGS UP. Rest your legs on the couch or on a footstool while you read or watch TV. You deserve the extra comfort, and keeping your legs elevated relieves pressure on your veins.

SUPPORT YOURSELF. Compression stockings, available over the counter or by doctor's prescription, give varicose veins the extra support they need and keep blood flowing through your legs smoothly and steadily.

Physical and Emotional Abuse

YOU DON'T HAVE TO TAKE IT ANYMORE

It looked like a scene from a soap opera. The young woman wearing cut-offs and a white T-shirt was screaming as her ex-husband dragged her from the convenience store sidewalk toward his car.

"Please!" the woman begged as her former spouse opened the car door and shoved her into the driver's seat. "Somebody help!"

An older woman who'd been about to walk into the store hesitated, then took a few steps toward the curb. When the young woman frantically jerked away from her ex and slid toward the passenger's door, the older woman took two swift steps toward the car and wrenched open the door.

The ex-husband grabbed his former wife's shirt and held on. But the two women were stronger. The shirt ripped and the older woman slammed the door on the ex's hand. The two women ran into the convenience store, past a half-dozen startled customers and into the employees' bathroom.

There they stayed, protected by a dead-bolted steel door, until the police arrived four minutes later.

The young woman was lucky. Most abuse takes place in the privacy of the home, where there is little help for the victim. But the problem has reached such epidemic proportions that today it spills out onto public streets and malls.

One-fifth to one-third of all American women will be physically assaulted by a current or former partner within their lifetime, reports the American Medical Association. Two million women will be assaulted each year, and nearly half of them will be beaten three or more times within a 12-month period. Thirty-three to 46 percent will be sexually assaulted as well.

These numbers are just the tip of the iceberg. Most violence against women is not reported, and little is done to uncover it. Women are afraid of retribution, and the doctors and police officers who come to their aid simply do not ask what caused their injuries, experts say. As a result, the abuse continues. Studies indicate that abused women represent one-quarter to one-third of all women requiring emergency room treatment and 50 percent of all women who are slain in the United States.

Who's at Risk?

Every woman is at risk of being abused sometime during her life. But women who were abused as children and women who witnessed their mothers being abused have the highest risk, experts agree.

Children who are spanked, beaten and belittled "learn abuse is acceptable, that abuse is part of love and that a woman who stays in an abusive relationship is powerless to stop it," explains Leah J. Dickstein, M.D., professor of psychiatry and behavioral sciences at the University of Louisville School of Medicine in Kentucky. And kids who grow up watching their moms being hit grow up with a distorted perception of gender roles and how family members relate to one another.

Girls absorb the message that you just grin and bear it when you're hit, while boys absorb the message that hitting by men may be appropriate behavior to show love and power in relationships.

Other than those who grew up in an abusive home, women who

are most likely to be abused are single, separated or divorced and between the ages of 17 and 28. They are more likely to be abused if their partner is jealous or possessive and if either they or their partner uses drugs or alcohol.

What Is Abuse?

Although most of us picture broken bones, black eyes and bruises when we think of abused women, abuse can be sexual or emotional as well.

Sexual abuse is intercourse without a woman's consent, penetration with objects, forcing a woman to have sex with other people or forcing a woman to watch pornography, says Charlotte Watson, a nationally known expert on abuse and executive director of My Sisters' Place, a battered women's program in Westchester County, New York.

Refusing to use or refusing to allow a woman to use prophylactics to protect herself against sexually transmitted diseases and unwanted pregnancy is also sexual abuse, as is sexual activity that occurs when a woman is not fully conscious.

Emotional abuse is more complex, adds Watson. Men who are extremely jealous or possessive or who insist on controlling household finances are emotionally abusive. Those who humiliate their partner through insults, criticism, constant interruptions, lying and refusing to listen are emotionally abusive. Depriving a woman of access to her children or to sleep, clothing, food or transportation is also emotional abuse, and men who play mind games or set up situations in which a woman tends to doubt her own perceptions are abusers.

The result? While physical and sexual abuse can land a woman in the hospital, the constant terror and self-doubt women experience from emotional abuse may result in serious health problems such as eating disorders, depression, anxiety, post-traumatic stress disorder, insomnia and stress-related rashes, muscle spasms and digestive problems.

It can also cause feelings of worthlessness, shame and self-loathing, which in turn may lead to suicide or drug and alcohol abuse as a desperate attempt to alleviate emotional pain.

Unfortunately, an abusive partner may encourage a woman to use drugs and alcohol as a way to keep her "calm."

Why Do Men Beat Women?

"Men don't learn to communicate vulnerable feelings verbally when they're little boys," says Dr. Dickstein. Instead some boys learn that aggression—hitting, cursing, shoving and pushing—often helps them get what they want. They learn that in the short term, bullying, threatening and hurting are the fastest and safest routes to immediate gratification and feeling powerful.

Beating a woman and putting her down indicates a pathological need to dominate and coercively control another individual, says Evan Stark, Ph.D., co-founder of the Domestic Violence Training Project in New Haven, Connecticut, and associate professor of public administration and social work at Rutgers University in Newark, New Jersey.

What's more, when men are abusive, friends and family often excuse his actions by sympathetically clucking, "He was under stress," or "She should have known not to make him angry," says Watson.

Watson believes that violence against women will never be quelled until this type of subtly destructive behavior carries the same social stigma that has gradually come to be associated with drunk driving: Only jerks do it.

WILL YOUR MATE BECOME ABUSIVE?

Men who batter often share similar backgrounds and attitudes about male entitlement and power, no matter what economic class or ethnic group they come from. Unfortunately, their battering tendencies may not show up until they begin living with a woman, says Ty Schroyer, men's program coordinator at the Duluth Domestic Abuse Intervention Project in Minnesota.

Still, there are several red-light behaviors that should alert any woman to the possibility that a guy has the potential for abuse. Here's what experts say they are.

Masterminding dates from start to finish. What may seem to be a romantic eagerness to impress you may actually indicate that a man is excessively controlling, says abuse expert Charlotte Watson, executive director of My Sisters' Place, a battered women's program in Westchester County, New York. When you're going out on a date, "you have to set up a test," says Watson. "Tell him, 'I don't want to see that movie. How about if we see another movie instead?'" Then "pay attention to how he reacts," says Watson. "If he has a temper tantrum or has to have his way when you express

How do you change an attitude? Whenever it's expressed, in word or deed, you challenge it, says Watson. "When the life of the party comes over and the brunt of all his jokes is his wife, you have to say 'You can't do that here.'"

Why Do Women Stay?

Historically, men were allowed to beat their wives as long as they used a stick no wider than their thumb, says Watson. It wasn't until about 20 years ago that abused women in the United States had the option of pressing charges against their batterers in criminal court. Clergy, courts and even the women's families believed domestic violence to be a private matter between husband and wife. Women who complained about being treated badly would be told by their families, "You made your bed, now lie in it."

"Women tend to minimize the violence they endure," says Julie Blackman, Ph.D., a social psychologist and forensic consultant in Mont-

a different preference or point of view," think again about continuing the relationship.

Harming pets. Anyone who beats and otherwise harshly punishes his pets is someone to stay away from, says Watson.

Poor impulse control. Punching walls or blowing his top when faced with long lines, traffic or a lack of parking may indicate a man cannot handle the inevitable frustrations and compromise required in an intimate relationship, warns Angela Browne, Ph.D., a psychiatrist at the University of Massachusetts Medical Center in Boston.

Substance abuse. Men who abuse drugs and alcohol have a higher-than-average risk of violence, reports the American Medical Association.

Other warning signs. If a man has a police record for violent crimes or sexual assaults, has a poor self-image or a father who abused his wife, or he pressures you for sex or shows a general dislike, fear or disrespect for women, he is a potential abuser.

clair, New Jersey. A woman may have many reasons to remain with a man who humiliates or degrades her, Watson says. She may believe she loves him, or she may need his paycheck to support her and their children.

Fear of repercussions is also a factor. "The system has been so non-responsive, women historically have seen no value in reporting their abuse. Or they think 'If I tell, it could get worse,'" Watson says.

What Can Women Do?

The only thing a woman can do in any abusive situation is leave, experts agree.

"Studies have shown mediation is a waste of time," says Dr. Dickstein. "It doesn't work." An abused woman may be afraid to discuss the problem with her partner because he might later become violent. And counseling with an assailant is potentially dangerous.

But leaving may also be dangerous. "There is a 75 percent increase in the likelihood of being murdered while a woman is in the process of leaving or has left," says Dr. Dickstein. That's why it must be planned with the utmost care. A woman who is parting from a man who uses drugs or alcohol, threatens to kill her or commit suicide, has or threatens to use weapons or flatly refuses to let her go should take special precautions to ensure her safety, suggest Ann Jones and Susan Schechter in *When Love Goes Wrong*.

Here are some steps you can take to safely free yourself.

SET UP A SIGNAL. Tell a sympathetic neighbor that you'll send a particular signal—a curtain that's normally open suddenly being shut, for example—to call police if you're in danger, experts suggest.

HOLD A FIRE DRILL. If you have children, give them a "fire drill" that will show them what to do if your batterer turns on you and explodes. The kids should be taught how to quickly get out of the house through a variety of exits and told to which neighbors or relatives they should run.

"People say doing this scares kids," says Watson. "But the kids are already scared. They feel more secure having a plan of action and knowing what to do."

HEED YOUR INSTINCTS. If you're feeling afraid and becoming isolated from friends and family, and you feel like you're walking on eggshells when he's around, it's probably time to get out, says Dr. Stark. Don't wait until the police have to take you to the emergency room, he advises. Women who have not yet been repeatedly abused are in better physical and emotional shape to help themselves.

ASSEMBLE A SAFETY KIT. It's also useful to surreptitiously put together a "safety kit" for a fast getaway. The kit should include school records for the kids, Social Security cards, copies of birth certificates, prescription medications, any money you're able to set aside and an address book with all your important phone numbers and contacts. Store it in a place you can get to once you leave the house. Some experts recommend keeping money and a spare set of house keys hidden somewhere in the car. But do this only if your abuser doesn't make a habit of sifting through things to check up on you.

FIND AN ADVOCATE. Before you leave, ask the local police department where you can find an advocate, which is the term used by social service workers to describe counselors who specialize in helping battered women. Advocates can help you find money, housing, emotional support and transitional shelters, says Angela Browne, Ph.D., a psychiatrist at the University of Massachusetts Medical Center in Boston. They also know their way around the judicial system, so they can help you gain custody of your children and preserve your rights toward any property you may own with your partner.

FIND A REFUGE. The addresses of women's shelters are not revealed to the public, so you should ask your advocate or police department for the location of one in your community. Be aware that you may encounter many frustrations—every bureaucracy has red tape, and abuse is so epidemic that sometimes shelters are full.

DOCUMENT YOUR ABUSE. Assemble a record of evidence regarding your abuse. Have a friend or preferably a doctor or hospital worker take pictures of any new bruises, black eyes and other injuries and write the date right on the photo. Even if you don't want to press charges against your batterer at the time, the evidence may come in handy at a later date.

HAVE YOUR BATTERER ARRESTED. You are the best judge of whether involving the police is likely to quell your partner's violence or escalate it. But research shows that arrest works best for men who have "something to lose," like a job or reputation.

"Sometimes arrest can be a miracle cure, particularly if the court and the district attorney give the same message," says Dr. Stark.

It gives the woman some space to make a decision about what to do next, and it gives batterers a message, that their behavior is illegal and intolerable.

If you have your batterer arrested, ask to speak to a police officer or supervisor who will help you find an advocate.

One caveat: If a woman is really in danger, she should be in a secret, safe shelter with her children before pressing charges.

JOIN A SUPPORT GROUP. Participating in a support group—usually offered free or on a sliding fee scale through local shelters—to talk about abuse issues is one of the best possible therapies. Talking to other women breaks down the isolation abused women feel, reassures women that they are not crazy and helps women learn from other women in various stages of recovery from violence, Watson says.

DON'T GO BACK. Most women leave several times before making a final break, says Watson. The first few times they may go back for emotional reasons such as wanting to "save" the family or because they hope their partner will change. The next few times they may not want to go back but fear that they can't escape without being found or that they may not be able to support themselves and their kids.

But no woman should return to an abusive mate once she's gotten away, experts agree. Instead, you have to recognize that in most cases, abuse follows a distinct cycle. In phase one, the male partner starts threatening the woman and pushing or shoving her around. She responds by trying to please him and keep him calm. It doesn't work. In phase two, the man begins to abuse the woman physically and/or sexually. Her life is in danger. In phase three, the abuser apologizes and tearfully promises to mend his ways. And he does—just long enough to get the woman home again.

You may doubt or regret leaving your partner, Watson says. But any woman who is battered must reconcile herself to the reality that it is very unlikely that a man who abuses women will change.

LEAVE GUILT TO THE GUY WHO ABUSED YOU. Everyone talks about what a wonderful, nurturing resource a family can be, but few dwell on how destructive it is when one member is abusive.

Don't feel guilty for "breaking up the family" if you leave an abuser, doctors say. The abuser broke it up long before you ever made a move, so let him bear the burden of guilt, not you.

Pneumonia

BEATING AN INSIDIOUS DISEASE

Pneumonia is serious: More than two million Americans get it each year, and from 2 to 4 percent die. While most of us don't think of pneumonia as all that common these days, it's the fourth leading killer of women of all ages, topped only by heart disease, cancer and stroke.

Although women are no more predisposed to pneumonia than men are, many of us have risk factors that more readily put us in the line of fire.

Smoking is one of them. "The incidence of smoking is growing in only one segment of the population: women," says Steven R. Mostow, M.D., chairman of the Influenza and Pneumonia Committee of the American Thoracic Society and professor of medicine at the University of Colorado in Denver. If you smoke, tar and nicotine reduce your lungs' capacity to handle oxygen and make lung tissue less flexible. This makes you more susceptible to pneumonia.

Another factor is single parenthood; more women than men are raising children alone. If you're a mother with small children, you know how often your kids come home from school or day care with a viral infection. Kids are exposed to an incredible range of bugs at school and, says Dr. Mostow, "children are incredibly efficient disseminators of virus."

Also, when a woman is pregnant, she has a much higher than normal risk for infection by group B streptococcus bacteria. Often the bacteria settle in the urinary tract or postpartum wound, but they may also cause pneumonia. There is no vaccine for group B strep.

Risk factors for pneumonia shared equally by men and women include underlying lung disease, heart disease, diabetes, asthma, cancer, immune deficiencies (such as AIDS), cystic fibrosis and alcoholism.

WOMAN TO WOMAN TAKING PRECAUTIONS PAYS OFF

Barbara L. Parks is assistant principal of Northern Valley Regional High School in Demarest, New Jersey. She has chronic bronchitis, and in 1984, when she was 40, she contracted pneumonia. Since then, she's developed ways to keep from getting it again. This is her story.

I've always had chronic bronchitis. Even as an infant, I was hospitalized with what they called croup at the time. As an adult, I never just get a normal head cold—there's usually a lot of infection in my chest and throat and lungs and head.

In the spring of 1984, I had what the doctor diagnosed as a bronchial infection. I had planned a trip to Florida, so I decided to go, but within a couple of days, I was so sick I flew home. It was on the plane home that I thought that I had pneumonia.

My doctor didn't believe it was pneumonia, but I asked for a chest x-ray anyway, and it showed viral pneumonia in my left lung. I was hospitalized for about a week. There was no pain, but I couldn't breathe easily, and I couldn't walk upstairs. Mostly I was just very, very weak.

I knew I had pneumonia because I know my own body—and I knew there was something seriously wrong. Also, because my father had it a few times, I knew that real deep hacking cough from way down in

The Causes of Pneumonia

Pneumonia is really an umbrella term for an acute infection in the lung. The infection can be caused by any one of a number of bacteria, viruses or fungi, or even tuberculosis. Whatever the cause, when you get pneumonia, an area of your lung becomes so infected and inflamed that it ceases to do its job of exchanging oxygen for carbon dioxide. Less oxygen in the blood leads to "air hunger" and the overwhelming fatigue that's characteristic of pneumonia.

Other general symptoms of pneumonia include cough, which may or may not produce phlegm, chills, fever, sweats, chest pain and shortness of breath. Most bouts of pneumonia come on suddenly, although some forms—like Legionnaire's disease—are preceded by seemingly unrelated symptoms such as diarrhea before respiratory symptoms actually develop.

---

the chest—and that's the way I was coughing.

I was out of work the whole month of May. When I went back, I still had to take it very, very slowly. It was a long time before I felt strong again.

I try to take precautions by keeping physically fit—I work out, try to watch what I eat to stay healthy and try to get enough sleep. Staying generally healthy is important because I work in a school, I'm around kids all the time, my office is right next to the nurse's office—it's the worst environment for respiratory problems.

I get the flu shot every year, and recently when I got sick, I was only out for two days. I felt like the antibiotics really got to it right away.

I go to the doctor a lot faster these days; I don't wait, not at all. Even if it's just that my throat is starting to go scratchy—that's the beginning, and I get violent headaches, and it's always on the left side. You can say, "Oh, this is just a head cold," but it never is with me. It always goes into something, at least bronchitis. I'm very careful to keep my head and throat covered in cold weather.

I personally think that my left side is more susceptible. I'm not sure, but I think sometimes I still can't breathe as deeply in that lung. Maybe that's just from remembering. I just have the feeling that if I let it go, it will get very bad. I haven't had pneumonia since, but I live in dread of it.

A few pneumonias have unique symptoms, says Dr. Mostow. "Young single women are at very low risk for pneumonia; however, when they get pneumonia, the most common cause is mycoplasma. It has a very specific presentation—a hacking, nonproductive cough and headache that is worsened by the coughing. It's the only pneumonia that causes headache."

What Kind of Pneumonia Is It?

Pneumonias are classified as either community-acquired or hospital-acquired. They're further identified in terms of their location as either lobar (in the lobe of a lung) or bronchial (in the air passages). Finally, they're categorized by the type of organism that's causing them, such as bacterial or viral.

"Whatever bugs live in the back of the throat are usually the bugs that cause pneumonia in a particular person," explains Steven W. Stogner, M.D., a pneumonia specialist who is director of intensive care and respiratory therapy at Forrest General Hospital in Hattiesburg, Mississippi.

But these bugs—which all of us have in our throats or mouths—aren't dangerous unless there is some change that weakens our bodies, such as stress, the flu, lowered immunity or an overgrowth of bacteria due to antibiotic therapy.

This is interesting because most pneumonias are treated—at least initially—without the results of any testing because it's important to stop it fast. Frequently the specific organism is not known, but the doctor makes assumptions based on your history, your symptoms and a chest x-ray and prescribes an appropriate antibiotic. If it doesn't work—because the doctor's educated guess about the kind of organism was wrong or the organism is a strain that's resistant to that antibiotic—another drug may be chosen. "If it's a really severe pneumonia or if it's not responding to therapy, we make a very gallant effort to determine the cause," says Dr. Stogner. Tests can include blood and sputum samples or a bronchoscopy, in which samples from the lung are gathered via a tube through the nose or mouth.

How to Prevent It

Though in most cases pneumonia is treatable, you're better off not getting it in the first place. Here are ways to avoid it.

TAKE CARE OF YOURSELF. Pneumonia is much more likely to get a foothold if you're run down, tired or fighting off another infection, so eat a balanced diet, get the vitamins, minerals and other nutrients you need, exercise and get enough sleep. "A very good general state of health is probably your best bet," says Dr. Stogner.

STOP SMOKING. "There would be little need for a pulmonary specialist if so many people didn't smoke," says Dr. Stogner. "Quitting is the number one thing you can do to avoid pneumonia." If you can't go cold turkey, ask your doctor about nicotine substitution systems, such as nicotine gum or the patch, and behavior modification programs. The good news about quitting smoking is that "within just weeks, lung tissue begins to heal," says Dr. Mostow.

DRINK MODERATELY. Alcohol abuse inhibits the function of cilia, the microscopic hairs in the lung that sweep out dust, pollen, bacteria and other unwelcome substances. "When you get drunk, the cilia get drunk, too," explains Dr. Mostow, "and they don't cleanse the lung of bacteria, smoke and dust." The bacteria get a chance to multiply and settle in—and you wake up the morning after closer to getting pneumonia.

GET YOUR SHOTS. Dr. Mostow recommends that women consider getting flu and pneumonia vaccines. "Don't wait for your doctor to suggest it—go in and ask if you are a candidate for the vaccine," he says, particularly if you have conditions that put you in a high-risk group, such as underlying heart or lung disease.

The pneumonia vaccine protects against the most common bacterial type of the disease—streptococcus pneumonia. It's needed only once in a lifetime and has virtually no side effects, according to Dr. Mostow.

Dr. Mostow also recommends flu shots for single working mothers and their children. This is because flu can weaken the lungs and body and open the door to pneumonia.

TAKE PRECAUTIONS WITH THE SICK. "If you're visiting someone in the hospital who has pneumonia, ask the nurses if you need to take any respiratory precautions," advises Dr. Stogner. Most pneumonias are not very contagious, so there's no need to be afraid to visit, but it's a good idea to check, he adds.

DON'T BE AFRAID TO CALL THE DOCTOR. If you catch a cold from a child or co-worker and have a productive cough with phlegm, says Dr. Mostow, you have a bacterial infection superimposed on the cold virus. That's the time to see your doctor, who will prescribe medication, probably an antibiotic. This precaution will greatly increase your chances of avoiding really serious illness.

Post-pregnancy Problems

CONQUER THEM
WITH COMMON SENSE

It's over. The doctor's gone, the nurses are gone, your husband's gone, the baby's asleep in a bassinet by your side, and your body's your own once again.

In fact, exhausted, bruised, stretched and stitched together though it may be, your body already has a lighter-than-air feel. But before you move even an inch, reality—a cramp—intervenes.

Arrrrgggh. Isn't this kind of stuff supposed to be over? Well, yes and no.

Aches and pains are a fact of life after delivery. But most women between the ages of 30 and 45 who are pregnant for the first time have fewer serious health problems than women under 20, says Stephen Fortunato, M.D., director of maternal and fetal medicine at Tulane University in New Orleans. That's because, he says, most of these women go into pregnancy in a bit better health and are more likely to have supportive husbands.

The Aftershocks of Delivery

Although each woman's experience is different, the most frequent postpartum problems are things like cramps, vaginal bleeding, vaginal dryness and pain from the incision (called an episiotomy) that your doctor may have made between the anus and vagina to prevent you from tearing during delivery, says Dr. Fortunato.

"The crampiness is just the uterus coming down to its normal size and stopping itself from bleeding," he says. "In most parts of your body, a clot stops the bleeding. But the way the uterus does it is to squeeze the blood vessels shut."

Every woman has uterine contractions to some extent, says Dr. Fortunato. They're usually more intense for women who are breastfeeding, because every time the baby suckles, their bodies release a burst of pitocin, the hormone that stimulates milk release and contractions in the uterus. That's why the uterus of a woman who is breastfeeding will shrink back into shape more quickly than that of a woman who isn't, says Dr. Fortunato.

Bleeding is also a sign that the body is healing itself, says Dr. Fortunato. "You'll have a discharge that is red, moving toward a paler color, for about three weeks after birth. The bleeding will stop, then somewhere around the fourth or fifth week after pregnancy, most women will shed the scar from the placenta, which is basically like a scab coming off. This resembles a menstrual period."

Women should wear regular menstrual pads to catch the drips—tampons are not a good idea because they can increase the likelihood of infection.

You Can Get Pregnant

This bleeding is not a menstrual period. When will your periods begin again? It can take six months, but since every woman is different, it's tough to say exactly, says Yvonne Thornton, M.D., professor of clinical obstetrics and gynecology at Columbia University College of Physicians and Surgeons in New York City and director of perinatal diagnostic testing at Morristown Memorial Hospital in New Jersey.

But don't think that you can't get pregnant if your periods haven't started up, cautions Dr. Thornton. You can—even if you're breastfeeding.

Most of us have heard that breastfeeding women don't ovulate, but that's not always true. That's why breastfeeding is not a reliable form of birth control, says Dr. Thornton.

Until a woman's menstrual cycle gets back on track again, she may also have vaginal dryness, adds Helen Kay, M.D., a specialist in maternal/fetal medicine and associate professor of obstetrics and gynecology at Duke University in Durham, North Carolina. Low estrogen levels after delivery, particularly if a woman is breastfeeding, can make the vagina so dry that intercourse is painful. Dr. Kay recommends taking time to heal or using lubricating jelly, like K-Y, until vaginal moisture returns.

Low estrogen levels can also make women feel like they're going through menopause, adds Dr. Fortunato. They can actually have hot flashes. The only cure for that is time.

To Cut or Not to Cut?

Probably the most common postpartum complication is pain from an episiotomy. It makes walking, sitting and going to the bathroom uncomfortable. In addition to helping to avoid tearing, an episiotomy is done to help prevent loss of muscle tone in the pelvic area that can lead to bulging of the rectum or bladder, says Dr. Fortunato.

But you may not need an episiotomy, so discuss it with your doctor. If you tell your doctor you don't want an episiotomy to begin with, many doctors will go along with this, says Dr. Fortunato.

If you do have one, however, here's how to avoid episiotomy pain.

GET A MIDLINE INCISION. There are two types of incision, Dr. Fortunato says. One goes through the vaginal lips; the other cuts down from the vagina to the rectum. With the second type, the big muscle tissue is not cut. Healing is more rapid and the likelihood of prolonged pain is reduced, he says.

TAKE A SITZ BATH. If you have an incision, sitting in a warm, shallow bath three or four times a day for the first week after delivery should reduce the pain of both the episiotomy and any hemorrhoids left over from pregnancy, Dr. Kay says. Soap is optional. Taking the bath after a bowel movement—or using a turkey baster to spray your bottom with warm water at that time—will also prevent infection of the incision.

USE ANESTHETIC SPRAYS. If the area is still painful between baths, pick up an over-the-counter anesthetic spray that contains benzocaine from your drugstore and use it to numb the area, says Dr. Fortunato.

The Problem with Infections

Although most postpartum difficulties are more aggravating than serious, there are two that can put you in danger: Infections of the uterus or breast.

"A uterine infection is much more common in cesarean deliveries than in uncomplicated vaginal deliveries, but before antibiotics were used regularly after all cesarean births, about 80 percent of women got infected," says Dr. Fortunato. Today, with antibiotics being given, the infection rate is down to somewhere around 10 to 30 percent after cesarean section.

MOMMY SINGS THE BLUES

After delivery, just about every woman has hormonal fluctuations that can take the sparkle off having a new baby. But approximately 7 percent of new mothers will actually become seriously depressed.

Having the blues is normal; being depressed is not, says Stephen J. Fortunato, M.D., director of maternal and fetal medicine at Tulane University in New Orleans. "Women who get postpartum blues will get sort of a sad feeling and burst into tears over nothing," he says. They'll sit with tears streaming down their faces and say that nothing's really wrong. It's just the way they feel.

"But with postpartum depression you'll have the feeling that you're in a pit and you can't climb out," he says. "There's nothing you can see to do and you have no energy. You have trouble going to sleep, and you may wake early in the morning. And everything in the body tends to slow down. You even tend to get constipated."

Get in touch with your doctor if you suspect you may be slipping into postpartum depression, says Dr. Fortunato. She can evaluate your condition and perhaps prescribe a medication to get you back on track.

Here's how women are infected, says Dr. Fortunato. "Membranes tend to protect the uterus and the fluid inside during pregnancy. But if they've ruptured during labor, you've been in labor for a while and you've had multiple pelvic examinations during labor, all of those things can introduce bacteria from the vaginal tract up into the uterus."

Breast infection, called mastitis, is another common problem, particularly for women who breastfeed, says Dr. Fortunato. It's caused by staphylococcus or streptococcus bacteria.

"A lot of times it comes from the baby's mouth through a cracked nipple," says Dr. Fortunato. "The first sign is a little red streak from the nipple out to the periphery. Other signs are redness, heat, tenderness, swelling, pain and fever, which may also indicate clogged milk ducts."

Frequently emptying the breasts can help head off an infection, and "if an infection is caught early, it can be treated with antibiotics and does not need to interrupt breastfeeding," says Dr. Fortunato. If you let the infection go, however, it will form an abscess that will have to be lanced and drained.

Here's how you can avoid both uterine and breast infections.

AVOID SEX UNTIL YOU STOP BLEEDING. "I usually tell people to wait a month or until bleeding has completely stopped, whichever occurs last," says Dr. Fortunato. "The reason for that is that the mucus plug in the cervix doesn't form for as long as you're bleeding. And the mucus plug is what protects you from getting an infection."

KEEP YOUR NIPPLES CLEAN AND SUPPLE. For women who breastfeed, "good nipple care will prevent them from cracking," says Dr. Fortunato. Wash the nipples with warm water after you feed— never use soap. If you think a breast cream would maintain the suppleness of your skin, ask a nurse or breastfeeding instructor which one to use, or try a lanolin ointment. Vitamin E oil is also popular.

FEED YOUR BABY ON A REGULAR SCHEDULE. "Emptying the breast helps prevent mastitis," says Dr. Fortunato, "since one of the things that promotes the infection is when the breast is engorged with milk." Bacteria thrives in stagnant milk no matter where it is, he adds. So if you're back at work or not able to breastfeed your baby frequently, express some milk. You can refrigerate or freeze it for later.

Post-traumatic Stress Disorder

How to Win the Battle

Brakes squeal, a flash of chrome slices through your peripheral vision, and an ear-splitting "BLAM!" says you've just been hit by another car.

The jolt knocks your vehicle onto the shoulder, where your tires slide over gravel. A headlight and fender crumple into the guard rail. Metal screams against metal, but eventually the car stops. And from within the sudden well of silence that surrounds the driver's seat, you dazedly look through the windshield to see what happened to the other guy.

It's a picture you'll never forget. After knocking you off the road, the other guy smashed into a pickup. And he wasn't wearing a seat belt.

Traumatic events such as rape, earthquakes, warfare and automobile crashes in which there are deaths or life-threatening injuries have a way of etching themselves on our consciousness and popping up to haunt us for weeks, months and perhaps years thereafter.

They can make us afraid to visit places that are somehow identified with the event, and they can make us short-tempered, irritable and jumpy. A mother who has witnessed the drowning of a child may never go near a pool. A cashier who was beaten and robbed may speak rudely to customers. Or a woman who escaped from a burning house may jump out of her skin every time someone lights a match.

These are some of the symptoms of post-traumatic stress disorder (PTSD). But vivid memories of a past traumatic event that affect behavior aren't always PTSD, says Naomi Breslau, Ph.D., director of psychiatric research at Henry Ford Health Sciences Center in Detroit and professor of psychiatry at Case Western Reserve University in Cleveland. PTSD is actually a psychiatric disorder defined by a cluster of six or more symptoms, including re-experiencing the trauma, emotional numbness, avoidance, depressed mood, sleep and concentration problems and nervousness. Symptoms must go on for more than one month and cause distress or impairment in social, work or other important areas of a person's life.

Only a small percentage of people will develop PTSD as defined in psychiatry. Often these people have other risk factors, which can include depression and anxiety, before the trauma occurs.

"The concept of post-traumatic stress disorder was first identified in war as 'shell shock' or 'combat fatigue,' " says Dr. Breslau. Men exposed to battlefield horrors in which they saw humans sliced, burned and blown to smithereens returned home jumping at shadows, unable to respond to their wives and kids and haunted by the battles left behind.

But today we know that PTSD is not limited to the battlefield or even to men. It can affect anyone who has witnessed, experienced or even heard about a violent event.

A Woman's Vulnerability

PTSD is not uncommon. Studies show that sometime in their lives, approximately 40 percent of all men and women experience violent events that can lead to the problem, and approximately 25 percent of them will subsequently develop the disorder.

In a study of more than 1,000 men and women in the Detroit area, Dr. Breslau found that 80 percent of those who had been raped developed PTSD. Twenty-four percent of those whose life had been threatened also developed the problem, as did 23 percent of those who had seen someone killed or seriously hurt, 22 percent of those who had been physically assaulted, 21 percent of those who had been told of the sudden death or accident of a close relative or friend and 11 percent of those who had a sudden injury or serious accident.

Women were most at risk.

"Even if you disregard rape, we found that women were twice as likely overall to react to traumatic events with post-traumatic stress disorder as men," says Dr. Breslau. And women who had been clinically depressed before the event were 11 times more likely to experience the disorder than those who were not.

"We don't know a whole lot about why women are more at risk," she adds. But "there might be some special vulnerability of women that we don't yet understand."

Trying to Forget

Although studies indicate that anywhere from one-third to one-half of all those who develop PTSD will get better within three to six months of the traumatic event without any help, that still leaves a lot of women in pain. And no one can figure out in advance whose symptoms will diminish and whose will get worse.

That's why Dr. Breslau suggests the following strategies should you find yourself the survivor of a traumatic event such as rape or assault.

GET PROFESSIONAL HELP. "If a woman has been raped or attacked, she should see a psychologist or psychiatrist right away," says Dr. Breslau. She can talk about the experience and clarify what happened. It will not only lessen the likelihood of developing the disorder, it will help keep her from getting into any of the avoidance behavior—avoiding people, places and things that are reminders of the event—that so often becomes a problem.

To find someone who specializes in treating PTSD, check with your local hospital, medical center or university for a clinic that is specifically set up to deal with anxiety disorders or trauma.

TREAT ANY COEXISTING PROBLEMS. Since women who have a history of depression are the ones most likely to develop PTSD, a key strategy in keeping the disorder at bay is to treat the depression through therapy or with antidepressants, says Dr. Breslau.

DON'T AVOID ANYTHING. Once you've either seen or experienced a traumatic event, it's natural to want to avoid places, people and situations that remind you of the incident or of your own vulnerability. But don't let yourself do it, says Dr. Breslau. Once you allow yourself to avoid one thing, you start avoiding others. The next thing you know, you're so afraid of everything that you spend your life cowering in your home.

INOCULATE YOURSELF AGAINST STRESS. Should you develop PTSD, there are several treatment strategies your therapist may suggest, including exposure, a technique in which you repeatedly relive the traumatic event from the safety of your therapist's office until you can think of it without getting upset, and stress inoculation training, a technique that includes correcting mistaken thinking, muscle relaxation and deep breathing.

A study at the Medical College of Pennsylvania in Philadelphia of 45 rape survivors who suffered from PTSD found that supportive counseling reduced symptoms by 26 percent. Nine therapy sessions using the exposure technique reduced symptoms 40 percent, and nine sessions of stress inoculation training reduced symptoms by 55 percent.

Three months later, women in the study who had used exposure techniques were found to have the fewest symptoms. In a later study, the combination of exposure and stress inoculation training was found to be more effective than either treatment alone. Three months after treatment, 90 percent of clients improved significantly.

Check with your therapist to see which technique—or combination of techniques—is right for you.

Premenstrual Syndrome
No Two Experiences Are Alike

Your breasts are tender, you feel bloated and achy, and your head's pounding something awful. You're also edgy and irritable. Actually, you're more than irritable. Your friend is going to be five minutes late for lunch—something that doesn't usually faze you, but today you're downright furious. If she doesn't hurry up and get here, you'll really let her have it.

You never used to feel this way. But lately the two weeks just prior to your period have been a struggle. Last month there were several days when you were in a bad mood before your feet even hit the floor in the morning. It felt like a black cloud was following you around. The month before that you felt anxious and edgy, like you wanted to jump out of your skin. Yesterday you snapped at your husband over a rather minor matter. And today you feel like you're going to lose it with your friend. Could this be PMS? Well, maybe.

The Problem of Definition

The term *PMS* has come to mean a lot of different things. If you mean premenstrual symptoms, like bloating or moodiness, that's one thing. Up to 90 percent of women in their childbearing years experience some premenstrual symptoms, of which there are over 150. In fact, the thirties and forties are often when symptoms first develop. It's also a time when they tend to get worse if you already had them. So there's a good chance you have premenstrual symptoms.

Premenstrual syndrome (PMS), on the other hand, is something more severe. Fewer women—between 3 and 5 percent—are thought to suffer from it.

PMS differs from milder premenstrual discomfort in that its symptoms are severe enough to interfere with a woman's personal, social and work life. Its symptoms occur regularly. That is, instead of occurring randomly—a month here and a month there—they occur frequently, in at least two out of every three menstrual cycles. Symptoms tend to appear somewhere between ovulation and the beginning of a period. And the time span when symptoms occur is followed by a time—usually the two weeks right after the start of a period—when the woman is symptom-free.

Whether you have premenstrual symptoms or PMS, you may be wondering what causes your feelings and behavior to shift in the two weeks before your period. That's hard to say exactly, but there are lots of theories.

Some researchers suspect that the mood changes and emotional shifts are related to the levels of progesterone and estrogen, reproductive hormones whose levels rise and fall during the menstrual cycle. The thinking is that the increased tension, anxiety and irritability of PMS may be due to a low estrogen-to-progesterone ratio. That is, levels of progesterone, a hormone believed to have a tranquilizing effect, may be lower than estrogen levels, and anxiety results.

Women in their thirties and forties are more likely to have been on and off the Pill or have gotten pregnant, and these hormonal changes may be what triggers the hormone shifts and the development of PMS, says Stephanie DeGraff Bender, director of the PMS Clinic in Boulder, Colorado, and author of *PMS: A Positive Program to Gain Control*.

Another theory is that PMS symptoms arise from shifting levels of neurotransmitters, the special brain chemicals believed to influence mood. In particular, the chemicals serotonin, norepinephrine and dopamine are thought to be involved. The change in neurotransmitter levels may be tied to changes in estrogen and progesterone levels, but just how isn't exactly clear.

There are also some indications that nutrition may play a role. In particular, magnesium, riboflavin, vitamin A, calcium and manganese deficiencies may contribute to the exacerbation of symptoms.

Stress may also play a role in the development of PMS and may be another reason that women tend to develop PMS in their thirties and forties. Women past 30 have more complex lives, says Nancy Fugate-Woods, Ph.D., of the Center for Women's Health Research at the University of Washington School of Nursing in Seattle. These women often have children or are working full time, or both. They may be single parents or supporting their parents, she says. They have a lot more stress at this phase of their life than they did when they were younger, and the development of PMS may be somehow related to that, she says.

The Link to Menopause

Some women find that their PMS gets markedly worse just before menopause, says Ellen Klutznick, Psy.D., a psychotherapist in San Francisco who counsels menopausal and perimenopausal women. And some experts say it can be a sign that a woman has entered perimenopause, the stage in which estrogen levels start to decline, women's periods begin to change, and menopausal problems like hot flashes, mood swings and weight gain arise. Just because you develop PMS doesn't mean you're entering menopause, but if your symptoms get markedly worse, that can be a sign, and it can't hurt to have your hormone levels checked, says Dr. Klutznick.

Living with PMS

Premenstrual syndrome can really take its toll on the women who have it.

Mood symptoms tend to be most troublesome, experts say. "The symptoms women are really concerned about are depression, anxiety, anger, sleeplessness and hopelessness," says Annette Rossignol, Sc.D., professor and chair of the Department of Public Health at Oregon State University in Corvallis. It's hard to say whether these are the symptoms women get most, but they are the ones for which they seek help most often, she says.

These emotional changes can affect relationships. Women may find themselves feeling and behaving differently. They may lose control with a friend or snap at a co-worker or at their children, says Bender. Then, feeling guilty afterward, they resolve not to let something similar happen the next month. But often it does, and the guilt over their behavior, combined with their failed attempts not to repeat it, causes their self-esteem to plummet, she says.

The impact of PMS can extend beyond the women themselves. "PMS is not just a woman's issue," says Dr. Rossignol. "It's a family issue." Often a woman's change in behavior can be difficult or confusing to partners and children. One month the kids may find Mom more than happy to have the whole softball team over, while the next month she snaps at the mere mention of the idea, explains Bender. And spouses may find their partners getting upset over things that never seemed to bother them before.

Finding Relief

Whether you suffer from premenstrual symptoms or PMS, there are some things you can do to make the two weeks prior to your period a little easier. Here are some suggestions.

KEEP A SYMPTOM DIARY. The first step in figuring out whether you have PMS is to start charting your symptoms. "Any expert will say you have to sit down and, for three or four months, document what you are experiencing on a day-to-day basis," says Suzanne Trupin, M.D., head of the Department of Obstetrics and Gynecology at the University of Illinois College of Medicine at Urbana-Champaign.

The idea is to track your symptoms to see if they occur in the latter half of your menstrual cycle. If they do, that's a clue you may have PMS. If your symptoms occur throughout your cycle, you may have some other health problem. If you have a lot of different symptoms and it's overwhelming to chart them all, "pick the top three symptoms that bother you the most and chart those," says Dr. Trupin.

CUT BACK ON CAFFEINE. Caffeine is a stimulant to the nervous system and can contribute to mood swings, feelings of anxiety, nervousness and edginess. Women with premenstrual symptoms and syndrome often find that cutting back on caffeine helps decrease anxiety. Aim to cut back a little at a time, says Dr. Trupin. "Progressively add decaffeinated coffee to your caffeinated till you're drinking all decaf," she says. It's unrealistic to think you can do it all in just a few weeks, she says. It may take a few months.

If you drink caffeinated soda, try the same thing: Mix decaffeinated soda with the caffeinated a little at a time until all you're drinking is decaf.

STAY ACTIVE. Exercise is very important for women with premenstrual symptoms or syndrome, says Marcia Szewczyk, M.D., assistant professor in the Department of Family and Community Medicine and director of the PMS Clinic at the Bowman Gray School of Medicine in Winston-Salem, North Carolina. "I encourage women to go out and do regular walking or jogging or to play tennis," she says. Exercise can help boost your mood because it stimulates the release of endorphins, the body's natural mood elevators.

DESALT YOURSELF. If bloating and water retention are major problems for you, try reducing your salt intake, experts say. Read food labels and look for ingredients that include the word *sodium*. And keep an eye out for high-salt foods when you dine out. Salad dressings in particular can be high in salt, so try opting for oil and vinegar.

WATCH WHAT YOU EAT. Fluctuating blood sugar levels can cause your energy level to swing up and down, making it harder to cope with any premenstrual symptoms you have, says Dr. Szewczyk. Maintaining a steady blood sugar level can make coping easier. So "eat frequent small meals," she says, and avoid sweets like cookies, candy and chocolate.

GO FOR CALCIUM. Getting more calcium in your diet may help decrease premenstrual symptoms, according to researchers at the Grand Forks Human Nutrition Research Center in North Dakota, part of the Agricultural Research Service at the U. S. Department of Agriculture. Calcium is believed to affect levels of hormones and neurotransmitters.

In a small study of women with premenstrual symptoms but not PMS, mood problems such as depression, anxiety, tension and loneliness were reduced when women increased the calcium levels in their diets, says James G. Penland, Ph.D., research psychologist at the Grand Forks center. Water retention, pain and concentration problems were also somewhat alleviated. Women with PMS may also benefit.

So aim to get at least 1,200 milligrams of calcium each day, says Dr. Penland. Two eight-ounce glasses of 1 percent milk (about 300 milligrams each) and one cup of low-fat yogurt (about 415 milligrams) will bring you close to what you need.

PUT YOUR CRAVINGS ON HOLD. When you get a craving for sweet foods—the cookies, candy and cake—try to put it off for half an hour, says Dr. Rossignol. You may change your mind about whether you really have to have them, she says.

PUT SOME PRESSURE ON. Try reflexology, a technique that involves applying manual pressure to specific areas of the ears, hands and feet. According to Terry Oleson, Ph.D., chair of the Department of Behavioral Medicine at the California Institute in Los Angeles, the first study on reflexology indicates that applying manual pressure to specific pressure points on the ear, hand or foot may relieve some of the symptoms women experience with PMS.

Applying pressure to points on the upper half of the ear tends to relieve symptoms in the lower half of the body, while pressure to the lower half works on the upper half of the body, for headaches. While trained reflexologists are available to perform the technique, women can try it on themselves, says Dr. Oleson. Gently pinch your ear between two fingers until you find a sensitive spot, he says. Once you locate one, gently apply pressure with the two fingers for 30 to 60 seconds, then release and repeat up to three times if you like, says Dr. Oleson.

COMMUNICATE YOUR TROUBLES. Find time when you do not have symptoms to talk with your partner about your premenstrual experience, says Bender. Changes in your moods and behavior can be confusing and even hurtful, and talking about what's happening may help him understand. Tell your partner how PMS makes you feel, how you might behave, how he can help you and what you are doing to address it, she says.

SHARE WITH THE KIDS. Premenstrual syndrome can be confusing to children, too, says Bender. Tell your kids that you have an imbalance in your body that may cause you to act different at times, she says. For younger children, try hanging a smiley face magnet on the fridge and use it to communicate how you're feeling, says Bender. On "PMS days" simply turn the magnet upside down. Kids usually get the picture, she says.

GET HELP. If you can't get your premenstrual symptoms under control on your own, seek medical help. A doctor will take a medical history, do a physical exam and psychological evaluation and ask you to fill out a symptom diary for three months in order to diagnose you.

Psoriasis

NOT CURABLE,
BUT CONTROLLABLE

If you could change one part of your body, what would it be? "If I could change one thing," says Donna Egan, "absolutely, it would be my skin."

Egan, a critical care nurse from Levittown, Pennsylvania, is one of about five million Americans with psoriasis. For her and others with the disease, life can become a series of restrictions. Some women stop wearing skirts, sleeveless tops and bathing suits. Some won't date. Others have been turned away from health clubs, supermarkets and hair salons. One woman cooked a dish for a pot-luck lunch, but her co-workers barely touched it, even though they knew her disorder was not contagious. Others are even shunned by loved ones, who won't touch them.

Psoriasis can range from mild—where a few small red patches appear on the elbows or feet—to severe, with unsightly scaly areas covering the entire body. It forms when skin cells mature too quickly—in about 4 days as opposed to 28—and pile up. It's unpredictable, unattractive and even painful. Experts don't know what causes it.

America's appearance-oriented culture makes psoriasis particularly difficult for women, says Joan Shelk, R.N., clinical administrator at the Leone Center for Dermatology and Psoriasis Treatment in Arlington Heights, Illinois, who has counseled psoriasis patients for 17 years.

"Two important issues for those with psoriasis are feeling unclean and feeling ugly," she says. "This is so counter to what most women are taught. We are taught, 'You must look beautiful. You must look clean.' But with psoriasis you can't." In the context of her own health background, Shelk's view is especially poignant. "I survived cancer. It was ovarian. And I would rather go through that whole ordeal again—the radiation therapy, the surgery, everything—than suffer with psoriasis. My cancer didn't show. This shows," she says.

WOMAN TO WOMAN LEARNING TO LIVE WITH LESIONS

Darcy Love, who works with special education students in Billings, Montana, was diagnosed with psoriasis when she was in her early twenties. It appears between her eyebrows, on her scalp, on her shins, on her elbows and on her cheeks. Now in her forties, she's learned to live with it. This is her story.

I can't say it's terrible, but when people ask, it's hard. They say, "What's that?" or they use one-liners like, "Oh, the heartbreak of psoriasis."

I've educated myself on what psoriasis is so when people ask, I can explain. I explain that it's not contagious. That's most important. And I also tell people, "It's too much of a good thing." And they say, "What do you mean?" Then I say that it's because the skin cells grow too fast.

I was diagnosed when I was 23. I already had two kids. I didn't know at the time it was hereditary. I didn't realize the kids could have it. My youngest son has it. He got it when he was 22 years old. His whole body is involved. We talk about it. I think he deals with it better than I do. He doesn't spend a lot of time messing with it. He deals with it well. It doesn't slow him down. He wears shorts in the summertime.

When I first found out that he had it, I felt guilty. I wanted it on

What It's All About

There's a genetic component to psoriasis, so both men and women run the risk of passing it on to their children, says Thomas Helm, M.D., a dermatologist in Williamsville, New York, and assistant professor of dermatology at the State University of New York at Buffalo, though the chance is less than 10 percent.

A woman's treatment options are often limited, explains Mark Lebwohl, M.D., director of the Division of Dermatology at Mount Sinai Medical Center in New York City. That's because some medications can cause birth defects, which means they're forbidden for women of childbearing age, he says. For instance, two drugs for severe psoriasis, etretinate (Tegison) and isotretinoin (Accutane), should never be taken by women who plan to have children. Another treatment, PUVA, combines a type of drug called a psoralen with exposure to ultraviolet A (UVA) light. It is also not advisable during pregnancy, but available data

---

me. I felt so bad. I really felt bad for two to three years. Now because he deals with it so well, it's easier. But anytime I hear about some remedy that may help control it, I tell him. I heard that Murphy's Oil Soap helps. So we use that when taking a shower.

Sometimes I think it's stress-related, so I handle that with my exercise program. I run every day. I used to smoke and I think that aggravated it. When I quit and started exercising, my psoriasis didn't seem as bad. I know a couple of times I got off my program and it was like a red flag . . . boom.

I also practice reflexology. That's where you work on the reflexes on the bottom of your feet to increase the oxygen in the bloodstream. My husband gives me foot treatments every other night. It takes about 15 minutes.

The one thing I would suggest is to read and educate yourself about it. I went to the library. I got information from the National Psoriasis Foundation and the doctor. Whatever information I got, I read.

And the National Psoriasis Foundation newsletter has comments from people who have it. They ask questions that you have or questions you may not be able to ask. It's a neat network.

When I get frustrated I tell myself I know it's going to get better. And the people I know know what it is and they're not affected by it.

suggest that in cases where it was administered inadvertently, there was no significant increase in birth defects.

Taking Care of Yourself

But psoriasis doesn't have to rule your life. The first step in controlling it is to try to prevent flare-ups. Here's how.

GREASE YOURSELF UP. Letting your skin dry out is just opening the door to an outbreak. Stay lubricated, says Michelle Fiore, M.D., a dermatologist and former director of the Psoriasis Medical Center in Palo Alto, California. "Use heavy moisturizers—the thicker and greasier the better." Among her over-the-counter favorites are Aquaphor, Eltra, Theraplex and Albolene. Even petroleum jelly will do the trick.

HEAD FOR THE SUN AND SEA. For many, sun is the solution, says Dr. Helm. Consult with your dermatologist about how much to get. And pay attention to cosmetics and moisturizers, says Shelk. Many contain sunscreens that may block the rays your psoriasis needs. And while your psoriasis needs sun, skin that's clear still needs to be protected. Use sunscreen on psoriasis-free areas to avoid burning.

SHAVE CAREFULLY. Any small trauma—a bump, bruise or scrape—can act as a starting place for psoriasis, says Dr. Fiore. For women that includes shaving their legs. "If you get a little infection of the hair follicle, that can act as the beginning of psoriasis," she says. To avoid this, shave with sharp, double-edged blades and allow moisture to absorb into the leg hair first. If you already have ingrown hairs, try shaving in the direction the hair grows, says Dr. Fiore.

TRY A SPORTS BRA. Friction from bras can trigger or aggravate psoriasis, so try a sports bra. "They're generally more comfortable, and the cotton ones are great," says Shelk. She suggests buying them one size larger than usual.

TAKE CARE OF YOUR NAILS. Nails can be a trouble spot, so if you're prone to psoriasis, keep them cut short, don't poke things underneath to clean them, and don't push or clip the cuticles too much, says Dr. Fiore. If you want to dress up your nails a bit, try a thin coat of clear polish. Stay away from false nails. They'll stick to and pull on your natural nail, and this aggravation can trigger an outbreak of psoriasis.

FIGHT THOSE FOLDS. Skin-fold areas, particularly under the breasts, are potential trouble spots for women. Experts say bacteria and yeast create by-products that can aggravate psoriasis. To keep skin-fold areas yeast-free, try over-the-counter preparations such as Lotrimin, or to keep folds bacteria-free, use antibiotic soaps, cleansers or creams like Bactracin and Neomycin, says Dr. Fiore. Another way to protect the area under the breasts is to reduce friction. Try applying your medication and covering it with a strip of flannel, says Shelk.

WATCH OUT FOR IRRITATION. Trauma to the skin from picking, scratching, sunburn or even surgery can aggravate psoriasis and cause spots to develop at the areas of injury, says Dr. Helm. Radio headsets, ski goggles and even eyeglasses can exacerbate psoriasis on places such as the ear. Ear piercing may also bring out psoriasis.

Getting Medical Help

Preventing a psoriasis outbreak is one thing, but dealing with one after it's happened is another. Try to avoid just camouflaging it, says Dr. Helm. "The real key is aggressively nipping a flare-up in the bud with treatment before widespread involvement occurs," he says.

Treatments for psoriasis run the gamut, says Michael Zanolli, M.D., director of clinical dermatology services at the Vanderbilt Phototherapy and Skin Treatment Center in Nashville. Women with mild cases can try moisturizers, over-the-counter medications, topical steroid creams, sunbathing, coal tar applications and anthralin, a prescription medication derived from tree bark.

If those don't work, doctors may recommend phototherapy with natural sunlight or ultraviolet B, PUVA or day treatment programs, in which various combinations of therapies are used over a period of several hours in a specialized treatment center. For severe psoriasis, your doctor may try potent prescription medications such as methotrexate (Mexate), which interferes with cell replication. Other drugs such as cyclosporine may also be prescribed.

Finally, a topical vitamin D application, calcipotriene (Dovonex), is another possibility. It doesn't cause the thinning of the skin that can occur with topical steroid creams.

BE CAREFUL WITH STEROID CREAMS. Women's skin can be thinner than men's, says Dr. Fiore. Potent topical steroid creams sometimes can cause additional thinning, so be on the lookout for increasingly fragile skin, particularly on your face and under your breasts.

GO FRAGRANCE-FREE. Wearing cosmetics or fragrance on your skin during light therapy may trigger irritation, says Shelk. Wait until after your treatment to do your beauty routine.

CONSIDER COMBINATIONS. Sometimes treatments work better in combination, says Dr. Helm, so ask your doctor about possible options.

DON'T DO IT YOURSELF. Tanning beds are not regulated in many areas, so the wavelengths and intensity of exposure can vary greatly from one treatment to the next, says Dr. Helm. See a professional for UVA treatment.

The Art of Coping

You've got it, you're trying to treat it. But you've got to get on with your life. How do other women with the disease manage?

TRY THE CAMOUFLAGE GAME. Cover milder psoriasis on the arms and legs with patches such as Actiderm or Restore Dressing, which may be available over the counter at your pharmacy, says Dr. Fiore. These patches can even be used under panty hose. If you can't find the patches, flesh-colored medical tape will do.

Camouflage makeup for birthmarks can also be used. Up close, the makeup will make the scales visible, but from a distance they'll look much better, says Dr. Fiore. DermaBlend Leg and Body Cover can also be used on the face. It can be particularly good, says Shelk, because it's waterproof, so it lasts in the pool and survives hot weather. And it doesn't have to be used with a setting powder base, so it's easier to use. Look for it at the cosmetic counter at your local department store.

WASH IT OUT. Frequent hair-washing is important to get rid of psoriasis scales. Over-the-counter medicated shampoos, especially those containing coal tar, selenium, zinc and salicylic acid, are helpful, says Dr. Fiore.

BOLSTER YOURSELF. A woman's self-esteem can really plummet during a psoriasis outbreak, says Barbara Cohen, a psychotherapist in Palo Alto, California, who counsels clients with psoriasis and has it herself. Concentrate on your strengths, she says, and if you can't pull yourself out of the dumps, consider therapy.

STAY ACTIVE. Participate in activities that bring you in contact with other people, experts advise. One study showed that employed people with the disease had better images of themselves and felt less stigmatized than those who did not work.

DE-STRESS YOURSELF. Many women feel their psoriasis is exacerbated by stress, says Elizabeth Abel, M.D., a dermatologist in Mountain View, California, and clinical associate professor of dermatology at Stanford University School of Medicine. Recognizing that stress triggers their skin condition can help people better address the problem, she says. Biofeedback and meditation are two stress-management techniques to consider.

Raynaud's Disease

Mostly in the Hands of Women

Mary Ann knows she lacks style at times. In early fall, the 50-year-old Philadelphia lawyer can be seen wearing big, fuzzy mittens and a large scarf wrapped around her head babushka-style. And when she entertains colleagues in her suburban home, she doesn't offer to fix the drinks. She asks her guests to do it themselves.

Not very chic, perhaps, but for Mary Ann the habits are a matter of self-defense. She has Raynaud's disease, a disorder in which the hands, and sometimes other body parts, respond abnormally to cold or stress. A slight drop in the temperature or contact with cold objects such as soda cans, water or ice can cause intense pain and color changes in the fingers. The pain may be so bad that any exposure to cold is intolerable. The only way to stop Raynaud's is to stay warm and avoid contact with cold objects.

What's Happening Here?

The body's protective device, the sympathetic nervous system, controls the opening and closing of blood vessels. When most people are exposed to cold, this system tends to constrict the blood supply to the extremities and direct it to the center of the body. With Raynaud's disease, the slightest hint of cold causes an exaggerated contraction of the blood vessels.

It's not clear why, says George Spencer-Green, M.D., associate professor of medicine in the connective tissue disease section at Dartmouth Medical School in Hanover, New Hampshire. Doctors speculate that it could be due to some interference with the sympathetic nervous system or to an abnormality of the vessel itself. They do know that Raynaud's disease is more common in women than in men and that the onset of symptoms is typically between the ages of 20 and 40. Some experts think that female hormones may be a factor, but it's not clear yet how.

You'll know for sure that you have Raynaud's when contact with the cold causes three color changes in your skin—to white, then blue, then red. But three changes are not always required for a diagnosis of Raynaud's, says Leslie Kahl, M.D., assistant professor of medicine in the Division of Rheumatology at Washington University in St. Louis. One color, white, may be enough, she says, but what's key is whether the color change occurs repeatedly. Numbness is another clue, but the best way to find out if it's Raynaud's is to see your doctor.

The Two Types of Raynaud's

Raynaud's comes in two forms. One is Raynaud's disease, which occurs in isolation. The other is Raynaud's phenomenon, which occurs in conjunction with other diseases, including scleroderma, a hardening and shrinking of the skin; lupus, a chronic inflammatory disease that affects the skin, joints, kidneys, nervous system and mucous membranes; and rheumatoid arthritis. Raynaud's phenomenon also commonly occurs in people who use vibrating or hammering tools or instruments.

Your doctor will do blood tests and examine your nail folds, the area right above the cuticle under the skin, to figure out which form of Raynaud's you have.

It's estimated that 5 to 10 percent of Americans have Raynaud's.

We're in the Majority

It's not known why more women than men have Raynaud's, but women get autoimmune diseases such as scleroderma and lupus more than men do, and Raynaud's often develops with these.

Also, smoking may contribute to Raynaud's because the nicotine in tobacco causes blood vessels to constrict. "People are more likely to develop a more severe case if they're smokers. And smokers whom I have convinced to quit have often noticed that their Raynaud's improves dramatically," says Dr. Kahl.

Other products that stimulate the sympathetic nervous system, such as diet pills and cold remedies, may contribute to the development of Raynaud's, says Dr. Kahl.

Medications that women take for other health problems may also contribute to or exacerbate Raynaud's. Women get migraine headaches more than men, and migraine medications, called beta-blockers, can trigger Raynaud's. Beta-blockers are also used to treat high blood pressure, and their use may worsen symptoms or make previously un-diagnosed symptoms more apparent, says Dr. Spencer-Green.

Finally, researchers say that there may be a link between women's hormone levels and Raynaud's, though they're not sure what the link is. "Mounting evidence supports the notion that there is a specific rela-tionship between hormones and the immune system," says Joan Merrill, M.D., assistant chief of rheumatology at St. Luke's–Roosevelt Hospital in New York City. "But it's not clear how that works yet," she says.

Our Special Concerns

There's no definitive answer on whether the birth control pill af-fects Raynaud's. Some doctors say that while there are no large studies to support it, a few of their patients have developed Raynaud's while on the Pill. And Rosalind Ramsey-Goldman, M.D., Dr.Ph., assistant profes-sor of medicine in the Division of Rheumatology at Northwestern University School of Medicine in Chicago, says some researchers be-lieve the Pill may exacerbate Raynaud's in some patients who have increased levels of antiphospholipid antibodies. These antibodies are sometimes associated with spontaneous abortions and other blood-clotting disorders. If you have Raynaud's and are considering the Pill, talk it over with your doctor.

The impact of Raynaud's on pregnancy is also unknown, experts say. Some doctors say women with Raynaud's may actually feel better during pregnancy due to increased blood vessel dilation, yet little re-search has been done to confirm this. And while pregnancy difficulties have been identified in women with lupus and other autoimmune dis-eases, less research has been done on Raynaud's phenomenon.

A study of 97 women conducted by Dr. Kahl looked at pregnancy in women with severe Raynaud's phenomenon. She found that women who had Raynaud's before their first pregnancy had smaller babies, although within normal range, and were more likely to have premature babies. "If a woman has severe Raynaud's, then it's fair to say there's a slightly increased risk of premature birth," she says. All women with Raynaud's don't need to be alarmed, though, she says. This study included women with very severe Raynaud's, so the conclusions can't necessarily be applied to women with milder forms of the disease.

There are no studies to prove that the severity of Raynaud's varies during the phases of the menstrual cycle, but some doctors say their patients report changes. The impact of Raynaud's on conception and fertility is also unknown.

Keeping Raynaud's Under Cover

Raynaud's isn't curable, but it is manageable. Here's what you can do.

BE PREPARED FOR TEMPERATURE CHANGES. Don't make drastic changes from warm to cold, says Dr. Ramsey-Goldman. Carry a sweater with you at all times, she says. And keep an extra sweater or leggings in a drawer at work. "People at work tolerate different temperatures, and you may not be allowed to adjust the thermostat," she says.

DON'T FORGET THE HAT AND SCARF. Bundle up in cold weather, and this means wearing a hat and scarf, too, says Dr. Kahl. "Women may be savvy enough to wear mittens, but not hats," she says. "Get into stylish hats. Make the hat your signature. Make it a positive instead of a negative," she says.

SLIDE INTO SILK. One key to keeping warm is to dress in layers, says Dr. Kahl. "Wear silk underclothing. It doesn't add to the bulk, but it will add to warmth," she says. The underwear doesn't have to be long-sleeved, she explains. Even a silk camisole will do. The key is to keep your core body temperature up.

QUIT SMOKING. There are lots of good reasons to give up smoking, but if you've got Raynaud's, now you've got another. Do what you can to quit or cut back.

USE A FRIDGE MITT. The less you subject your hands to cold, the better, and that includes the cold from the refrigerator. "If you're taking something out of the fridge, wear an oven mitt," says Dr. Ramsey-Goldman. Some women even take gloves or mitts to the grocery store with them.

TRY BIOFEEDBACK. Biofeedback is effective for some

women, says Dr. Ramsey-Goldman. "By touching the hands with a temperature probe, women can learn to raise the temperature in their fingers by as much as one degree," she says. There are also techniques where patients immerse their hands in cold water and then, through a visualization technique, learn to bring back the circulation in their hands. Ask your doctor about biofeedback possibilities.

NOTE YOUR RESPONSE TO DRUGS. Certain drugs such as beta-blockers and blood pressure medications can either trigger Raynaud's or exacerbate it. So watch your response to these drugs. Be a good observer and note any changes in your Raynaud's, says Dr. Kahl. You might want to keep a three-day diary and rate each attack on a 1-to-5 scale in terms of severity. If you notice increased severity, tell your doctor.

CONDITION YOUR HANDS. You can fool your blood vessels into staying open by using a technique developed by the Cold Research Division at the U.S. Army Research Institute of Environmental Medicine in Natick, Massachusetts. The method helps increase blood flow and decrease symptoms in nearly all Raynaud's patients, say researchers there.

To use this technique at home, you'll probably have to wait for cold weather. Take two containers large enough to fit both hands in and fill them with hot water, about 104° to 107°F. Put one container in a cold area, around 32°F, and one in a warm area. While dressed for indoors, immerse your hands in the warm water in the warm room for two to five minutes. Then wrap your hands in a towel and go to the cold area. Immerse your hands in the warm water there for about ten minutes. Then go back indoors and repeat the warm-water submersion for two to five minutes. Repeat this method three to six times a day every other day until you've done 50 cycles of three dips each.

STEER CLEAR OF FROSTBITE. Avoiding frostbite is really critical, says Dr. Kahl. Frostbite can damage blood vessels and contribute to the development of Raynaud's. Watch for signs of frostbite such as numbness or your skin turning white or pale.

INVESTIGATE MEDICAL OPTIONS. Raynaud's can often be controlled without medication, says Dr. Spencer-Green. But in severe cases that are difficult to manage, doctors may recommend prescription medications such as nifedipine (Procardia), diltiazem (Cardizem Tablets) and generic reserpine, which can help control symptoms but are not considered "cures" for the disorder. Topical agents, such as nitroglycerin ointments (Nitro-Bid ointment), are effective in controlling symptoms in some patients.

Repetitive Strain Injury

STIFLING THE PAIN IN A PINCH

Repetitive strain injury is the reason secretaries are wearing wrist splints and hairdressers are having hand surgery.

The injuries—which generally involve muscles and tendons pinching nerves in the neck, shoulder, elbow, wrist or hand—are the result of repetitive actions usually related to on-the-job activities such as typing and cutting. These motions frequently interfere with the body's normal movement, and they can cause chronic pain.

How common are these problems? In a series of studies by the National Institute for Occupational Safety and Health, researchers found that repetitive strain injury (RSI) occurred in as many as 40 percent of newspaper workers who work at computers. People who use keyboards or calculators, assemble small parts, cut fabric and package small items are at increased risk, as are welders, musicians and truck drivers.

The common denominator is that the jobs these workers do generally involve the execution of fine motor movements of the hands and arms at a pace that is not natural.

RSI is increasing at a rapid rate, experts agree. Possibly caused by the increasing number of jobs that require repetitive motions such as keyboarding, these injuries now account for 50 percent of all occupational illnesses reported in the United States.

The Tunnel of Pain

Of all the repetitive strain injuries that can occur, carpal tunnel syndrome is the most common in women. Smaller bone structure and hormones put women between the ages of 30 and 45 at twice the risk of men for this injury, experts say.

The carpal tunnel is just that—a tunnel that's formed by the carpal bones of the wrist and a ligament. Through the middle run nine tendons and the median nerve, a sensitive structure that provides feeling to the thumb, index finger, part of the middle finger and half of the ring finger.

Normally the nerve has plenty of room inside the carpal tunnel, and feeling and function in the hand are normal. But when the nerve gets pinched by swollen tendons as it passes through the tunnel, blood flow to the nerve is reduced, the nerve swells, and scar tissue begins to form. The result is the tingling, numbness, weakness and pain that lead to a diagnosis of carpal tunnel syndrome.

The major symptoms of carpal tunnel syndrome are pain and numbness that awaken you at night, although when the syndrome is severe, it can cause loss of grip strength and weakness in the hands that results in clumsiness. Half of all patients who get carpal tunnel syndrome eventually get it in both hands.

What's behind It

Carpal tunnel syndrome is believed to be caused by activities that involve repetitive upward and downward motions of the wrist and those in which the wrist is placed continually in a cocked or bent position. Upward and downward motions cause the tendons to become inflamed and swollen. A cocked or bent position narrows the carpal tunnel, compressing the median nerve.

Typing on a computer keyboard, working on an assembly line, cutting hair or keying on a calculator or cash register are the kinds of repetitive activities that can cause carpal tunnel syndrome. And so can home activities and hobbies such as kneading bread or knitting, says Karen Piegorsch, an ergonomist and clinical specialist in orthopedic physical therapy in Columbia, South Carolina. In a study conducted by researchers in Colorado, for example, 15.9 percent of 552 individuals visiting a doctor for the first time for carpal tunnel syndrome were homemakers.

Body size is also believed to play a role. Because the average woman's body is smaller than a man's, it may predispose her to carpal tunnel syndrome. Decreased carpal tunnel size (along with sex differences related to hormones) contribute to the development of the condition, says Richard Katz, M.D., medical director of SSM Rehabilitation Institute in St. Louis. The tendons and nerves in a woman's hand may be similar in size to those of a man, yet her bones, which support the hand, may be much smaller. This means they have less room in which to operate and are more in danger of becoming compressed, says Amy Ladd, M.D., a hand surgeon and assistant professor of functional restoration in the Division of Hand and Orthopedic Surgery at Stanford University School of Medicine.

A woman's smaller body size in relation to the large equipment and tools she operates at work may also make her more susceptible, says Piegorsch. That's because tools designed for a man may force her to work with equipment that is too high, too heavy or at the wrong angle.

What Hormones Can Do

Many women also develop carpal tunnel in the second and third trimesters of pregnancy because of hormonal changes, says Dr. Ladd. Studies indicate that between 2 and 25 percent of pregnant women have it. During pregnancy there is more fluid retention, and as the body swells, so do the structures in the carpal tunnel. Researchers believe that the change in the estrogen/progesterone balance may be responsible for fluid retention, says Dr. Ladd.

The hormonal shifts of menopause also put women at high risk for carpal tunnel syndrome, researchers say, as do birth control pills in women who retain fluid, says Dr. Ladd.

And premenstrual water retention may increase pain in women who have the syndrome, says Alan Bernstein, M.D., chief of neurology at the Kaiser Permanente Medical Center in Hayward, California. "Premenstrual swelling affects everywhere in the body," he says. "If tendons swell, it doesn't take a lot to pinch the nerve."

Having long fingernails is another factor. Often women with long nails who use keyboards a lot hold their fingers in an unnatural position, which places excess stress on their fingers and wrists, according to Piegorsch.

The syndrome can also plague women who have thyroid disease or rheumatoid arthritis—two diseases that cause swelling and affect more women than men.

Playing It Safe

Women may be more susceptible to carpal tunnel than men, but there are things you can do to lower your risks. Here's how.

SIT PROPERLY. When you sit at a keyboard, make sure your chair is adjusted properly. When sitting, your back should be well-supported and your feet should be flat on the floor. Your knees and hips should be bent to 90 degrees, and your shoulders should be over your hips.

Be especially aware of the angle of the keyboard and the height of the chair relative to the keyboard. When you're seated in a chair that's properly adjusted, your wrists can gently flex upward with no extreme bends in either direction, says Piegorsch. "The goal is to adjust your workstation to allow your body to be in a balanced posture," she says.

WARM UP AND STRETCH. If you're going to use part of your upper body repetitively, be sure to warm up and stretch, says Dr. Katz. For example, start with slow typing, then speed up later.

TAKE BREAKS. Rest periodically throughout the day. Change to a less repetitive activity or one that allows you to use a different set of muscles, says Piegorsch. A good plan is to take a 30-second break every half-hour to change positions or get up and move around.

WATCH YOUR NECK AND SHOULDERS. Since the nerves and blood vessels that pass through the carpal tunnel originate in the neck and shoulder area, poor neck and shoulder posture can contribute to the development of carpal tunnel syndrome, says Piegorsch. Be aware of your posture while working in the kitchen, too. Counters are often too high for shorter women and cause them to hunch their shoulders while chopping and cutting, she says. If your counters are too high, work on a lower surface or stand on a low stool.

TRIM YOUR NAILS. Keep your nails at the length that allows you to type with the tips of your fingers in a natural position. That's probably less than an eighth of an inch.

Tackling the Hurt

If you're suffering from the pain of carpal tunnel, here are some coping mechanisms.

CHANGE THE WAY YOU WORK OR PLAY. If you're doing activities with a lot of repetitive wrist motions, try cutting back. A woman who types for a living might want to limit the amount of knitting she does after work, for example, while someone who uses a screw-gun on an assembly line might want to give hedge-clipping chores to another family member.

Also take a look at your workstation and see if it's right for you. For help, call the federally sponsored Job Accommodation Network at 1-800-526-7234. The people there can suggest ways to modify your work area to help deal with repetitive strain injuries and other disabilities.

VIE FOR VITAMINS. Vitamin B_6 may help reduce carpal tunnel pain, says Dr. Bernstein. Experts believe that B_6 helps increase serotonin, a chemical messenger in your brain that can decrease pain. But since vitamin B_6 can cause nerve damage in some people, he adds, check with your doctor about how much you should take before you try it.

SEE A HEALTH PROFESSIONAL. When pain starts waking you up at night, it's time to see a doctor, says Dr. Bernstein. Find an orthopedic surgeon or neurologist who specializes in carpal tunnel syndrome. She might suggest a splint to keep your wrist in a neutral position. Night splints can be useful, says Dr. Bernstein, because we often flex our wrists while we sleep. Using splints on the job is often ineffective, however, since the patient may end up fighting against the splint, which may cause further injury to the wrist and lead to other problems such as tendinitis.

CONSIDER SURGERY. If your wrist still hurts eight weeks after you've tried rest, stretching, splinting and new work habits, it might be time to talk to your doctor about surgery. Surgery can alleviate pain and prevent further injury to the nerve by literally dividing the carpal ligament that runs through your wrist, thus releasing the bear hug it's got on your median nerve. Once free, the nerve begins to recover and stops sending pain messages to your brain. The whole area can then get back to business.

Rosacea

ARE YOU SEEING RED?

It's been *years* since you've had anything even resembling a zit. In fact, you went through high school practically unscathed, while classmates suffered interminably. Now here you are, over 30, with these pimplelike things on your face. They're unsightly and embarrassing and you never know when they'll appear. "What's going on here?" you wonder.

Sound familiar? If so, you may have rosacea (pronounced *roe-ZAY-shuh*), an unpredictable skin disorder that can get progressively worse with time.

Never heard of it? You're not alone. A Gallup survey indicated that almost three-fourths of Americans are unaware of the disease. Yet it seems to be on the rise as the Baby Boom generation enters middle age. It often first appears in adults during their thirties and forties.

Rosacea can resemble acne, with papules (small red bumps) and pustules (pus-filled bumps) appearing on the forehead, nose and cheeks.

The whiteheads and blackheads well-known to those with acne are absent. But it can also appear as flushing and redness of the skin, either on the cheeks or the tip of the nose, which is how it usually begins. Later, spiderlike networks of broken capillaries may appear. In severe forms, rhinophyma—the bumpy, bulbous, W. C. Fields–type nose—shows up, although this occurs more often in men than in women. Rosacea may also affect the eyes, causing redness and flakiness around the eye, inflammation of the iris and a bloodshot appearance.

Women and Rosacea

Some of us are more prone to rosacea than others, experts say. Fair-skinned, fair-haired people, those with a tendency to blush, and people of Northern European descent are at greatest risk. Aside from the genetic link, though, experts aren't sure what causes it.

And it's hard to say how many people get rosacea, because many people don't see their doctor about it, says Jonathan Wilkin, M.D., director of the Division of Dermatology at Ohio State University Medical Center in Columbus. A fair estimate, he says, is 5 percent of Americans. Most experts believe rosacea occurs more often in women, though no precise figures are available.

Several drugs used to regulate the menstrual cycle can cause hot flashes that can trigger or exacerbate rosacea. And women may experience flare-ups during premenopause, menopause and some phases of the menstrual cycle.

Dr. Wilkin says that many women experience premenopausal hot flashes as early as their midthirties. With the hot flashes come sweating and flushing, and it's the flushing response that triggers rosacea.

How You Can Curb Rosacea

There's no cure to date, but rosacea is controllable through lifestyle changes. Here's how to fend it off.

Go sting-free. Avoid products that cause your face to flush and sting, such as astringents and toners. These include some sunscreens, says Dr. Wilkin. "Many sunscreens come in alcohol-based gels that sting the face," he says. Sunscreens for babies are usually the safest bet, he says.

Spray your hair only. Be careful not to get hair spray on your face. It can irritate the skin, says Dr. Wilkin.

Minimize sun exposure. Excessive sun exposure triggers rosacea outbreaks in some individuals, so keep it to a minimum, says Dr. Wilkin. Besides using sunscreen, wear a hat and go for the shady spots.

BE GENTLE TO YOUR FACE. Treat your face gently, says Dr. Wilkin. Don't get aggressive facial peels. Wash gently with a mild soap such as Dove, use lukewarm water and pat your face dry. Also protect your face from the cold and wind with a scarf.

WATCH YOUR MEDICATIONS. Certain drugs can spur a rosacea-like reaction, says Jerome Z. Litt, M.D., a dermatologist in Beachwood, Ohio, and assistant clinical professor of dermatology at Case Western Reserve University School of Medicine in Cleveland. The biggest offenders are strong, prescription fluorinated corticosteroid creams and ointments such as Temovate, Ultravate, Psorcon, Lidex and Diprolene.

The prescription form of niacin, used to control cholesterol, can also cause strong flushing reactions, adds Dr. Wilkin. Don't stop taking it—just take aspirin before the niacin and that should shut off the flushing reaction, he says. (Be sure to check this with your physician first.) Also, calcium channel blockers such as verapamil (Calan) and nifedipine (Adalat), generally used for high blood pressure, can contribute to rosacea.

FORGET HOT, HOT, HOT. Let hot beverages and food cool. They can cause you to heat up and flush, which will exacerbate rosacea, says Dr. Helm.

COOL DOWN AFTER EXERCISE. It's best not to overheat, so after exercising, cool down quickly. "If you get beet-red, wrap a cool, wet towel around your face and head. Or hold ice chips in your mouth and suck on them," says Dr. Wilkin. And when possible, get yourself into a cool shower as quickly as possible.

GO EASY ON ALCOHOL. Keep your alcohol intake to a minimum. Choose drinks with a low alcohol content. "If you're going to drink wine, the last thing you want is red wine. Go with white instead, " says Dr. Wilkin. The coloring in red wine comes from grape skins, which contain chemicals that contribute to flushing, he says. If you're considering distilled liquor, go with gin or vodka. Like white wine, they contain fewer chemicals, so you won't flush as much. "The best ploy, of course, is to avoid alcohol altogether," he says.

WATCH THE COFFEE. While many people say the caffeine in hot beverages is the culprit behind rosacea flare-ups, it's actually the heat that's responsible. And going cold turkey on caffeine can actually cause a flushing response, says Dr. Wilkin. So if you plan to kick your caffeine habit, wean yourself slowly.

REDUCE STRESS. Stress can provoke rosacea outbreaks, so do what you can to minimize it. Biofeedback, a relaxation method that helps you learn to control how your body responds to stress, is effective for some people, says Dr. Wilkin.

USE MAKEUP MAGIC. Try non-oil-based makeups; they'll irritate your face less. The National Rosacea Society recommends makeup that is non-oil-based and contains no alcohol. And on days when your nose is lit up with redness, try cosmetics or foundations with a green tint; they'll neutralize the redness and camouflage the problem.

KEEP A JOURNAL. Take note of when you break out and try to identify the cause. "You have to be the detective. Keep a journal and see if there's a pattern, " says Dr. Litt.

How to Treat It

Is an outbreak already in swing? Experts advocate treating it initially with both oral and topical medications. "Some women are so discouraged by their skin problem that seeing improvement the first few weeks of treatment can help build confidence," says Dr. Helm. "A topical product may not bring the rapid results they need, so I try to control the condition quickly with oral medication and later rely on topical products alone to control the condition." Oral medications generally include tetracycline (Andromycin), erythromycin (E-Mycin) and minocycline (Minocin), and a popular topical agent is MetroGel, which contains the antibiotic metronidazole.

Severe cases of rosacea, in which blood vessels stand out or the nose has become enlarged, may be helped with laser treatments. Electrodestruction, a procedure that makes problem vessels less visible by sealing off their blood supply, is another choice. So is plastic surgery.

Sexually Transmitted Diseases

For Us, a Bigger Price to Pay

As women, we often share our health woes with each other. Without a second thought we'll tell each other we have PMS, pump-bumps, hay fever or a headache.

We'll even share the news that we have an ovarian cyst, are having trouble with our menstrual cycle or have been diagnosed with breast cancer.

But there's a topic that's still pretty much taboo, and that's sexually transmitted diseases (STDs). We just don't openly admit to having them.

But the fact of the matter is, many of us do. Women are infected more readily than men when it comes to some STDs, and the consequences they suffer are often greater, too, says Jeanne LeVasseur, R.N., a family nurse-practitioner who teaches at the University of Connecticut School of Nursing in Storrs.

Why We're at Greater Risk

An estimated six million American women contract STDs each year. While that's about 50 percent of all sexually transmitted diseases, women are twice as likely as men to get certain types, namely gonorrhea and chlamydia, and half again as likely to get syphilis.

That's due in part to the way we're built. When an STD is introduced into a woman's body, it's basically an internal inoculation with an infection, says Linda Alexander, R.N., Ph.D., director of the Women's Health Program at the American Social Health Association in Research Triangle Park, North Carolina.

In addition, the lining of the vagina is a mucous membrane, which is thin and particularly susceptible to infections. Also, women can be exposed to the infecting organisms for longer than men because semen and infecting organisms can pool in the vagina.

STDs in women are also more difficult to diagnose, says Dr. Alexander. Part of the reason is that STD infections often have no symptoms. And even when lesions or signs are present, they are often located inside the vagina, where women can't see them.

LIVING WITH HERPES

The women who often have the most emotional response to being diagnosed with an STD are those with herpes, says Jeanne LeVasseur, R.N., a family nurse-practitioner who teaches at the University of Connecticut School of Nursing in Storrs.

These women often worry that their sex lives are over, she says. "Particularly for a young woman who isn't married or in a relationship that's stable and continuing, she wonders how she's ever going to find another man who will love her," says LeVasseur.

"These women need to take the healing process one step at a time," she says. "First there is going to be this physical healing, right now, of this area of the body that is infected. And over time they will come to terms with it emotionally."

In the year after the first outbreak of herpes, a woman will learn how her body is going to respond to the virus, explains LeVasseur. About one-third of women have recurrent outbreaks, a third have infrequent outbreaks, and another third never have another outbreak, she says.

Infertility and Other Consequences

STDs are a crucial issue for women because they can have serious long-term complications, says Judith Wasserheit, M.D., director of the Division of STD/HIV Prevention at the Centers for Disease Control and Prevention in Atlanta. "Those complications disproportionately affect women's lives," she says.

First, STDs can lead to infertility. Some infections, such as chlamydia, invade the upper genital tract and progress into pelvic inflammatory disease (PID). This can scar and block the fallopian tubes, making it difficult if not impossible for sperm to reach an egg to fertilize it. More than one million PID infections occur in women every year, and often they're a result of an STD, primarily gonorrhea or chlamydia. As many as 150,000 of those women may become infertile due to STDs.

STDs can also complicate pregnancy, says Dr. Wasserheit. Scar tissue from PID can sometimes allow sperm to get through to the egg but then not permit the fertilized egg to move down the fallopian tube into the uterus. This is known as an ectopic pregnancy, which is a medical emergency and can be life-threatening to the mother.

"There can be more outbreaks in the first year than in subsequent years, which I think offers some hope that if they can get beyond the first year, they will get to a place where things are more stable for them," she says.

One of the most effective treatments is the prescription antiviral drug acyclovir (Zovirax), which shortens outbreaks, she says.

The thing that women are often most concerned about with herpes is how they will be able to find a partner and fall in love when they have this disease, says LeVasseur. How will they tell him? "I remind them that right now they are thinking about an imaginary partner that they do not know or haven't met yet. And the idea of discussing it seems impossible or insurmountable with this imaginary figure. I remind them that when they do get to that point, that will be a real person and they will be discussing this with someone that they care about and who cares about them, and the discussion will be easier because of that."

Finally, STDs often cause women to lose their pregnancies through stillbirth or spontaneous abortion or to deliver either premature or low-birthweight babies, says Dr. Wasserheit.

STDs can also increase a woman's chances of developing other diseases. The human papillomavirus (HPV), which is more commonly known as genital warts, for example, has more than 70 strains, and two types have been linked to risk of cervical cancer, says King Holmes, M.D., Ph.D., director of the Center for AIDS and STDs at the University of Washington School of Medicine in Seattle. Some STDs, such as chlamydia, gonorrhea and perhaps trichomoniasis, appear to increase a woman's chance of acquiring HIV, the virus that causes AIDS, if she's exposed sexually to a man who is HIV-positive.

In addition to the physical repercussions, there is often emotional fallout for women with STDs. Research indicates that the emotional

CONCERNING CONDOMS

It's not always easy to talk with your partner about sex, your sexual histories, sexually transmitted diseases and condoms, but there are some things you can do to make it easier. Try these suggestions.

TAKE YOUR TIME. First, go slowly with the relationship so that you feel you know the person better, says Jeanne LeVasseur, R.N., a family nurse-practitioner who teaches at the University of Connecticut School of Nursing in Storrs. "Get to the point in the relationship where you have some emotional intimacy before you have sex," she says.

BE DECISIVE. "You need to make up your mind before you begin the discussion that you will use a condom," says LeVasseur. "You have to all of a sudden decide and be completely resolved that this is the only way that you will have sex. The women that I've talked to who use a condom and are most successful at using it see it as a nonnegotiable issue. They expect to use them. They value their bodies and their lives and view protected sex as the only possibility."

SET THE STAGE FOR CONVERSATION. When you are ready to talk about sex and condoms, pick a quiet and private time responses of women to STD infections are different from those of men. A survey of patients infected with genital warts and herpes, conducted by the American Social Health Association in North Carolina, found that women are initially more angry, humiliated and embarrassed than men are when they find out they have an STD, says Dr. Alexander. "And their feelings tend to last for years afterward," she says. "The emotional burden is significantly higher for women than it is for men."

The Six Most Common Offenders

Sexually transmitted diseases can be avoided if your partner uses a condom and if you're careful about whom you have sex with. And prevention is essential. Here's a brief look at what's out there.

Chlamydia, a bacterial infection, is currently one of the most common STDs, but it can be cured with antibiotics if it's treated early. As

---

to talk about it, a time that's separate from when you would have sex, says LeVasseur.

STRESS THE GOOD STUFF. If your partner has reservations about using condoms, stress both the positive aspects of the relationship and the positives about condom use, says LeVasseur. Tell him that they offer safety and that they will protect both of you, she says.

ACKNOWLEDGE YOUR PARTNER'S FEELINGS. If your partner says he doesn't like condoms for a particular reason, value his feelings and recognize them in your response, says LeVasseur. For example, if he says he doesn't like condoms because he has less sensation when he wears them, acknowledge that there may be some loss of feeling, but then move on and say you hope the two of you can get used to it.

USE "I" STATEMENTS. When talking about condoms, emphasize your thoughts and feelings and try not to blame your partner, says LeVasseur. For example, instead of saying "You make me angry/nervous/upset when you refuse to wear a condom," try "I feel nervous when we don't use condoms, and I can't relax. I would feel more comfortable if . . ."

many as 75 percent of the women who get it, and 25 percent of the men, have no symptoms. When chlamydia does cause symptoms, they usually include abnormal discharge, pain during urination, lower abdominal pain or pain during intercourse.

Gonorrhea is a bacterial infection that can invade the cervix, urethra, rectum, eyes or throat, and it often coexists with chlamydia. With gonorrhea you may have vaginal discharge or burning and itching when you urinate, or you may have no symptoms at all.

Human papillomavirus, also known as HPV or genital warts, is one of the most common STDs in the United States. As its name indicates, it's a virus, so once a woman is infected, the disease is with her for life. When warts develop, they can be on the outer genital area, in the vagina, on the cervix, in the anus or even in the throat.

Treatment for genital warts includes freezing them through a procedure called cryotherapy, zapping them with laser therapy, removing them surgically, or applying chemicals to them. Once treated, genital warts may reappear later on. Some strains of the virus are associated with cervical cancer, so it's important for women who have had a bout of HPV to have a Pap smear at least once a year. For active infections, more frequent Paps are recommended.

Genital herpes, or herpes simplex type 2, is spread by skin-to-skin contact with an infected area. Symptoms usually begin as mild itching or burning, pain in the genital area, legs or buttocks, or vaginal discharge. Then painful, sometimes open sores appear in the genital area, buttocks, anus and perhaps elsewhere on the body. They heal in several weeks, but many individuals suffer with painful outbreaks.

Herpes cannot be cured, but prescription antiviral drugs—such as acyclovir (Zovirax), which is most effective—are available. These drugs can reduce how often outbreaks occur and how bad they are. But herpes can lead to severe complications during pregnancy.

Trichomoniasis, or trich, is an infection caused by a parasite. Symptoms may include vaginal discharge, discomfort during intercourse, pain during urination and an offensive vaginal odor. It's possible for individuals, particularly men, to have trich and not know it, because often there are no symptoms. Since it's a parasite, trich can be cured with antibiotics.

Syphilis is a bacterial infection that can invade the heart, eyes, brain, bones and nervous system in its advanced stages. In the initial phase, syphilis usually appears as painless sores in the genital area, usually ten days to three months after exposure to an infected partner.

How to Safeguard Yourself

Since STDs pose such significant dangers, here's what you can do to safeguard your health.

SEE YOUR DOCTOR. Visit your health-care practitioner to be screened to be sure you are free of any STDs. Just because you're symptom-free doesn't mean you're in the clear, says LeVasseur.

Some general guidelines for whether you should be screened are whether you've had more than one partner in a year and whether you've engaged in intercourse without a condom, she says.

DON'T WAIT TO BE ASKED. Ask your doctor directly about STDs and screening, says Dr. Alexander. Don't assume that your annual gynecological exam screens you for everything. Most don't.

LEARN YOUR PARTNER'S HISTORY. Before you engage in sexual activity, find out whether your partner is or ever has been infected with an STD, and which one. Since not all STDs produce symptoms, the best way to be sure a new partner you're considering having sex with is disease-free is to ask him to be screened.

DECIDE ON CONDOMS. If you're going to have sex with someone you don't know for sure is STD-free, do your best to have him use a latex condom that contains the spermicide nonoxynol-9. Research shows that latex condoms cannot be penetrated by microscopic viruses such as HIV, and the spermicide nonoxynol-9 works to kill both sperm and many infectious organisms.

CONSIDER THE FEMALE CONDOM. A condom for women, marketed under the name Reality, offers a form of protection for women whose partners refuse to wear condoms. The female condom consists of a polyurethane sheath with two rings, a smaller springlike ring that fits against the cervix like a diaphragm and a larger ring that remains outside the vagina and through which the penis enters. The condom was designed to provide women with a condom over which they have control and which is protective against STDs.

PUT UP OTHER BARRIERS. While latex condoms are the best line of defense against STDs, says Lisa Hirsch, M.D., assistant professor of obstetrics and gynecology at the University of California Medical Center at Irvine, the next best is a diaphragm. The spermicidal jelly, foam or cream used with a diaphragm can help kill certain STD bacteria, and the diaphragm itself can prevent STD organisms from migrating into the upper genital tract.

BE CAREFUL WITH ORAL SEX. Having oral sex doesn't necessarily protect you from STDs, says Dr. Hirsch. While most women think it's safer, you can get herpes, gonorrhea, syphilis, hepatitis and HIV through oral sex. So again, be sure to practice safe sex.

If You're Infected

If you think you might have an STD, here are some things to remember.

DON'T WAIT. If you think you may have contracted an STD recently or that your past sexual behavior may have placed you at risk, get tested and treated as soon as you can. The longer you wait, the greater the potential consequences.

GO FOR THE FOLLOW-UP. "If a patient has gonorrhea or chlamydia or syphilis, she should definitely return for follow-up," says Dr. Hirsch. Even if you didn't finish your medications, go back and see your doctor. The infection may have been cured, but if it hasn't, the doctor may prescribe other drugs you can take, she says.

CONSIDER A MORE FREQUENT PAP. Medical research shows that there's a 20 percent false-negative rate in the reading of Pap smears, says Dr. Hirsch. In other words, your Pap can incorrectly tell you there's nothing wrong. The current recommendation is to have a Pap smear once a year, but women who are not in monogamous relationships should consider having a Pap smear twice a year, says Dr. Hirsch.

WAIT TILL YOU'RE CLEAR. If screening reveals you have a bacterial STD, abstain from all forms of sex until you are treated and free of the infection, says Dr. Hirsch.

BANISH THE GUILT. A woman isn't a bad person because she gets an STD, says LeVasseur. "An STD is an infectious illness just like all infectious illnesses that don't carry the additional freight of intimacy and sex," she says. "Getting an STD may mean you are more willing to take risks or less willing to protect yourself, but it doesn't mean you are bad or dirty," she says.

PREPARE AHEAD FOR PREGNANCY. If you've got a viral STD and are planning a pregnancy, talk to your doctor ahead of time. Certain STDs can be transmitted to a fetus during childbirth, so find out if you can be treated or if it's better for you to have a cesarean rather than a vaginal delivery.

Sinusitis

MAKE BREATHING EASY

When God was handing out noses, most of us probably hoped for something attractive—a stylish Roman or a cute little turned-up version. Who thought about mucus drainage and discharge?

Well, according to Nelson Gantz, M.D., chairman of the Department of Medicine and chief of the Division of Infectious Diseases at the Polyclinic Medical Center in Harrisburg, Pennsylvania, form should follow function. With apologies to God, Dr. Gantz suspects that the reason that sinusitis is a common health problem in the United States is that the sinuses aren't very well designed. "The sinuses should really have better drainage," Dr. Gantz says.

Although sinusitis is a common condition, it isn't as common as the complaints about it would indicate. "People frequently think they have sinusitis when they actually have bad colds, allergies or tension headaches," says Donald Leopold, M.D., associate professor of otolaryngology/head and neck surgery at Johns Hopkins University in Baltimore. Strictly speaking, sinusitis is a bacterial infection that swells the sinuses, causing headache, facial pain and sometimes fever and other symptoms.

The sinuses are eight hollow compartments located behind your cheekbones and eyes, like little bedrooms tucked off the nose's main hallway. No one pays much attention to them until they start to hurt. But then, oh, brother! The symptoms of sinusitis—thick, yellowish-greenish mucus that keeps draining and makes breathing through your nose a battle, severe headache with facial tenderness centered around the cheeks and eyes, a dry cough and sometimes a fever—can make you miserable.

Design defects may be part of the problem, but it takes a catalyst to infect and inflame the sinuses. The common cold is frequently the culprit. Colds cause congestion, which makes it harder for the cilia, tiny hairlike projections that line your nasal cavity, to sweep out germs in the air you breathe. Congestion from a cold or a bout with seasonal allergies flattens the cilia, giving bacteria a chance to accumulate in the nasal passages and infiltrate the sinuses. Only 1 cold in 200 actually develops into sinusitis, but because women catch an average of three or four colds each year, the odds are that most of us will suffer the pain and discomfort of a sinus infection at least once in our lives.

Pregnancy and Other Causes

Except when they're pregnant, women are no more likely than men to have sinusitis. During pregnancy, hormones secreted to thicken the uterus also thicken nasal passages, causing nasal congestion, which in turn can increase the incidence of sinusitis. "Some women say they never want to get pregnant again," says Howard Levine, M.D., director of nasal and sinus surgery at the Mount Sinai Nasal-Sinus Center in Cleveland, "because they have so much trouble breathing that they can hardly sleep or eat."

Sinusitis is seldom the most troublesome symptom that pregnant women face. But when it does develop, especially in conjunction with asthma or allergies, it can make breathing—never a simple task when a fetus is pushing on your ribcage—a major challenge. Physicians may prescribe antibiotics and often recommend steam treatments and other home remedies, but pregnant women should consider avoiding decongestants, which can elevate their blood pressure.

Pregnant women aren't the only ones at special risk for sinus problems. Anyone who has asthma or seasonal allergies is vulnerable, too.

People with vasomotor rhinitis, a condition that makes them exceptionally sensitive to airborne pollutants such as perfume and cigarette smoke, are also more apt to develop sinusitis.

Low humidity and polluted air set the scene for all kinds of respiratory problems that could lead to sinusitis, says Stanley Shapshay, M.D., chairman of the Department of Otolaryngology/Head and Neck Surgery at Tufts University School of Medicine and otolaryngologist-in-chief at the New England Medical Center Hospital, both in Boston. "As air quality deteriorates, doctors are seeing much more airway disease," he says.

How to Keep Your Nose Clear

Because an acute attack of sinusitis is such a dreadful experience, anyone who's endured it once wants to avoid future episodes. If preven-

SORTING THROUGH THE SINUS DRUGS

Choosing the right medication for congestion can be a complicated business. Decongestants containing pseudoephedrine and phenylpropanolamine usually work, but they can make you jittery and keep you up at night, says Donald Leopold, M.D., associate professor of otolaryngology/head and neck surgery at Johns Hopkins University in Baltimore. Antihistamines aren't good for sinusitis—they can worsen congestion, making mucus even thicker and harder to expel. Antihistamines will work, however, when your nasal passages are plugged up due to allergies.

Decongestant nasal sprays are okay for short-term use—no more than three to five days at a time. But if you use them longer or too frequently, they can have a rebound effect, according to Howard Levine, M.D., director of nasal and sinus surgery at the Mount Sinai Nasal-Sinus Center in Cleveland. Instead of opening up your sinuses, they'll worsen congestion.

The best over-the-counter medication if you have a lot of thick nasal mucus may actually be cough medicine. Look for brands like Robitussin, which contain guaifenesin, a mucus-thinning agent. Follow the label directions for dosage, says Dr. Levine.

tion is the key, steam is the first line of defense. Taking a hot shower, for example, opens up the sinuses. Decongestants may also be taken at the first sign of cold congestion, because if nasal passages stay blocked long enough, they will inevitably get infected. And although antihistamines may seem like a good idea, they're not. They're great for relieving allergic symptoms, but they dry up mucous membranes and increase congestion.

The best advice, says Dr. Levine, is don't catch cold. "Most colds are spread by hand-to-hand contact," he says, "so it helps to wash your hands frequently." If you manage to get a cold anyway, here are some tips to keep your sinuses from swelling.

GET HUMID. Invest in a humidifier, says Dr. Levine, but be sure to keep it clean. Humidifiers are great for adding moisture to the air, but they're also great at growing mold and mildew. Using distilled water helps, but you should also clean your humidifier weekly. Empty the tank and scrub it out with a half-cup of household bleach or vinegar mixed with a gallon of water. Rinse well before you use the humidifier again. By the way, it doesn't matter whether you buy a warm-air or cool-air humidifier: It's the water itself that creates the climate for mold and mildew.

DRINK CHICKEN SOUP. "Grandma was right," says Dr. Levine. "The heat from the soup is mucus-thinning, and the garlic is, too." For best results, drink your chicken soup—or any other hot liquid, such as hot tea with lemon, Chinese hot-and-sour soup or even hot water—from a cup so that the steam rises right up into your nasal passages.

BREATHE DEEP. Fragrant herbal steam not only relieves congestion, it also soothes the soul. Place a drop or two of eucalyptus, pine or tea tree pure essential oil (available at health food stores) into a large pot of boiling water. Remove the pot from the heat. Hold a towel over your head and the pot and breathe in deeply for ten minutes. Rosemary Gladstar, an herbalist in East Barre, Vermont, and author of *Herbal Healing for Women*, recommends doing this two or three times a day, using eucalyptus, sage or pine oil.

SPICE UP YOUR LIFE. Treat yourself to fiery Mexican, Chinese or Indian food. Horseradish, cayenne, curry, jalapeño and chili seasonings help unblock sinuses. These fiery foods seem to stimulate nasal secretions to loosen up and pour out. Horseradish works particularly well, says Gladstar, who recommends grating it fresh and eating it on toast, with soup or on rice. It's almost painful to eat, she says, but it clears congestion and thereby helps the body fight infection.

STAY MOIST. "With noses, the big thing is humidity," says Dr. Leopold. "If your nose gets dry, bad things happen." When nasal passages dry out, you're more susceptible to nosebleeds. The mucus blanket thickens, the cilia can't move, and you're more likely to get infections.

There are several alternatives for moisturizing the nose, according to Dr. Leopold. Drink lots of water. Use saline nasal sprays, which are simply purified salt water in spray bottles and are available in drugstores. On drugstore shelves, you can also find moisture creams such as petroleum jelly or Eucerin lotion. Put a little on a cotton-tipped swab and lightly coat your nostrils. Also ask your pharmacist about gel-mist sprays for keeping your nose moist.

EXERT PRESSURE. Acupressure works wonders for sinus symptom relief. Traditional Chinese medicine practitioners use pressure points in the web of flesh between the thumb and forefinger to relieve sinus headaches and a point just above the bridge of the nose, between the eyebrows, to relieve congestion, says Harriet Beinfield, a licensed acupuncturist and co-author of *Between Heaven and Earth: A Guide to Chinese Medicine.* You may also apply pressure to your cheeks (along the ridge of the cheekbones) and temples and along the sides of the nose. Look for tender or sensitive spots in the crease between the nostrils and the cheeks.

When you've found the right spot, you'll know. You may feel a twinge or a tingle. You may feel some relief right away. Press gently but firmly, using your knuckle or fingertip (with a short nail), using a rotating motion in a tight circle. Continue massaging for 30 seconds to five minutes, as you wish. Repeat as often as it feels good, says Beinfield.

WATCH WHAT YOU CONSUME. When you have a sinus infection, avoid coffee, tea, cola and alcoholic beverages, says Dr. Levine. The caffeine in coffee, tea and colas is a diuretic, and alcohol dehydrates you. Stay away from dairy products and chocolate, too; they thicken congestion.

Skin Cancer

IT's 99 PERCENT PREVENTABLE

The mole is getting larger.

You first noticed it on your face a couple of months ago. It was just a small mark, light brown, with irregular edges. It was too small and pale for anyone else to really notice, but every morning when you put on your moisturizer, you noticed that it seemed to be getting a little darker. And now it's gotten bigger.

What could it be?

Every woman gets tiny freckles, moles, bumps, blisters and marks on her skin at one time or another. Usually they come and go. Any one of these can be a perfectly innocent dot of color—or the beginning of skin cancer. But since the rate of skin cancer has doubled in both men and women over the past 20 years, every mark that changes its appearance over time needs to be checked by a physician.

Three Kinds of Cancer

"There are three major types of skin cancer—basal cell carcinoma, squamous cell carcinoma and melanoma," says dermatologist Jean L. Bolognia, M.D., director of the Pigmented Lesion Clinic at Yale University School of Medicine.

"Basal cell carcinoma is the most common of the three in both men and women. It's seen primarily in the head and neck region, although it can occur anywhere on the body. It can begin as a pearly bump or a scab," says Dr. Bolognia. The chances it will spread elsewhere are extremely low—less than 1 in 10,000, she says.

Squamous cell carcinoma is more serious than basal cell carcinoma, says Dr. Bolognia, because it is more likely to spread, particularly to regional lymph nodes. These tumors can look like warts or a single area of eczema that just doesn't go away. They're found on sun-exposed areas such as the back of your hand or forearm or in the head and neck region.

Basal cell and squamous cell carcinoma affect about 700,000 men and women every year, according to the American Cancer Society (ACS). But that's just a ballpark figure, says Joann Schellenbach, national director of media relations for the ACS. "This stuff is so prevalent that nobody counts it. Doctors just cut it off and throw it out."

Melanoma, however, is a different story.

"Melanoma is a malignancy of melanocytes, which are the pigment-producing cells of the skin," says Dr. Bolognia. "It can develop within a mole or in normal skin. It's characterized by asymmetry in the majority of cases—if you draw a line down the middle of the lesion, the right doesn't look like the left, either because of an irregularity of color or an irregularity of the border, or both.

"The major exception to that rule," adds Dr. Bolognia, "is a melanoma that arises quickly and looks like a black bump on the skin. This type of melanoma is referred to as nodular."

The most common locations for melanoma in women, she says, are the calf and shin, followed by the upper back. (In men, the most common location is the back.)

Detecting It Early

Fortunately, all forms of skin cancer are easily treated on an outpatient basis if they're caught early, says Nancy R. Matus, M.D., head of dermatology at Easton Hospital in Pennsylvania and clinical assistant professor of dermatology at Hahnemann University in Philadelphia. The majority of all skin cancers are removed by surgical excision or other procedures, including electrosurgery, freezing or lasers.

Although squamous cell carcinomas can spread to other places in the body, treatment of early (thin) lesions generally means cure. With basal cell carcinoma, it's less likely that the cancer will spread, but the problem may recur in the same area.

The overall five-year survival rate for people with melanoma that's caught early (before it invades to a depth greater than one millimeter) is over 90 percent. It's somewhat better for women than for men, according to Dr. Bolognia, but no one is certain why. Women do see their doctors earlier and tend to have thinner lesions, she notes, but that doesn't completely explain their better survival rates. "For some unknown reason, they just do better."

Scoping Out Risk

What puts women at risk for skin cancer?

Excessive sun exposure and a fair complexion are major risk factors for basal cell and squamous cell carcinomas. With melanoma, these factors plus a large number of moles and a family history of melanoma increase the risk, says Dr. Bolognia.

Dermatologists usually classify people into six different skin types, explains Dr. Bolognia. "Classified as Type I are the people who never tan. Type II is the person who doesn't tan well. Types III and IV are people who tan well. Type V individuals have brown skin, and Type VI people have black skin." It's primarily women with skin types I and II who develop skin cancer, according to Dr. Bolognia.

Researchers have found that two kinds of ultraviolet (UV) rays in sunlight can cause skin cancer. Ultraviolet-A (UVA) rays are the longest rays: They predominate in the solar energy that reaches the earth. With relatively long exposure, these rays can cause tanning and burning, and they contribute to premature aging and wrinkling of the skin as well as skin cancer. The other types of rays are ultraviolet-B (UVB), which are believed to be the primary cause of sunburn, photo-aging and skin cancer.

Artificial lights used in suntanning parlors also emit ultraviolet rays, and for this reason, dermatologists are adamantly against them. Originally tanning salons used UVB light, until it was proven beyond a shadow of a doubt that it causes skin cancer. Then they switched to UVA. The problem is that UVA causes aging of the skin and enhances the cancer-causing effects of UVB.

"Dermatologists hate suntanning parlors," says Dr. Bologna. "We'd like to see the government pass laws against their use."

Screening Sunlight

Since the ultraviolet rays in sunlight play such a big part in causing skin cancer, the best prevention is to avoid exposure to sunlight. But that's easier said than done for most of us, especially if we relish year-round outdoor activities.

But you can cut your risks to a fraction if you take sun-protective action. These tactics are especially important between the hours of 10:00 A.M. and 3:00 P.M., when UVB rays are the strongest. Protection is also super-important when you're at high elevations, where there's less atmosphere to block the sun's skin-endangering radiation. Here's what doctors recommend to ban the rays.

BLOCK THE A'S AND B'S. Since both UVA and UVB rays can contribute to skin cancer, you should look for types of sunscreen that shield against both. "Most sunscreens are very efficient at filtering UVB and short-wave UVA rays. The UVA protector that's usually used is benzophenone or oxybenzone. Unfortunately, in this country, we don't have a big choice in terms of broad-spectrum UVA protection," says Nicholas J. Lowe, M.D., clinical professor of dermatology at the University of California at Los Angeles School of Medicine and director of the Skin Research Foundation of California in Santa Monica. Although it can be hard to find, one ingredient to look for that protects against the longer UVA rays is Parsol 1789.

LEVEL OFF AT 15. "I recommend an SPF of 15," says Dr. Bologna. There are sunscreens with SPFs (sun protection factors) as high as 50, but doctors say they really don't do an appreciably better job than those with an SPF of 15. And they're more expensive. So save your money and buy plenty of SPF 15 sunscreen. It is more important that you slather it on generously and frequently whenever you're in the sun.

If your skin develops a rash or feels irritated when you use a sunscreen, try a chemical-free sunscreen, says Dr. Bologna. This type contains zinc oxide and titanium dioxide, which will protect your skin with less chance of an allergic reaction. Unlike the zinc oxide that once adorned lifeguards' noses, this product goes on clear.

GET READY, GET SET. The chemical ingredients in sunscreen have to be absorbed by the skin before they can go to work for you. So apply a sunscreen at least 30 minutes before you go outside.

DRY, AND REAPPLY. If you're basking on the beach or lounging by poolside, be sure to put on more sunscreen after you go in swimming. Even waterproof sunscreen can use a boost after you've toweled dry.

MIND YOUR MEDICINES. Medications that can make your skin extra-sensitive to the sun's rays include ibuprofen, antihistamines such as dimenhydrinate (Dramamine) and diphenhydramine (Benadryl) and tranquilizers such as perphenazine (Trilafon) and trifluoperazine (Stelazine). Some others that can make you sun-sensitive include tetracycline products (Minocin, Declomycin), oral contraceptives such as levonorgestrel (Triphasil) and norethindrone/ethinyl estradiol (Ovcon), tretinoin (Retin-A) and some diabetes drugs such as chlorpropamide (Diabinese, Glucamide).

USE MAKEUP WITH SUNSCREEN. "Try makeup and moisturizers that contain a sunscreen," says Dr. Bolognia. That way applying sunscreen becomes a part of your morning ritual, and you can't forget to use it. And if you're using a tanner, you should select one that has sunscreen in it.

USE A WRINKLE STICK. Sunscreen that creeps into your eyes can be painful, but using a wax-based stick—sold at cosmetic counters as a "wrinkle stick" or a "moisture stick"—can prevent the problem, says Dr. Bolognia. Just use it to apply wax around your eyes. It will establish a protective barrier between your eyes and the sunscreen in your makeup or moisturizer.

WEAR CLOTHING THAT SCREENS YOUR SKIN. Not all sun protection is in chemical form, says Dr. Bolognia. "There are tightly woven T-shirts and windbreakers you can buy. Some examples are Frogwear and Solumbra. The material is quite light, and water evaporates quickly." They provide an SPF of 30. (Call 1-800-328-4440 to order Frogwear and 1-800-882-7860 for Solumbra.)

WEAR A BROAD-BRIMMED HAT. A broad-brimmed hat not only lends you an air of nineteenth-century rose-garden nostalgia, it also keeps the sun off your face and neck.

DON'T GET A SUNLIGHT SIZZLE. Unlike the sunlight shining through your car windows, which is less damaging because it comes at you from an angle, rays from above may be intense enough to damage your skin. If you spend a lot of time under a skylight, don't forget your sunscreen.

Mole Patrol

Since early detection of skin cancer is so important, doctors recommend that you keep an eye on your skin—especially moles and dark patches. Here's what experts suggest to help you stop trouble before it begins.

WATCH FOR CHANGES. "A mole is a benign tumor of pigment cells," according to Dr. Bolognia. But moles are likely to change as you age. "As you get older your moles go from dark and flat to flesh-colored, raised and soft," she says. When a mole gets raised and firm or changes in color or size, it needs to be checked by your doctor.

PREGNANT? DOUBLE-CHECK YOUR MOLES. The high-estrogen state of pregnancy can cause melanocytes (cells that make pigment) to work overtime, says Dr. Bolognia. And although it's a good idea to point out any changes in moles to your doctor at any time, it's an especially good idea during pregnancy. There is evidence that the thickness of melanomas detected during pregnancy tends to be greater than that of those in women who are not pregnant.

KEEP COUNT. The average person has approximately 30 moles, says Dr. Bolognia, so you don't need to see a dermatologist unless there are changes. But the person who has more than 50 moles, dark or irregularly shaped moles and/or a family history of melanoma should see a dermatologist regularly. Once a year is recommended if the moles stay the same, but go more often if you are continuing to develop new moles.

Smoking

PUT OUT THE FIRE FOR GOOD

Ah, the power of the smoke-filled room. The allure of the smoky jazz club. The sophistication of the actress Bette Davis, a plume of smoke rising from the cigarette resting between her long, glamorous fingers.

Not anymore. Smoking is definitely out. The list of places where smoking is taboo continues to grow, from restaurants to offices to public buildings, particularly as the dangers of second-hand smoke become more well-known.

Indeed, these days, if you're one of the 22.2 million women who still smoke, it may seem as if the whole world is against you.

Although the number of men and women who smoke has been steadily decreasing, the rate of decline has not been nearly as sharp for women as for men. In 1965, 52 percent of men and 33 percent of women smoked; today the rate is 28 percent for men and 25 percent for women.

Moreover, "there are no grounds for complacency about smoking trends in women," says researcher Ellen R. Gritz, Ph.D., chairman of the Department of Behavioral Sciences at the University of Texas M. D. Anderson Cancer Center in Houston and former director of the Division of Cancer Control in the Jonsson Comprehensive Cancer Center at the University of California at Los Angeles.

Although more adult women may be quitting, teenage smoking rates—as measured among high school seniors—have not declined appreciably since 1984. In 1993, 19 percent of teenage boys and 18 percent of teenage girls continued smoking on a daily basis.

How Smoking Spells Trouble

The American Cancer Society (ACS) calls smoking the most preventable cause of premature death in America, adding that tobacco use is responsible for more than one in six deaths in the United States. That's more than 400,000 deaths a year.

In addition to being responsible for 87 percent of lung cancers, smoking also causes up to 90 percent of emphysema cases in women, says Norman Edelman, M.D., consultant on scientific affairs to the American Lung Association (ALA). Smoking is also a major cause of heart disease and has been linked with everything from gastric ulcers and colds to chronic lung diseases such as bronchitis, as well as cancers of the mouth, pharynx, larynx, esophagus, pancreas, kidneys and bladder.

For women, smoking has additional consequences. It has been implicated in miscarriage and lower birthweights, as well as bleeding during pregnancy and fetal deaths. And a study by the National Institute of Environmental Health Science in Durham, North Carolina, found that the fertility of women smokers declines by approximately 30 percent in any given menstrual cycle.

Additionally, women smokers over 35 who are on the birth control pill increase their risk of heart attack by 20 times.

Studies show that the risk of sudden infant death syndrome (SIDS) is two to four times higher among newborns whose mothers smoked during pregnancy than among infants whose mothers did not smoke. The occurrence of SIDS also rises when mothers resume smoking after quitting during pregnancy. Also, breastfeeding mothers who smoke tend to produce less milk.

Female smokers also face an increased risk of certain forms of cervical cancer, along with urinary incontinence and cataracts.

And that's not all. "On average, women smokers go through

menopause four to six years earlier," says Terry Pechacek, Ph.D., associate professor of medicine at the State University of New York at Buffalo and former chief of smoking research at the National Cancer Institute in Bethesda, Maryland. "Earlier menopause means damage to the bones and an increased likelihood of osteoporosis," he says. Also, with early menopause comes increased risk of heart disease, further elevating the risk of women who smoke.

To add insult to injury, just as smoking subtracts years from your life span, it adds them to your looks. Smoking reduces the oxygen that reaches the skin and leads to skin damage from the poisonous chemicals in cigarettes, explains Dr. Pechacek. Plus, smoking damages the ability of skin cells to repair themselves. "This leads to more rapid drying and aging of the skin."

Why It's Hard to Quit

Chances are if you're a smoker, you've tried to quit. But of the 17 million men and women who try each year, only 10 percent make it stick for longer than six months. And the success rate is lower among women than among men.

One reason for this may be that women report more depression when they quit smoking. In studies, depression has been shown to make it more likely that you'll go back to smoking, says Douglas E. Jorenby, Ph.D., coordinator of clinical activities for the Center for Tobacco Research and Intervention at the University of Wisconsin Medical School in Madison.

Women may also have more difficulty quitting because, paradoxically, even as nicotine raises blood pressure and increases heart rate, it smooths out and softens difficult feelings. "Women still have more difficulty acceptably expressing their anger than men do," says Gary DeNelsky, Ph.D., head of the Department of Psychology at the Cleveland Clinic Foundation in Ohio and director of the clinic's Smoking Cessation Program.

If you've tried to quit before but haven't yet made it, be assured that it's never too late. "Persistence seems to be the most important determining factor," says Dr. DeNelsky. "Each time you slip, don't view it as a failure but rather as a learning experience."

According to the Atlanta Centers for Disease Control and Prevention's Office on Smoking and Health, female smokers who quit in their late thirties add an average of three years to their lives. Even if they quit in their late sixties, they'll add a year to their lives.

There's more good news: After you've been off cigarettes just a year, the risk of heart disease attributable to smoking is reduced by half. After 15 years of abstinence, the risk is similar to that of people who never smoked.

A Little Help from Some Friends

The average cigarette contains ten milligrams of nicotine, of which between one and two milligrams is delivered to the lungs when the cigarette is smoked.

When you do decide to quit, be prepared for some unpleasant times. But don't let your fears stop you from acting. "Withdrawal symp-

---

WHAT HAPPENS WHEN YOU STOP

The stories about what smokers go through when they try to kick the habit are legendary—and sometimes apocryphal. Here's the truth about what could happen to you, so you'll know what to expect.

The burning desire. Crave, you will. Nicotine levels drop rapidly. Within two hours you'll develop the desire for a cigarette, says Mitchell Nides, Ph.D., a psychologist and researcher at the University of California at Los Angeles. "Emotionally you may long for your 'friend,' the cigarette. You may even dream of cigarettes. You have to realize that will happen."

The bad mood. Physicians call it dysphoria. You—and your spouse, children and friends—will call it other, less formal names. "You'll be more on edge and irritable, more likely to snap or be hostile to other people," says Terry Pechacek, Ph.D., associate professor of medicine at the State University of New York at Buffalo and former chief of smoking research at the National Cancer Institute in Bethesda, Maryland. And you may feel depressed or anxious. The good news is that the number of dark days should be no more than ten, with the first few the worst.

The weight gain. It's true that you'll probably gain a little weight, since smoking works to suppress the appetite. Here, too, your fears may be exaggerated: The average gain is about five pounds, and even this weight can be managed.

toms can be highly individualistic," says Dr. Pechacek. "Asking others what is going to happen is not realistic. The only way to know is to quit yourself." If you're prepared for the craving and the tantalizing situations that will arise, he adds, "it won't be as bad as you fear."

The woman who is most likely to quit is the woman who uses both a doctor and a program simultaneously, says Joann Schellenbach, national director of media relations for the ACS. Your doctor should be able to refer you to stop-smoking programs in your area. Or you can check with your local hospital's social services department or the local chapter of the ACS, the American Heart Association or the ALA to find the stop-smoking program nearest you. A good program is one with a quit rate of 20 percent, Schellenbach observes. Anything higher and they're probably fooling around with their numbers.

Schellenbach recommends that you talk to your doctor about whether you're a good candidate for nicotine gum or the nicotine patch. Both can help gradually reduce your physical addiction to nicotine.

Nicotine gum usually contains two milligrams of nicotine, and as many as 30 pieces may be chewed a day. The gum costs about $20 per box of 96 pieces, and you may go through up to four boxes in the course of three months. Your physician will give you the proper precautions, but make sure you've completely stopped smoking before you start chomping; otherwise you'll be putting too much nicotine into your system.

The patch provides larger doses of nicotine—anywhere from 7 to 21 milligrams—over longer periods of time, from 16 to 24 hours. Patches run about $90 per month, and you may need to use them for three months. It's also dangerous to smoke when you're wearing a patch because you can overload your body with nicotine, so make sure you've stopped completely.

Neither of these aids should be viewed as a "magic bullet," says Dr. Pechacek. "They only deal with half of the addiction, the physiological side." You're responsible for learning the other half: dealing with emotional and situational challenges like stress, anger, boredom and alcohol.

Meeting the Challenge

Before embarking on any program to stop, be realistic about the challenge of quitting an addictive habit. Here are some tips to help ease the pangs.

PAY ATTENTION. Identify the times when you find smoking particularly enjoyable, Dr. Pechacek suggests, because that's when you are most likely to relapse. Be on the lookout for ritual and social cues, like smoking with that first cup of coffee, when you're in a bar or nightclub where alcohol is being served or while chatting on the telephone. Firm up your resolve during those times, and find something else to do—like chewing gum or avoiding the situation altogether.

KNOW WHY YOU WANT TO QUIT. "Most smokers primarily want to quit for health reasons," says Mitchell Nides, M.D., a psychologist and researcher at the University of California at Los Angeles. Other smokers feel increasing social pressure to snuff out their cigarettes, he says, adding, "it's the reverse of the pressure they got as kids to begin smoking." Social pressure isn't as likely to keep you off cigarettes as concerns about your health are, he says.

GET READY. "Make sure you're picking the right time, that you've told all of your friends and have gotten rid of all of your ashtrays and cigarettes," Dr. Nides suggests. Ask your friends and family to support your effort by not smoking in your presence.

USE THE "FOUR Ds." Michael Cummings, Ph.D., director of the Smoking Cessation Clinic at the Roswell Park Cancer Institute in Buffalo, New York, suggests that smokers use the "four Ds": Delay, deep breathe, do something else and drink water.

If you can delay the urge to smoke for a few minutes, that gnawing feeling in the pit of your stomach will subside. The same with deep breathing and distracting yourself when you become bored, a time when many people light up simply for lack of anything better to do. Drinking one or two extra glasses of water whenever you have the urge to smoke will flood your system and cleanse it of nicotine and other chemicals.

LOSE WEIGHT LATER. "Don't be discouraged about weight gain while you're quitting," Dr. Cummings cautions. "Most smokers gain a few pounds after quitting, but it doesn't have to be excessive." If gaining weight worries you, get some exercise—take a walk, go to an aerobics class or ride your bike.

WRITE ALL ABOUT IT. Put together a letter to someone you care about, explaining why smoking is more important than your life, says Robert Van de Castle, Ph.D., professor emeritus of behavioral medicine at the University of Virginia Medical Center in Charlottesville. He says his patients feel so guilty when they've done this that they're motivated to stay on the wagon.

STAY UPBEAT. Try to view your withdrawal symptoms as recovery signs, says Dr. Nides. You should talk to your doctor about withdrawal and how to interpret it, he says. "If you have an increased cough," he says, "that's a way of the lungs clearing themselves."

Stress

FIGHTING THE FALLOUT FROM LIFE

At 37, Fran Davis was the quintessential Philadelphia lawyer. She worked 80 hours a week, traveled from one case to another all over the country, worked on some of the biggest and hottest cases in corporate America and loved every minute of it.

"I was a born litigator," says Davis. "I have a real go-for-the-jugular thing about lawyering. It's exciting and it's exhilarating. Yes, it's stressful. But I don't look at stress as a negative word. I need a certain amount to do what I want to do, to be competitive."

Unfortunately, she adds dryly, "it tends to get out of hand." Stress can build until, rather than giving you an edge, it becomes destructive. You lose your concentration, forget things and start to get disorganized.

All this happened to Fran Davis. But she's not the only woman to let stress get out of hand.

Seventy-five percent of women and 70 percent of men between

the ages of 25 and 44 say they experience "a lot" or a "moderate amount" of stress in their lives, according to a survey conducted by the National Center for Health Statistics in Hyattsville, Maryland.

And a study by the Northwestern National Life Insurance Company in Minneapolis reported that more than half of the workers in high-stress jobs suffer from physical or mental problems such as exhaustion, insomnia and headaches. Further, women seem particularly affected. Not only are they more likely to report stress-related illness, they are more likely to feel burned out and think about quitting.

In a survey by the Families and Work Institute in New York, 40 percent of women said they found it hard to get up and face another day at work every morning, and 42 percent said they feel "used up" by the end of the day.

Why are so many women burned out, used up and stressed out? Hormones, evolving social roles and a national marketplace that's reinventing itself are some good guesses. And unlike Fran Davis, who reduced her litigation work, cut her hours in half, moved to the country and worked from home, most women—particularly those with families to support—can't take such radical steps to reduce stress.

The Survival Advantage

The way our bodies respond to stress is preprogrammed. It's an ancient survival mechanism, genetically transmitted from generation to generation, that has kept our species on the alert for centuries.

When the senses perceive any threat to our existence, the brain triggers a flood of chemicals throughout the body—primarily epinephrine, norepinephrine and adrenocorticotropin—that will prepare it to fight or flee. The heart beats faster, more oxygen gets to the muscles, energy from fat and sugar is released, blood clotting speeds up and immune responses slow down.

In turn, adrenocorticotropin also triggers the release of the hormone cortisol, which essentially maintains this turbocharged state as long as the threat exists.

But although a woman's stress response works in much the same way as a man's, there are some major factors that make her response to stress far stronger, says researcher Eva Redei, Ph.D., assistant professor of pharmacology and psychiatry at the University of Pennsylvania in Philadelphia.

"Women naturally have higher levels of cortisol than men," she explains. Dr. Redei's animal studies indicate that the female hormone estrogen also increases a woman's chemical response to stress. Significant changes in levels of progesterone, another female sex hormone, alter the stress response the same way that cortisol does. Our levels of progesterone increase eight to ten times just before we menstruate.

"These changes in stress responses are like riding a roller coaster," says Dr. Redei. They give women a survival advantage in terms of their ability to sense danger and react within a heartbeat. The problem is that a woman's stress response system can't tell the difference between a deadline-intense project at work, an injured child at home and a marauding dinosaur. It just goes to full alert at the drop of a hat—raising our levels of stress and dampening our immune system just enough to make us vulnerable to everything from colds, cancer and heart disease to inflammatory bowel disease, diabetes and asthma.

Let Jack Do It

Although studies indicate that the complexity of women's roles— worker, wife, mother, daughter, friend—actually acts as a buffer against stress from any single role, trying to deal with the sheer number of tasks that are involved in these roles can produce enough stress to sink a ship.

But do we ask for help?

Not on your life. "We think we need to do it all on our own," says therapist Mandy Manderino, Ph.D., associate professor at the University of Missouri in Columbia.

Not only do we need to be the perfect wife and Mom, we need to be the perfect employee as well. And that's not fair, she adds—to anyone.

"It is important for women to stop overfunctioning and ask for help," she adds. "Some women are beginning to discover they need not do it all. However, other women continue to try to be everything to everyone. It is these women who are at high risk for stress-related problems."

She also points out that women may be able to get more help from their spouses than they have in the past. "Because greater numbers of women have joined the workforce, men are beginning to share in the cooking, cleaning and child-care responsibilities. This is not only liberating for women but for men as well," says Dr. Manderino.

Here's what you can do to get some much-needed help.

SET YOUR PRIORITIES. Of all the myriad tasks demanding your attention, ask yourself which is the most important. Your daily to-do list should be based on your personal goals, says Dr. Manderino. "Is an absolutely spotless toilet bowl a top priority for you?" she asks. "Or is it more important to go out in the yard and play baseball with your kids or perhaps finish your college degree?"

GET OFF THE BACK BURNER. "Oftentimes women put themselves last or leave themselves out entirely when setting priorities. They have difficulty making time for themselves," says Dr. Manderino. They can just never get to the gym or find a half-hour to soak in the tub. "They say, 'Well, I'd like to, but all these other things come first.'

"But if you're giving away energy, there's got to be a way to get back energy," she points out. "There has to be some 'me' time. And if that constantly gets moved to please someone else, you're going to continue to be stressed."

Pick a time every day and set it aside to do things just for yourself, says Dr. Manderino. Play, relax, exercise—do anything you like. But it can't be unpleasant work, and it can't be for anybody else but you.

RE-ENERGIZE. Fight stress by renewing your personal energy with some type of relaxation exercise, says Dr. Manderino. Do yoga, t'ai chi or meditation—whatever works for you.

"I'm a really active person and I can't meditate," says Dr. Manderino. "I can't sit still. So I do a walking meditation. I walk and focus on the 'now.' I anchor myself in the present by trying to notice the wildflowers, the smell of the damp ground and the trees."

LET GO OF TENSION. "Once in the morning and once in the afternoon, I like to close my eyes and take in a nice, deep breath, and as I do, become aware of any tension in my head, scalp and neck," says Dr. Manderino. "Then I let out the air and release any tension that I might have. I take in another breath, become aware of any muscles that might be tight in my head, scalp, neck, shoulders, arms, chest, abdomen and legs, then, as I breathe out, let it go."

SHORT-CIRCUIT NEGATIVE THINKING. "Sometimes I create stress by talking to myself in a way that's critical," says Dr. Manderino. "I'll say, 'That was stupid!' or 'How in the world did you ever get this job?'"

When that happens, "I try to catch myself and correct it immediately. I say, 'Wait a minute—you've had a really busy day, you're really stressed out, no wonder you forgot such and such.' In other words, I take the time to say something in response to my negative thoughts and actually dispute them with a positive statement."

DITCH THE BLOODSUCKERS. "Sometimes because women have been brought up to make relationships work, we stay in relationships that aren't very good for us," says Dr. Manderino. "And the relationship becomes a stressor.

"As women, all of us can name people who suck the life's blood right out of us. They are energy drainers, and it's very important to set limits with them. In some instances, we may have to leave them out of our lives entirely.

"Focus instead on people who are good to you and give you energy," says Dr. Manderino. Spend time with people who are nurturing rather than toxic.

The Workplace Revolution

Although there are no reptilian dinosaurs roaming the workplace today, there are tremendous changes there that many workers perceive as equally threatening.

Fueled by global economic expansion and the tremendous economic changes of the 1990s, some American corporations are abandoning antiquated management theories left over from the time when no worker was trusted to work on his own and a "supervisor" was the guy who flogged the slaves.

The result? "Midlevel management as we know it is going away," says organizational psychologist James Campbell Quick, Ph.D., professor of organizational behavior at the University of Texas at Arlington and editor of the *Journal of Occupational Health Psychology*. It's being replaced by workers who have been organized into teams and "empowered" to work on their own.

Team members at corporations such as Texas-based Chaparral Steel and the Ford Motor Company in Detroit take responsibility for finding the best way to get a job done, then they do it on time and with the quality expected by the rest of the workforce, says Dr. Quick. Critical feedback and approval are furnished by team members as well as supervisors, and there are procedures to help keep everyone on track. And of course, should the odd employee slack off or not do his job, there are consequences. Management has not abandoned the power to hire and fire.

In corporations where this type of organization has been in place, results have been positive, says Dr. Quick. "Stress levels of both management and workers go down. As one management friend said after he relinquished his authoritarian role, 'My stress level dropped 1,000 percent when I turned in my title as ruler of the world.'"

Unfortunately, any major workplace changes cause uncertainty among the workforce, and uncertainty causes stress, says Dr. Quick. So although a team-oriented organization will reduce stress in the long

STRESS

run, in the short run it can produce one of the problems it's designed to solve. Here are some of the ways a woman can prevent as much stress as possible from a changing workplace.

BUILD A NURTURING NETWORK. One of the key elements in reducing workplace stress is to build a support system that will nurture you, says Dr. Quick. And for women, that can mean pulling together a group of women with common problems and concerns.

In-depth interviews with top male and female executives conducted by Dr. Quick and his colleagues attempted to find out what these highly successful CEOs and CFOs did to reduce stress.

"We looked at everything," says Dr. Quick. "And we found that they didn't all relax, they didn't all play, they didn't all exercise, and they didn't all pray. But what they all *did* do was build social support both in and out of the office."

In particular, female managers got their support from the women who worked for them, says Dr. Quick. The managers formed the nucleus of a group of women that gave the managers the honest feedback and emotional caring they needed. In return, the managers helped the other women develop their work skills. The result was a sense of support for all members of the team—manager and workers alike.

TAKE CONTROL. The less control you have over your work, the more stressed you're likely to feel, says Dr. Quick. But be realistic about what you can and cannot control in a corporate setting. "You can control your own behavior, thinking and response," he says. But you cannot control whether the economy improves, a building starts going up or orders for steel start pouring in.

SORT OUT YOUR RESPONSIBILITY. Figure out what you are and are not responsible for and don't let people dump unrelated tasks on your plate, says Dr. Quick. Refer them to someone else.

At the University of Texas, for example, Dr. Quick is known as the "stress doctor." So even though his responsibility is studying and teaching about organizational stress, students come to him during office hours and outside class to talk about their personal problems— marriages that aren't working out and the like.

His solution? He refers them to campus and community counselors, ministers and rabbis, not because he doesn't care or because he doesn't want to help but because he knows that in order to keep his own stress levels low, he can take responsibility for his students' learning but not for their personal lives.

STAY AHEAD OF THE STEAMROLLER. As the economy

continues to evolve over the next decade or so, so will your workplace, says Dr. Quick. And the best way to keep your stress levels low is to position yourself to take advantage of the changes.

"Try to understand what's going on and figure out how you're going to fit into the new structure," says Dr. Quick. "Ask yourself, 'How can I add value to the new organization? Do I need new skills?'"

Then go out and equip yourself to meet the workplace's evolving needs by taking courses, attending workshops or even playing around with new technology related to your field.

KNOW WHEN TO GO. When you begin to sense that it's time to move on, do. Otherwise you'll create high stress levels in yourself and those around you. "Most people know intuitively when it's time to go," says Dr. Quick. "But the number one behavior to look at is performance." When the work environment stays pretty much the same but you no longer meet your own performance expectations—you didn't sell as much product as you expected this year, for example—then you know it's time to leave.

USE A CHAIN SAW. People who have become dead limbs on the corporate tree should be cut off, says Dr. Quick. If you're in a position to do so, "get rid of them or move them into a position where they can become revitalized." It may sound heartless, but the stress they cause in others can create major meltdowns—of organizations and other folks.

How do you know it's time to get out the chain saw? "You get a sense that they're roadblocks," says Dr. Quick. Instead of percolating with new ideas and welcoming new ideas from others, they're locked into doing things the same old way. So the people who work for them are constantly having to figure out how to do end runs around them, and that causes major stress.

"There are also performance indicators," says Dr. Quick. Each corporation has its own that are specific to its particular business. For example, "faculty are dead when they get bad student evaluations or produce no new research, or students refuse to take their classes."

He chuckles. "Am I dead yet?" he asks, then answers, "Not according to my provost."

Stroke

Be Aware of Your Risk

The 31-year-old woman had delivered a healthy baby only months before. Now she was lying pale and listless on a gurney as a neurosurgeon tried to figure out whether he could halt a progressing stroke.

It's true that 31-year-old women are not supposed to have strokes. But in 1992, stroke claimed the lives of over 1,600 American women between the ages of 25 and 45—making it the seventh leading cause of death for women in this age group. And what's even more alarming is the fact that, in contrast with other age groups, stroke among younger women has not declined, says Marie-Germaine Bousser, M.D., professor of neurology at St. Antoine's Hospital in Paris and a recognized expert on stroke in women.

Still, stroke is far more prevalent among older women. Nearly 7,000 women between the ages of 45 and 65 died of stroke in 1992. But in the same year, strokes claimed the lives of nearly 79,000 women over the age of 65—outnumbering the under-65 group by nearly ten to one.

Strokes caused by blocked arteries—called ischemic strokes—account for 80 percent of strokes that occur in men and women. (The majority of these come from hardening of the arteries, or atherosclerosis.) They can also be triggered by irregular heart rhythms or abnormalities of the heart valves.

Hemorrhagic strokes, which are responsible for the other 20 percent of strokes, occur from ruptured blood vessels either inside or on the outer surface of brain tissue. They can be triggered by high blood pressure, congenital weaknesses in arterial walls or even injuries to the head.

Even infections are a risk, researchers report. A study at the University of Heidelberg in Germany found that 23 percent of people who experienced a full-fledged stroke or a transient attack—a "mini-stroke" that leaves no apparent damage—had an upper respiratory infection during the previous four weeks.

A Woman's Special Risks

Although men are more likely to have strokes than women, certain kinds of stroke are more prevalent among women. For instance, women are more likely than men to experience one type of hemorrhagic stroke in which an artery bursts and bleeds into the space between the skull and brain tissue. The good news is—though no one knows why—that women also have a smaller chance of experiencing a second such stroke than men.

What causes a stroke in women? High blood pressure; pregnancy; migraine headaches; cigarette smoking; lupus, a chronic inflammatory disease that affects the skin, joints, kidneys, nervous system and mucous membranes; ulcerative colitis; Type II, or non-insulin-dependent, diabetes; and the use of estrogen in oral contraceptives or hormone replacement therapy put women at increased risk, statistics show. And while stroke hasn't been proven to run in families, researchers suspect that some of the risk factors for stroke—such as high blood pressure and diabetes—may be inherited.

Studies indicate the risk of stroke is 4 times greater for women with high blood pressure, and a pregnant woman is 13 times more likely to experience a stroke than a woman who isn't pregnant. A woman who experiences migraine headaches is 4 times more likely to have a stroke, and the risk is 3 times higher for a woman who smokes. And the risk of a woman with Type I diabetes is 3 times that of someone without the disease.

Despite the knowledge about what causes stroke or increases its probability, however, doctors cannot identify the cause of stroke in up to 50 percent of women, says Dr. Bousser. Their best guess is that it could be a combination of risk factors.

Pregnant and at Risk

Pregnancy in particular has drawn a lot of attention from researchers. For one thing, it triggers chemical changes in a woman's blood that cause the body's natural clot-busting mechanisms to take a nine-month vacation. For another, it stimulates production of several substances that actually encourage artery-blocking clots to form.

But most strokes that occur during pregnancy are caused by eclampsia, a condition in which spasms in the blood vessels can cause artery-popping high blood pressure.

Although scientists don't really know what causes eclampsia, says Dr. Bousser, they do know that high blood pressure causes stroke. The relationship is so strong, doctors say, that your risk of stroke jumps 50 percent every time the diastolic (bottom) measurement of your blood pressure reading goes up five points.

How dangerous is stroke during pregnancy? In a study at the University of Texas Southwestern Medical Center at Dallas of patients admitted to one hospital with pregnancy-related strokes, 20 percent died, while 40 percent of the survivors had neurological damage that caused paralysis or even blindness.

Popping the Pill

Although pregnancy puts women at risk for stroke, oral contraceptives can, too. Various studies indicate that stroke is one to six times more likely among women who use oral contraceptives, says Dr. Bousser. "The risk is increased primarily among women over 35 who have additional risk factors—smoking being the most important one."

Nobody knows exactly how much estrogen in a birth control pill it might take to increase stroke risk, nor do they know the effect of adding other hormones such as progesterone to the newest contraceptive formulations.

While high-dose estrogen contraceptives are known to increase stroke risk, studies show that low-dose contraceptives—the type currently used—do not themselves significantly increase the risk of stroke. They may, however, boost the risk from other factors, particularly high blood pressure and smoking, and should be avoided by women who are otherwise at risk for stroke.

Migraine and Cigarettes: A Risky Match

Migraine and cigarette smoking are two other factors that significantly increase women's risk of stroke.

In a study of 212 men and women between the ages of 18 and 80, Dr. Bousser and her colleagues found that women under the age of 45 who suffered from migraine headaches were four times more likely to have a stroke than women the same age without migraine.

If you have migraines and also smoke, your risks rise sharply, research has shown. In Dr. Bousser's study, "women with migraines who

---

WOMAN TO WOMAN NOT TOO YOUNG FOR A STROKE

Shari Kemper is a dispatch supervisor for the *Oregonian* newspaper in Portland, Oregon. In 1992, just months after the birth of her son Bryan, Shari had a stroke. An operation by a pioneering neurosurgeon saved her life. This is her story.

I was recovering from surgery at Good Samaritan Hospital, several months after the birth of my child, when I had the stroke. My husband had come to the hospital after work to have dinner with me. We were sitting there talking when the phone rang. It was my mom. I started to say "Hi," when all of a sudden I began seeing stars in my right eye. My left hand started to hurt.

I tried to tell both my mom and my husband, but my speech got slurred. I hung up. I think I passed out.

My husband thought I'd had an overdose of medication. He ran to get a nurse and practically pulled her into the room to show her that there was something wrong.

The nurse took one look at me and called the doctor on call, who was a neurologist. He sent me for a brain scan. I'd had a massive stroke. The whole left side of my body was paralyzed, and the left side of my face drooped.

smoked were *ten times* more likely to suffer a stroke than women who had neither of these risk factors," according to Dr. Bousser.

How to Prevent a Stroke

Because we know so much about what causes strokes in women, we also know how to prevent them.

DON'T SMOKE. Add this to your reasons to call it quits. In the Harvard Nurses' Health Study, an ongoing study begun in 1976 of more than 100,000 nurses who were then between the ages of 30 and 55, scientists found that a woman's risk of having a stroke increases every time she lights up. Compared to women who didn't smoke, reported the researchers, those who smoked 1 to 4 cigarettes per day had a little over three times the risk of a stroke, while women who smoked 5 to 14 cigarettes per day had nearly four times the risk.

My mom found out about a surgeon at Oregon Health Sciences University who had been helping stroke patients. I was transferred to that hospital and placed under the care of Dr. Stanley Barnwell. Dr. Barnwell told my family there was one option—an operation in which he put a catheter in my leg and threaded it all the way up an artery, past my heart and on up into my brain. My family said to go ahead.

The operation took over five hours. Dr. Barnwell went all the way up to the clot that caused the stroke and—this is the amazing part—he broke up the clot and just opened up the blood vessels that had already shut down in my head.

The next thing I knew, I woke up in the intensive care unit with my family all around. Now I had feeling on my left side and movement in my left arm and leg.

I left the hospital ten days later. Over the next year, I went from a wheelchair to a cane to being on my own. I had to learn how to read again, and how to make decisions. It wasn't easy, especially for my family. There were a lot of starts and stops—but I just kept telling the doctors, "My left side has to get better—I want to hold my baby!"

Now I can. And I'm also back at work again.

And it pays to quit. The researchers also found that women who quit smoking can reduce their risk of stroke in two to four years to a point nearly identical to that of someone who never smoked.

TAKE CARE OF YOUR HEART. "You can protect your brain by protecting your heart," says Linda A. Hershey, M.D., Ph.D., professor of neurology at the State University of New York at Buffalo School of Medicine and chief of neurology at the Veterans Administration Medical Center in Buffalo. That's because the same artery-clogging factors that cause heart disease—mainly a high-fat diet and a sedentary lifestyle—also can cause a stroke. About 20 percent of all strokes are caused by a blood clot that originates in the heart, then moves toward the brain. (For tips on keeping your heart healthy, see page 248.)

KEEP A LID ON YOUR BLOOD PRESSURE. Lowering your diastolic pressure by as little as 6 points reduces your risk of stroke as much as 25 percent in as little as two years, neurologists say. (For tips on controlling blood pressure, see page 276.)

EAT VEGETABLES. In the Nurses' Health Study, researchers have found that women who eat carrots five times a week can lower their risk of stroke 68 percent. Women who add five servings of spinach every week can lower their risk 43 percent. Both vegetables are rich in beta-carotene, researchers say.

DRINK—MODERATELY. A glass of wine once a day may also have a protective effect, but any more than that has been found to increase your risk of stroke. And your risk goes up sharply if you drink the equivalent of a bottle of wine or five ounces of whiskey during an evening. According to researchers at the University of Helsinki in Finland, drinking that amount of alcohol increases the risk of stroke 7-fold in women between the ages of 16 and 39 and 15-fold in women 40 to 50. So limit yourself to one drink a day.

TREAT INFECTIONS PROMPTLY. Researchers at the University of Helsinki have discovered that upper respiratory infections accompanied by a fever can put women at increased risk of stroke. "Don't suffer through an infection when you have a fever," advises Markku Kaste, M.D., chairman of the Department of Neurology at the university and one of the study's authors. "See your doctor immediately."

BRUSH YOUR TEETH. Dr. Kaste's study also revealed that women with dental decay and poor oral hygiene were at increased risk. Scientists haven't quite figured out how it works, explains Dr. Kaste, but it may involve bacteria that have been allowed to build up.

Dr. Kaste advises women to brush and floss twice a day and to see their dentist regularly for preventive checkups.

TAKE ASPIRIN OR TICLOPIDINE. Since wandering blood clots are responsible for about 80 percent of strokes, doctors try to prevent clots from forming in individuals at risk for stroke by "thinning" the blood. Aspirin and the prescription drug ticlopidine (Ticlid)—both of which have the ability to keep red blood cells from clumping together and forming clots—have been found to reduce the risk of strokes in women by 25 to 30 percent.

Studies indicate that for those at risk, three or four 325-milligram tablets of aspirin a day will provide maximum protection against stroke, says Mark L. Dyken, M.D., professor emeritus in the neurology department at Indiana University School of Medicine in Indianapolis and editor of the journal *Stroke*.

Some doctors prescribe a lower dose, adds Dr. Dyken, but studies have revealed that some people may not respond to the smaller dose of aspirin.

To avoid the potentially irritating effects of aspirin on your digestive system, says Dr. Dyken, make sure you take the coated kind, and take it only after meals. If the aspirin still irritates your stomach or if you have ulcers, your doctor might wish to prescribe ticlopidine.

EAT A BANANA. According to researchers at the University of California at San Diego, one of the simplest ways to prevent death from stroke is to add a single serving of potassium-rich foods to your diet every day. In a study that included 503 healthy women, for example, researchers found that the daily addition of a single serving of a potassium-rich food—a banana or potato, for example—could reduce the women's risk of death due to stroke by about 40 percent.

GET GOOD PRENATAL CARE. See your doctor or a certified nurse-midwife as soon as you suspect you're pregnant. Set up a regular schedule of visits so that any stroke-related problems such as high blood pressure can be spotted and treated.

Temporomandibular Disorder

A JAW BREAKER YOU DON'T NEED

It can make some of the best things in life—like eating a meal, talking to a friend or kissing your husband—feel like more trouble than they're worth.

Doctors know it as temporomandibular disorder (TMD), a malfunction of the temporomandibular joints, which are the two hinges that connect the jawbone to the bones at the temples. Those who have it know it as a real pain in the neck—or the face or the head or the ears.

People with TMD may wrestle with headaches, earaches and facial pain on a daily basis, often with no idea what's causing their discomfort. Some also experience neck pain, tingling sensations in the tongue and a clicking or popping noise when they eat, talk or move their jaws. And it can get worse: Some people with TMD can barely open their mouths.

"Research shows that anywhere from 40 to 80 percent of the population has some minor TMD symptoms, but less than 2 to 5 percent need to be treated," says Andrew Kaplan, D.M.D., director of the TMD/Facial Pain Clinic at Mount Sinai Hospital and associate clinical professor of dentistry at Mount Sinai School of Medicine, both in New York City.

Researchers don't know why, but that 2 percent includes a disproportionate number of women in their twenties, thirties and forties. In fact, female patients outnumber men by about five to one.

What makes women so much more susceptible to TMD than men? "One theory is that structurally, the joint is weaker in women, but it hasn't been proven," says Dr. Kaplan.

It's also possible that men and women get TMD in equal numbers, but women are more likely to seek treatment. "Women may be more aware of symptoms, which might make them more likely to report TMD problems," says William Greenfield, D.D.S., professor of oral and maxillofacial surgery at the New York University College of Dentistry in New York City.

The Causes of TMD

Some TMD cases are hereditary, resulting from a structural abnormality in the joint. Others are caused by an injury to the jaw. "If a boxer gets punched in the chin, or if you're in an auto accident and you slam forward into the dashboard with your chin, you experience direct trauma to the joint," says Dr. Kaplan. The joint can also be damaged by whiplash, he says: "As the head snaps back, the lower jaw stays put, so you actually get excessive opening of the jaw for a split second."

But most TMD cases are actually muscular problems resulting from the everyday strain we place on our jaws. Habits like gum chewing or tooth grinding put undue stress on the joint and muscles and can lead to TMD, causing persistent soreness in front of the ears and around the temples, according to Dr. Kaplan.

Another possible cause is poor posture. "It hasn't been proven, but one theory is that somebody who sits in front of a computer screen all day may crane her neck forward, which overworks the muscles in the neck and shoulders and may cause soreness in the jaw," says Dr. Kaplan. Carrying a heavy shoulder bag can also throw your body alignment out of whack, putting a strain on your neck and jaw muscles.

Is There a TMD Personality?

These straightforward physical causes may not be the only factors that determine who gets TMD. Many experts have speculated that psychological factors like chronic stress, tension and depression might play a role in the disorder.

In a study of 2,033 Taiwanese university students, those with TMD symptoms tested higher for stress, anxiety and anger than those who had no jaw problems. Other research shows that chronic TMD patients have many of the same psychological characteristics as other chronic pain patients.

"One school of thought says that unless you address the emotional problems that are causing bad habits like tooth grinding, you can't really get rid of TMD," says Dr. Greenfield. Behavioral therapy—using a combination of counseling, relaxation exercises and biofeedback—is often helpful for patients with stress-related TMD.

First Stop: The Dentist

To get help for TMD, start with your family dentist, suggests Dr. Kaplan. She will palpate the muscles of your head and neck, listening for joint noises. She may also measure how far you can open your mouth and how far the jaw can move from side to side. She should also examine your teeth for wear to determine whether your symptoms are caused by tooth grinding, also known as bruxism.

Your dentist may refer you to a physician, oral surgeon, psychologist, physical therapist or pain center, often found at university-affiliated or other large teaching hospitals.

If your symptoms are due to tooth grinding, your doctor may prescribe a muscle relaxant or recommend an appliance, a plastic mouthpiece that's worn at night to keep the upper and lower teeth from touching each other. "If a patient wakes up with jaw or muscle soreness and headaches and her teeth show signs of wear, she's probably a candidate for an appliance," says Dr. Kaplan. "The appliance reduces nighttime muscle activity in about 80 percent of patients."

Treatments for TMD can be much more invasive, according to Dr. Kaplan. Surgery, tooth capping and orthodontic braces used to be the remedies of choice to realign the bite and jaws. "Sometimes it has to be done as a last resort," he says, but he advises patients to try nonsurgical and reversible kinds of therapy first. "If you go for an initial consult and right off the bat your doctor recommends surgery or having your teeth capped or getting braces, you should definitely seek a second opinion."

Surgery to repair or remove displaced cartilage can sometimes help patients who don't respond to other treatments. "Surgery is only an option if there's something to fix, so it really doesn't apply to muscular problems," says Dr. Kaplan. "But if you've got displaced cartilage and it's painful and debilitating, if you can't open your mouth more than one or two fingers' worth, and if appliances, physical therapy or psychological interventions like relaxation or biofeedback training don't help, then you may be a candidate for surgery."

Coping with TMD

Minor TMD symptoms can often be managed at home with a few simple techniques.

REST YOUR JAW. "Probably the best thing people can do is to stick to soft foods for a while," says Dr. Kaplan. "It's like walking with a cane if you've sprained your ankle: A soft diet is like staying off your jaw." This means no chewing gum or ice, too.

CHANGE YOUR SLEEP POSITION. Lying on your back—with one pillow supporting your neck—may help to prevent a headache in the morning. If you can't sleep on your back, try lying on your side with pillows under your head, shoulder and arm, says Dr. Kaplan.

LEND A HAND. Brace your jaw by placing your fist under your chin whenever you feel the urge to yawn, suggests Dr. Kaplan. This will keep you from stressing the joint by opening your mouth too far. Your jaw will thank you.

EASE THE PAIN. An ice pack or hot water bottle relieves pain around the jaw, in front of the ears or near the temples, says Dr. Kaplan. "Try both and use whatever works best for you." But you can't use the ice pack for as long—or as often—as you use a hot water bottle.

If you're using a hot water bottle, apply it for about 20 minutes, then fill it with hot water and apply it again. (To prevent burns, be sure the water is not too hot.) You can do this as often as necessary.

An ice pack should never be used for more than 20 minutes, and you should wait at least an hour between applications. Severe skin damage can result from prolonged exposure to cold. If you make your own ice pack, make sure you put a towel between it and your face to protect your skin.

TAKE A LOAD OFF. If you carry a shoulder bag, keep it light and switch it periodically from one shoulder to the other, says Dr. Kaplan.

Tendinitis and Bursitis
TREATMENTS FOR TENDER JOINTS

We've all heard the expression "too little, too late." But the opposite—doing too much too soon, or too often—is what brings on tendinitis and bursitis.

Tendinitis develops when tendons, which connect muscle to bone, become inflamed. Similarly, bursitis occurs when bursa, the fluid-filled sacs designed to decrease friction in joints throughout the body, become irritated. Both problems are caused by overuse or misuse, either from athletic activity, workplace tasks or hobbies that require repetitive motions.

When Exercise Is the Cause

There are two ways to develop tendinitis and bursitis from exercise, says Edward G. McFarland, M.D., director of the Section for Sports

Medicine at Johns Hopkins University in Baltimore. The first can happen when you go from relative inactivity to a new activity. "You make a quantum leap from doing nothing to something. Instead of doing it in gradual increments, you do a real sudden burst of activity that's larger than what you're use to," he says. The second can occur "if you are in shape and you decide to increase your activity, but you make too big a jump," he says. "The big key to prevention is a gradual increase in the intensity of your workouts," says Dr. McFarland.

How Women Are Affected

No one can say whether women get more or less exercise-induced tendinitis and bursitis than men do. But doctors do know that in women, the three most common forms of sports-related tendinitis occur in the shoulder, knee and Achilles tendon, says Dr. McFarland. Women also develop tendinitis in the elbow, commonly known as tennis elbow. Areas where women commonly get bursitis include the shoulder, knee and hip, doctors say.

Preliminary research at Ohio State University in Columbus indicates that bursitis and tendinitis show up frequently in people with fibromyalgia, a condition characterized by fatigue and joint and muscle pain. Early results, based on research on 40 factory workers, showed that people with fibromyalgia were three times more likely to have bursitis and tendinitis than people who didn't have it. Fibromyalgia affects more women than men.

Trouble Spot: Shoulders

Shoulder pain is often called swimmer's shoulder, a combination of tendinitis and bursitis that can develop from doing the backstroke, crawl and butterfly strokes, says Cheryl Rubin, M.D., an orthopedic surgeon in Suffern, New York. More female swimmers tend to develop the problem than male swimmers, says Dr. Rubin. One theory is that we have to do more strokes to cover the same distance and therefore place more stress on our shoulders. Another theory says it's due to greater laxity in women's shoulders. Since our shoulder joints are looser than men's, the joint is more unstable, or more likely to move out of normal alignment. Such deviation can cause trauma to structures in the joint.

Women in their thirties and forties also develop bursitis in their shoulders from tennis. "Tennis is a major culprit," says George Waylonis, M.D., clinical professor of physical medicine and rehabilitation at Ohio State University in Columbus.

Trouble Spots: Hips, Knees and Feet

Women develop hip bursitis and knee tendinitis from doing step aerobics or high-impact aerobics, says Lynn Van Ost, R.N., clinical specialist at Jefferson Sports Medicine Center in Philadelphia.

Aerobics can also cause Achilles tendinitis and heel bursitis. So can running. The Achilles tendon can become aggravated when women have poor foot alignment or exercise on improper surfaces such as banked roads or gym floors not suited for aerobics. Training errors, such as doing too much exercise before you're in proper shape or exercising at too high an intensity, can also cause Achilles problems. It's unclear why, but women runners appear to be less susceptible to Achilles tendinitis than men.

Problems from Everyday Activities

Tendinitis and bursitis can also develop when a woman's work at home or in the office requires tasks involving repetitive motions.

Activities that can cause tendinitis in the wrists and hands include working at computer terminals or performing repetitive motions required in factory work, says Janet Edmunson, immediate past president of the Association for Worksite Health Promotion in Northbrook, Illinois. Assembly-line workers and postal workers—male and female—who use their wrists a lot can also get it.

Housework can also result in overuse injury. Kneeling for long periods of time, for instance, can irritate the bursa between the skin and the kneecap. This type of bursitis is less common than it used to be, says Dr. McFarland, but at one time it was commonly known as housemaid's knee.

Activities such as gardening and sewing can also cause tendinitis, says Carla DeWald, a physical therapist at the Physical Therapy Center of Blue Bell in Pennsylvania.

"You have to watch repetitive motion, whether it's in your hobby or your job, or a combination of the two," says DeWald.

Fending Off Pain

Tendinitis and bursitis can be prevented. Here are some tips for keeping yourself pain-free.

REMEMBER TO STRETCH. Warm up and stretch before you exercise. This will loosen up your muscles and joints and prevent them from sudden overload during physical exertion. "Stretching shouldn't be bouncy. It should be a long, steady stretch," says Dr. McFarland. For whatever stretch you do, a good rule of thumb is to hold the stretch for 15 to 30 seconds, relax, then stretch again. Stretch for about five to ten minutes before you exercise, says Dr. McFarland, and again at cool-down. For tendinitis of the wrist or hand related to work activities, stretch your fingers and arms periodically, says Edmunson.

GO GRADUAL. Whatever the exercise you choose, begin gradually. "First start out doing the activity for only 10 to 15 minutes maximum," says Dr. McFarland. Then increase initially every other day, with rest in between, until you are at the level that you want to achieve.

EASE INTO AEROBICS. If you're a beginner and haven't been getting any exercise, take it easy at those first couple of aerobics classes. "Go to the first class with the intention of not completing the class," says Dr. McFarland. "Participate until you are fatigued, but don't force yourself to finish the workout."

Women doing step aerobics can develop tendinitis of the knee, just below the kneecap, says DeWald. "Progress gradually," she says. And consider staying at a lower step height, says Dr. Rubin.

VARY YOUR ACTIVITY. Try different types of activities instead of the same exercise every day. Mix swimming with running or aerobics with cycling, for instance. "Cross-training allows you to exercise every day but not stress the same muscles and joints," says Dr. McFarland. Also, try variety within your sport. If you're having trouble with your shoulders while swimming, try a kickboard workout. Or if you're having difficulty with those overhead tennis shots, hit ground strokes.

LAY OFF THE HAND-WEIGHTS. If you're experiencing shoulder or elbow pain, it may be caused by the hand-weights you're using during aerobics or while you're running, so consider giving them a rest.

"When people use heavier weights (more than one pound), they can stress the joints, especially the elbows, back and shoulders," says Carol Garber, Ph.D., clinical professor of medicine at Brown University in Providence and director of the Human Performance Laboratory at Memorial Hospital of Rhode Island in Pawtucket. Laying off the weights probably won't affect your workout too much. Studies show that the aerobic benefit of hand-weights is pretty minimal, says Dr. Garber. "People can get the same aerobic benefit by doing vigorous arm motions without the weights," she says.

GET SOME GUIDANCE. Get good instruction from someone who knows the new sport you plan to try, says Dr. McFarland. This will help you avoid mistakes that can lead to injury.

HEED POSTURE AND POSITION. Prevent tendinitis from work-related tasks by paying attention to your posture and chair position, says Edmunson. "Make sure you are doing the movement properly. Your seat needs to be the right height," she says. Adjust your seat so your wrists aren't cocked up but instead are in the neutral position, she says.

Also talk to your company's medical or safety department for advice on how to position your chair or perform a work task properly, she says. If there is no one to consult where you work, try calling the occupational health department of your local hospital. Many hospitals conduct community health workshops.

PAY ATTENTION TO PAIN. If you feel pain, don't ignore it. If you have continuous pain without activity, pain that prevents you from doing other activities, pain that wakes you up at night or pain that is not relieved with ice or aspirin, see your doctor—you may have tendinitis, bursitis or another problem, says Dr. McFarland. Beginners in particular should consult a physician, because they often can't distinguish the good pain of muscle soreness from the bad pain of injury, while more experienced athletes usually can.

ICE IT. When you feel pain, use ice, not heat, says Dr. McFarland. One technique is called ice massage. Put water in a paper cup and freeze it, then peel away the top part of the cup and rub the ice on the area for 10 to 15 minutes or until it's numb. It's okay to massage ice directly on skin, but ice packs should have a protective cloth between the pack and your skin. If you have diabetes or poor blood flow to an extremity, however, do not use ice.

LET YOURSELF REST. If you have tendinitis pain, resting the part of your body that hurts will help. "People underestimate the value of rest," says Dr. McFarland. "People are afraid to rest. Rest is very beneficial. By and large most of us can afford to take a day or two off," he says. The rest recommendation applies to work, too. "Take a break from what you are doing," says Edmunson.

GIVE YOUR BODY RELIEF. Pay attention to the pain that you feel. If it's tendinitis or bursitis, you can treat it with anti-inflammatories like aspirin or ibuprofen combined with ice therapy for a brief period, says Dr. McFarland. If that doesn't work, then cut back on your activities, he says. If the pain doesn't subside with rest, see your doctor.

Thyroid Disease
RESETTING YOUR
BODY'S THERMOSTAT

Nancy Lambrechts, a Boston travel agent, was having the time of her life: A successful career, active participation in her tennis league, romantic weekend visits to her fiance in Belgium.

But by early 1990, she was feeling "worse and worse and worse." Nancy, then in her late thirties, had a hard time walking the five minutes to the train, let alone picking up a tennis racquet. Her pulse raced. Her weight dropped. Blood tests confirmed what her doctor suspected: an overactive thyroid.

Like 3.7 million Americans—90 percent of them women—Nancy had hyperthyroidism, the most common form of thyroid disease. Her thyroid gland, a butterfly-shaped organ nestled at the base of the throat, was pumping out too much of the powerful hormones that regulate metabolism, heart rate and temperature. The gland was going haywire because it was under attack by her own immune system.

"You burn up so much energy it makes you tired. It's like the inside of you is exercising while you're sitting still," says Nancy, who tried anti-thyroid pills and finally radioactive iodine to control her condition. "Now I'm feeling pretty good."

From Rundown to Overwrought

Like the thermostat in your car, your thyroid gland is something you don't notice—unless it malfunctions. Then it can pour an overload of hormones into your bloodstream or cut production to almost zero. Thyroid hormones affect virtually every metabolic process. Too much or too little can wreak havoc, causing, respectively, nervousness or depression, weight loss or gain, insomnia or constipation, bursts of energy or episodes of exhaustion. Untreated, thyroid diseases can lead to menstrual problems, pregnancy complications, infertility and even coma and death.

"But it's so easy to treat," says James J. Figge, M.D., chief of the Division of Endocrinology at Albany Medical College in New York. "If you watch for symptoms and ask to be tested, the disease can be controlled. And the difference in someone's life can be like night and day."

For reasons researchers don't understand, women get thyroid disease ten times more often than men do. Of the 5 million adults who know they have thyroid trouble, 4.6 million are women. Of those, 3.2 million have hyperthyroidism and 1.4 million have its opposite, hypothyroidism, in which too little hormone is produced.

"People don't have a clue why women have more thyroid disease," says David S. Cooper, M.D., director of endocrinology at Sinai Hospital and associate professor of medicine at Johns Hopkins University School of Medicine, both in Baltimore. "We do know that most forms of thyroid disease are autoimmune diseases, where the body produces antibodies that attack tissues." And autoimmune diseases are more common in women.

Getting an Early Warning

Thyroid disease cannot be prevented. But because it's often inherited—Nancy Lambrechts, for instance, discovered that her aunt and cousin also had overactive thyroids—doctors recommend blood screenings for early detection in women over 40 who have a family history of thyroid or autoimmune disease.

Dr. Cooper also suggests that pregnant women have this test, because 1 in 20 has thyroid difficulties in the months after delivery. Sometimes it's a brief bout of hyperthyroidism that subsides on its own.

But thyroid hormone levels can also plummet, leading to depression, memory loss and difficulty concentrating. The symptoms are often overlooked or wrongly attributed to postpartum depression.

"It turns out you can predict who's going to get the problem with a blood test," says Dr. Cooper. "If a woman has certain antibodies in her blood, there's a 50-50 chance she'll have this problem. It won't prevent it, but at least you'll be on the lookout for it and you can treat it."

Of course, screening is also vital if you have any warning signals of thyroid disease. Yet these red flags are often vague or misunderstood. A specialist may treat one symptom—like depression or constipation—without finding the underlying cause. In fact, hyperthyroidism often looks like something else. And hypothyroidism's symptoms—like fatigue and sluggishness—especially in postmenopausal women, are often dismissed as simple signs of aging.

"It can be very subtle, but the symptoms to look for are those that go on over a period of time, not something that happens one day and not again," says Dr. Figge. "The key is, if you're starting to develop a pattern of muscle cramps or loss of energy or gaining weight for no apparent reason, it's time to have it checked out."

There's also no cure for thyroid disease, but doctors have an arsenal of treatments ready to control it.

A "Grave" Problem

If it's hyperthyroidism—a common condition of another hormonal problem called Graves' disease—your metabolism roars into permanent high gear. You can see it and feel it: Typical symptoms include nervousness, sweating, heat intolerance and weight loss. When former president George Bush and his wife, Barbara, both developed Graves' disease, he was bothered by heart palpitations, while she had vision problems and bulging eyeballs.

"The metabolism just revs up," says Dr. Figge. "People with hyperthyroidism burn calories rapidly. Sometimes you can feel the heat radiating off their skin like a radiator."

Seventy-five percent of Americans are treated with radioactive iodine to damage some of the thyroid cells that produce too much hormone.

"Some people are uncomfortable about getting any form of radiation," Dr. Cooper says. "But there have been many studies following women for 15, 20 and even 40 years, and certainly there is no evidence it's harmful in any way. It does not affect fertility."

But almost everyone who takes radioactive iodine or undergoes a surgical procedure to remove all or part of the thyroid later develops an inactive thyroid and can expect to take synthetic thyroid hormones once a day for life.

Another option for hyperthyroidism is drugs that make it harder for the body to produce hormones. The drawbacks are that these drugs can cause allergies and lower resistance to infection.

Running on Empty

Before iodine was added to table salt in the 1920s, iodine deficiency was a prime cause of hypothyroidism in the United States. Today an autoimmune condition called Hashimoto's disease is the cause of most underactive thyroids. With Hashimoto's, a small goiter or thyroid enlargement develops, which often subsides with treatment.

Other factors that can slow down your thyroid include taking lithium, a drug used to treat manic-depressive illness, and receiving neck x-rays to treat cancer. Oddly, eating too much iodine-rich food—such as kelp—may also knock the gland out of commission. And many people with hypothyroidism started with an overactive thyroid that became underactive due to treatment.

Hormone levels drop with hypothyroidism. Your body responds by functioning more slowly. The results include fatigue, constipation, feeling chilly, gaining weight, mental sluggishness, hearing loss, dry skin, coarse hair and a puffy face and hands. Treatment is usually a daily tablet of levothyroxine (Levoid), a synthetic thyroid hormone that is identical to what your body produces. Levothyroxine can be taken during pregnancy.

Coping with Thyroid Disease

You can't prevent it or cure it, but doctors say there's plenty you can do to cope. Here are some suggestions.

GET CHECKED. If you have a family history of thyroid disease or autoimmune disorders, or if you have any symptoms that lead you to believe that your thyroid might be out of whack, ask your doctor to do a blood test. The sooner the problem is identified and treated, the better, doctors say.

ASK ABOUT TREATMENT. If you have hyperthyroidism, ask your doctor whether drugs or radioactive iodine is best for you. Discuss the effectiveness and side effects of each method. With your doctor, you should talk over the possibility that you'll need to take synthetic hormones later on, after you've taken the iodine or drugs. If tests reveal mild hypothyroidism, ask about hormone supplements, says Dr. Cooper.

Some doctors prefer to monitor patients with very low-level thyroid problems, however. "My bias is, patients should be treated," says Dr. Cooper. "Some of the mild symptoms may not even be recognized by the patient. But after treatment, the patient says, 'Gee, I didn't even realize I felt tired. I feel better now.' And there's no downside to being treated. There is no harm to taking hormones to normalize your thyroid, if you're taking the proper dose."

BUY THE BRAND NAME. If you take levothyroxine for hypothyroidism, ask your doctor or pharmacist for a brand-name form of the drug. "The generics aren't reliable," says Dr. Figge. "Absorption in the body is not as well-controlled, and so the dose that you really get may not be precise. And brand names aren't that expensive—about $10 a month. So there's really no excuse not to use them."

BE PATIENT. Once treatment begins, those troubling symptoms won't fade overnight. Depending on the type of thyroid disease you have, you may feel sluggish—or on pins and needles—for several weeks, says Dr. Cooper. "It's important not to be impatient with how you're feeling. These things take time," he says. "With hypothyroidism, you might not feel back to normal for more than a month. And with hyperthyroidism, the blood tests could look normal, but you may still be feeling nervousness, anxiety or a rapid heartbeat."

CHECK THE DOSE. Your doctor should give you a blood test annually to ensure that your hormone levels are on target. "Once a year is the minimum," says Lawrence C. Wood, M.D., president and medical director of the Thyroid Foundation of America and a thyroidologist at Massachusetts General Hospital in Boston. "You will also need it checked at menopause and if you suddenly go on a medication that contains a lot of iodine, like some vaginal douches do."

Women who take synthetic hormones for hypothyroidism may need up to 45 percent more when pregnant, so ask your doctor to check your thyroid levels every two months during pregnancy.

MIND THE MIX. If you take thyroid hormone pills and then decide to use birth control pills, your thyroid dose may need to be increased. "A woman should ask for a test about a month after starting the Pill," says Dr. Wood. "In some people, the estrogen in birth control pills seems to increase the need for the thyroid hormone."

STOP SMOKING. Researchers in the Netherlands say smoking may bring on Graves' disease in people predisposed to it. They don't know what it is about smoking that encourages the disease, but they say that kicking the habit could save you from it.

Ulcers

PREVENTABLE AND CURABLE

Debbie Childers, a 40-year-old suburban Philadelphia mother of three, felt the pain just as she was going to sleep. It hit right smack in the middle of her stomach—above the belly button, below the ribs and a hand span from her heart.

At first she felt the pain one or two evenings a week. Then it was every night.

She tried to ignore it. But the pain began to wake her around 2:00 A.M. Then at 4:00. And by the time Childers finally consulted her doctor, the pain was occurring pretty much all the time: before breakfast, during work, after lunch, before dinner, before bed.

The cause?

Debbie Childers had become one of the 25 million Americans who at some point in their lives will develop a peptic ulcer—a tiny hole in the lining of the stomach or upper intestine.

Not for Men Only

Twenty years ago, a peptic ulcer was a symbol of male power. It was the ubiquitous trophy of the hard-driving executive who worked 18-hour days, smoked like a chimney, made pots of money and lived in a suburban mansion he hardly had time to notice with a family he rarely had time to see.

The ulcer, doctors said, was a side effect of his success. The same adrenaline that pumped him up for the corporate kill also took out his stomach.

Today that kind of thinking has disappeared, along with the notion that ulcers are for men only.

"Today doctors know that there's as much ulcer disease in women as there is in men," says John Walsh, M.D., director of the Center for Ulcer Research and Education at the University of California at Los Angeles.

Neither gender has any special proclivity for the disease, nor any special protection, but there are some minor differences. Both are equally likely to develop a type of peptic ulcer, called a gastric ulcer, which is located in the stomach. But men are somewhat more likely to develop a duodenal ulcer, which is located in the upper intestine. And both are equally susceptible to a major cause of ulcers: spiral-shaped bacteria that set up housekeeping in the stomach or upper intestinal wall, what doctors call the duodenum. Both men and women feel the effects of everyday painkillers that can lead to ulcers, but more women than men take them—to relieve muscle aches, menstrual cramps, headaches and arthritis.

An Infectious Invader

Most ulcers are caused by a common type of bacteria called *Helicobacter pylori*, scientists say. No one knows exactly how the bacteria do their work, but scientists suspect that they interfere with the secretion of naturally protective gels and antacid in cells lining the digestive tract.

The bacteria are apparently often transmitted in childhood. For example, *H. pylori* might be transmitted when kids forget to wash their hands after they go to the bathroom, then put their hands in their mouths, says John Kurata, Ph.D., associate adjunct professor at the University of California at Los Angeles and director of research and policy analysis for the San Bernardino Medical Center.

The bacteria bore through the protective gel lining the digestive tract and settle in the stomach or duodenum. In most people they simply cause a minor inflammation that no one ever notices, says Dr. Kurata. In others they cause an ulcer.

Why does one woman get an ulcer and another does not? It's likely that one woman has a stomach or duodenum that is genetically predisposed to produce more acid than normal or is regularly exposed to a major irritant like smoke or alcohol, says Dr. Kurata.

Studies indicate that smokers are twice as likely as nonsmokers to develop an ulcer. The tobacco simultaneously impairs the digestive system's protective gel and stimulates acid secretion. And solutions of 80-proof alcohol applied directly to the protective gel in the stomach and duodenum have been shown to cause bleeding and ulceration. The effects of lower concentrations of alcohol found in beer and wine have not been studied carefully.

Here's how you can fight off an ulcer that's caused by bacteria.

AVOID IRRITANTS. "Eliminating tobacco smoke and alcohol will make a major difference" in preventing ulcer formation, says Dr. Walsh.

SEE YOUR DOCTOR. Any kind of stomach pain needs to be evaluated by a physician, doctors agree. If your doctor suspects an ulcer, she may order a blood test, breath test or endoscopic exam to determine whether you have the *H. pylori* bacteria.

Fortunately, the blood and breath tests are more accurate than the invasive endoscope in determining the presence of *H. pylori*, according to a panel of ulcer experts convened by the National Institutes of Health (NIH) in Bethesda, Maryland.

TRY TRIPLE THERAPY. If you do have the bacteria and an ulcer, the NIH panel recommends that you take antimicrobial drugs for two weeks.

The drug regimen that is most likely to eradicate the bacteria is generally referred to as triple therapy. It includes the antibiotics tetracycline (Vibramycin) and metronidazole (Flagyl) plus bismuth subsalicylate, an antibacterial preparation that is the major ingredient in Pepto-Bismol. A medication to reduce stomach acid may be added for those who are experiencing ulcer pain.

Why three different drugs? "Triple therapy is the most effective," says Dr. Walsh. Studies show that triple therapy will eliminate the ulcer-causing bacteria in 90 percent of those who have an ulcer. The ulcer will heal and will be far less likely to recur than if an acid-reducing drug were used alone.

In a study conducted at Baylor College of Medicine in Houston, David Graham, M.D., chief of gastroenterology, and his colleagues separated 109 men and women with recently healed ulcers into two groups.

They gave the acid-reducing drug ranitidine (Zantac) to one group, while the second group received triple therapy plus ranitidine.

The result? Within two years, ulcers had recurred in 74 to 95 percent of those who took the acid-reducing drug. In those who used triple therapy plus ranitidine, ulcers recurred in only 12 or 13 percent.

The Painkillers from Hell

Most of us pop over-the-counter painkillers without giving it much thought: We strain a muscle and limp over to the medicine cabinet or get a headache and reach for the aspirin.

But although both over-the-counter and prescription painkillers may relieve our pain in the short term, in the long term some of them may cause ulcers.

"There are no good statistics on this, but I would guess that up to one-half of women's ulcers are caused by taking nonsteroidal anti-inflammatory drugs," says Dr. Walsh.

Studies show that nonsteroidal anti-inflammatory drugs (NSAIDs) such as aspirin, ibuprofen, naproxen (Anaprox), sulindac (Clinoril) and indomethacin (Indocin) increase the chances of developing an ulcer tenfold. They reduce the natural gels and antacid secreted by cells lining the digestive system so that stomach acid eats through the stomach or duodenum to form an ulcer.

And although no one knows how much of these drugs must be ingested before they cause an ulcer, studies show that ulcers occur in 15 to 30 percent of those who use NSAIDs over a long period of time—even though the ulcers may not always cause symptomatic pain.

Fortunately, there are ways to reduce your risk of ulcers caused by anti-inflammatory drugs. Here's how.

GO LIGHT ON NSAIDs. For pain relief, take less potent anti-inflammatory drugs and at minimal doses, suggests Dr. Graham. The best ones to use are a 200-milligram tablet of ibuprofen, two tablets of aspirin or the new low-dose naproxen (Aleve). All will deliver just as much pain relief as other anti-inflammatories, says Dr. Graham, but their reduced anti-inflammatory capabilities will spare your digestive tract some heavy chemical insults.

KEEP THE HEAVY HITTERS IN RESERVE. Save high-potency anti-inflammatories like piroxicam (Feldene)—a prescription drug— for conditions like arthritis that specifically demand a medication that fights inflammation, says Dr. Graham. This drug has strong anti-inflammatory properties at the dose that gives pain relief, and it is far more likely to cause an ulcer than those that offer excellent pain relief but low anti-inflammatory levels.

USE PROTECTION. It's best to avoid anti-inflammatory drugs altogether if you've had an ulcer in the past, says Dr. Graham. But if you've had an ulcer and you simply must take these drugs to alleviate a serious problem like arthritis, ask your doctor if you can take them with misoprostol (Cytotec), a prescription drug that will protect the cells lining your digestive tract.

In a joint study based at Baylor College of Medicine, Dr. Graham and his colleagues separated 643 men and women who were taking nonsteroidal anti-inflammatory drugs into two groups. One group was given 200 micrograms of misoprostol four times a day for 12 weeks, and the other group received a placebo.

The result? The placebo group developed 40 ulcers, while the group that took misoprostal developed only 8.

Unwanted Hair
CUTTING BACK ON THE GROWTH

When people praise a woman's beautiful hair, they're referring specifically to scalp hair. Hair on a woman's chin, chest, thighs and forearms is considered unbecoming.

Nevertheless, many women have such hair. How many? Medical experts can't agree on a number because the social stigma of "unfeminine" hair keeps many women from seeking medical help.

Although unwanted hair is certainly a cosmetic problem, it may be a medical problem as well, depending on what causes it. Doctors differentiate between hypertrichosis—excess hair anywhere on the body that is generally short, fine and light in color—and hirsutism, the conversion of normal hairs to dark, heavy hairs at body sites such as the chin, cheeks, chest, the inside of the thighs and the back and belly, where women don't normally have such hair, but men do.

Hypertrichosis is inherited, according to Jerome Z. Litt, M.D., assistant clinical professor of dermatology at Case Western Reserve University School of Medicine in Cleveland. "Everyone goes to the grave with the same number of hairs she is born with, but that number is genetically determined. People of Mediterranean heritage appear hairier than Asians. White people are much hairier than black

---

WOMAN TO WOMAN AN EXPERIMENTAL DRUG CHANGED HER LIFE

Naomi Courtney is a customer service representative for QVC in San Antonio, Texas. She started missing menstrual periods in high school and first noticed coarse, dark hair on her cheeks and chin in 1987, when she was 21. As her condition worsened, she sought medical advice, but to no avail. Then one evening in the fall of 1992, as Naomi sat in a hospital lounge waiting to visit a friend and flipping idly through a discarded medical newsletter, she happened to see an article describing a pilot drug study for women with her constellation of symptoms. This is her story.

I had a beard—coarse, curly, dark hair on my cheeks and under my chin. I was going for a year without a period—every month, I'd be a little grumpy and have breast tenderness for a few days, but no period. My weight had ballooned to 225 pounds and was distributed like a man's— a big, solid lower belly.

I'd go to doctors and say, "I'm not having my period, I have all this hair on my face, I've never used birth control but I can't get pregnant— what's wrong?" They all told me the reason was that I was overweight, but that didn't make any sense. I had been a size 12 in high school, not fat, but I was having symptoms even then.

Still, I tried losing weight, but it didn't work. Then I picked up that article by gynecologist and researcher Dr. Karen Elkind-Hirsch describing her experimental treatment program for this disease—polycycstic ovary disease (PCOD)—and I said, "That's me!"

I enrolled in the treatment study. First they did a sonogram that showed that my ovaries were covered with cysts and about twice their normal size. The cysts had caused the ovaries to put out male hormones instead of the normal female hormones, which they confirmed with blood

people." Hypertrichosis may also occur in women with anorexia nervosa or hypothyroidism.

Hirsutism, on the other hand, is caused by an imbalance of the male hormones that are present in every woman's body. One of two things can happen: Either a woman's ovaries or adrenal glands begin

---

tests. The effect was almost as if I were taking steroids. I have the same amount of hair everyone else has, but because my body was putting out the wrong hormones, the hair changed.

I started taking Lupron (a synthetic gonadotropin-releasing hormone that suppresses the production of male and female hormones) for six months and went into a state of artificial menopause. At the same time, I took a low-dose birth control pill to start replacing the estrogen that my body wasn't manufacturing.

Very slowly, things started to change. I began to lose weight, gradually at first, and the hair started to disappear.

I'm off the Lupron now, but I continue to take the birth control pill, which seems to keep the PCOD under control. The weight is dropping off steadily at the rate of about four pounds a month without any changes in my diet. I still have dark hair on my face, but only about a third of what was there before I started the study. Dr. Elkind-Hirsch explained that it might take as long to go away as it did to develop.

When I look in the mirror, I can see that my skin texture has changed, the hair on my face has changed, even my body shape has changed.

I carry that article in my wallet—it's in shreds now, but it's my talis-man—and anytime I see a young woman who's overweight and has dark hair on her face, I ask her to please read it. If I can get one woman to go to her doctor and raise Cain—and believe me, you have to raise Cain, be-cause they all tell you it's because you're overweight—get the proper blood tests and the right medication, I may be able to save that woman from the misery I've gone through and to make one more doctor aware of what this disease is. I don't mind being an advocate for that.

producing an excessive amount of the male hormone androgen or her hair follicles become hypersensitive to normal amounts of androgen. It's androgen that converts a woman's normal fine, light-colored, short body hair to thick, dark, long hair, says Karen Elkind-Hirsch, M.D., Ph.D., associate professor of obstetrics and gynecology and a researcher in reproductive endocrinology at Baylor College of Medicine in Houston. "The most important thing to remember about hair is that androgens stimulate hair growth, diameter and color, while estrogen decreases pigmentation, growth and thickness. We all make male hormones, but men normally make more than women do. If a woman makes higher levels of male hormones, the hair that is hormone-dependent will grow."

Why It Happens

A number of things can cause your body to produce excess androgen, among them certain drugs for treating seizures, high blood pressure and cancer. By far the most common cause, however, is polycystic ovary disease (PCOD), in which a woman does not ovulate and cysts that form cause a hormonal imbalance that could lead to hirsutism. Other possible causes are adrenal or ovarian tumors; Cushing's syndrome, which is characterized by obesity and muscular weakness caused by excess hormones; and medications that contain androgens or corticosteroids.

Unwanted hair isn't necessarily inevitable or untreatable. Here's what you can do to prevent it or rid yourself of it.

TAKE CARE OF YOURSELF. If you're in general good health, your body is less likely to respond to stress by hypersecreting male hormones, says Dr. Litt.

WATCH YOUR WEIGHT. Some medical authorities believe that fat cells convert estrogen to androgen, causing excess hair to grow.

PRACTICE RELAXATION TECHNIQUES. "We know that stress, worry, anxiety and tension will stimulate the adrenal glands to put out more male hormones," according to Dr. Litt.

SEE A DOCTOR. Most of the causes of hormone-dependent hair growth are treatable with drugs or surgery. Particularly if you have other symptoms that might signal a hormone imbalance—such as missed periods, the inability to get pregnant, a change in body shape, deepening of your voice or acne—you should seek medical help. Some underlying causes of hirsutism can lead to serious health problems. With PCOD, for example, according to Dr. Elkind-Hirsch, there can be mild symptoms, such as occasional missed periods and the appearance of a few dark hairs, or such problems as infertility, diabetes, cardiovascular disease and precancerous lesions of the uterus.

GET HELP EARLY. As soon as you notice definite symptoms, consult a doctor, preferably a reproductive endocrinologist, says Karen Bradshaw, M.D., assistant director of the Division of Reproductive Endocrinology at the University of Texas Southwestern Medical Center in Dallas. Many conditions that cause hirsutism can be detected within a few years of puberty. "We have an adolescent clinic; we feel it's important to start therapy early to prevent overvirilization of the hair follicles," she says.

The longer you wait to treat the condition, the longer it will take to reverse it. Excess androgen production can often be stopped with birth control pills and sometimes an anti-androgen drug. "If it's recognized early and oral contraceptives are begun early, you can count on stopping the progression into more severe forms," says Dr. Bradshaw. But, he says, a 35-year-old woman who has had 15 years of unwanted hair growth will take longer to treat than a 20-year-old.

BY ALL MEANS, ELIMINATE IT. Whatever the cause of unwanted hair, doing something to get rid of it—shaving, waxing, bleaching, using depilatories or getting electrolysis—may help you feel less self-conscious. Electrolysis is the only method that completely destroys the follicle so that the hair will not grow back. It's expensive, however, when large areas are done, and it's frequently painful and can require several sessions to kill the follicle. Many women think that if they shave, more hair will grow, but that's not true, according to Dr. Bradshaw.

STICK WITH IT. The majority of treatments for androgen-dependent hirsutism take six to nine months to show results, but gradually, the hair disappears.

Vaginal Infections

MORE TO WORRY ABOUT
THAN YEAST

Most of us are familiar with vaginal infections. Either we've had one or know somebody who has.

Vaginal infections are so common that American women make an estimated four million visits to doctors each year because of them. Gynecologists say they hear more about vaginal infections than any other problem.

You might think yeast is the culprit in these infections, but it's not always. There are two other types of vaginal infections—bacterial vaginosis (BV) and trichomoniasis—that are not yeast-related at all. BV, in fact, is even more common than yeast infections—every year, there are twice as many cases of BV as of yeast. Both BV and trichomoniasis can have serious health consequences.

It's a Matter of Balance

Bacterial vaginosis may be sexually related and is the most common type of vaginal infection. Between 50 percent and 60 percent of women with multiple sexual partners get it, experts say. It's also estimated that among college-educated women who consider themselves to be in monogamous relationships, approximately 8 percent will get BV, says Sharon Hillier, Ph.D., research associate professor at the University of Washington School of Medicine in Seattle. But sex isn't always the bad guy: In one study, 2 to 5 percent of college women who'd never had sex were found to have BV.

BV develops when the natural pH balance of the vagina is disturbed by a douche, ejaculate or some other irritation, according to Dr. Hillier. Normally a woman's vagina contains an appropriate level of good bacteria called lactobacilli. When the pH balance is upset, the level of good bacteria gets too low and the level of bad bacteria gets too high. BV can be the result, and it can be hard to re-establish the normal levels, Dr. Hillier says.

Doctors say the thing women notice most about BV is a fishy odor, which can be particularly strong after sex. Often they have a discharge from the vagina. While some women have a lot of discharge and odor, others do not. And despite reports that some women who have it show no signs, a woman with BV will experience some change in discharge or odor from what is normal for her, says John Alderete, Ph.D., professor of microbiology at the University of Texas Health Sciences Center in San Antonio.

The Trouble with Multiple Sexual Partners

By multiple sexual partners, doctors mean several partners within a couple of months, as opposed to several long-term relationships in a row. "Women usually get it when they have a new sex partner," says Dr. Hillier. But women who think they are in a monogamous relationship who develop BV should not jump to the conclusion that their partner has been unfaithful. She may have had BV before and her vaginal ecosystem may not have recovered completely, or there may be another cause, such as douching.

Douching disrupts the natural ecosystem of the vagina by washing away the fragile good bacteria, says Dr. Hillier.

There is an increased risk of BV among women who use IUDs, says Dr. Hillier, but condoms may have a protective effect by keeping ejaculate out of the vagina.

It's Serious Business

If you think you have BV, you need to take care of it quickly because it can cause upper genital tract infections, including pelvic inflammatory disease (PID). If you're pregnant, there are other dangers. Studies show that pregnant women with BV have a 40 percent risk of premature delivery, says Edward Newton, M.D., professor of obstetrics and gynecology at the University of Texas Health Sciences Center at Houston. They are also at risk for amniotic fluid infection, infection of the placenta and, after delivery, an infection known as endometritis, he says.

Trich: Risky Business

Trichomoniasis, also known as trich, is caused by a parasite, the *Trichomonas vaginalis* organism, and the only way you can get it is from

---

TO DOUCHE OR NOT TO DOUCHE?

That is the question for many women who've grown up believing douching is good. Their mothers did it, and the ads said it would give them that "fresh and natural" feeling. But the latest message from medical experts is that douching may not be the best thing for you.

Experts say there hasn't been any scientific evidence to show that douching does any good. And many doctors say there's no reason for a woman to douche.

"The vaginal ecosystem is a self-cleaning, self-perpetuating, good ecosystem. There is absolutely no reason, ever, for a woman to douche. Ever," says Sharon Hillier, Ph.D., research associate professor at the University of Washington in Seattle.

Many douche products contain chemicals and preservatives that not only wash away the good along with the bad bacteria in the vagina but in some cases cause irritation of the vaginal wall, says Dr. Hillier. In addition, the pressure created during douching may force infectious organisms into the upper genital tract, where they can cause pelvic inflammatory disease (PID), she says. Douching may also be related to ectopic pregnancy, bacterial vaginosis and the loss of normal vaginal flora.

According to one study of 425 women, 42 percent of

an infected partner, says Dr. Alderete. While the parasite survives on moist surfaces such as toilet seats or towels, there are no documented cases of its being transmitted that way, says Philip Heine, M.D., assistant professor in the Department of Obstetrics and Gynecology at the University of Pittsburgh's Magee Women's Hospital.

Of the three types of vaginal infections, trichomoniasis occurs the least often; it's estimated that three to six million women get it every year. But the true rate is probably higher, maybe even double, says Dr. Alderete, because 50 percent of women with trichomoniasis go undiagnosed or misdiagnosed.

As with BV, symptoms of trichomoniasis vary from woman to woman. Generally, there will be a discharge that is white, grayish-green or yellow and is frothy and malodorous.

women with PID reported recent douching, compared with 25 percent of women who didn't have PID. And the more often women douched, the greater their risk for PID. Another study showed that douching increased the risk of ectopic pregnancy in women who'd had more than one lifetime sexual partner.

"Women are taught every night as they watch the ads that if they smell bad or if they don't feel fresh, that's a hygiene problem. That's absolutely ludicrous. If women don't smell good it's because they have an infection," says Dr. Hillier. "Women are taught endlessly that the only way to feel clean is to clean out this orifice that doesn't need cleaning. We don't clean out our rectums every day."

Women who have douched a lot in the past but have stopped are probably not at increased risk for infection, adds Phillip Heine, M.D., assistant professor in the Department of Obstetrics and Gynecology at the University of Pittsburgh's Magee Women's Hospital. The vaginal bacteria regenerate, he explains.

What can women who are used to douching do instead? "Wash thoroughly into the vagina with the fingers using just water," suggests Stanley Marinoff, M.D., director of the Center for Vulvovaginal Disorders in Washington, D.C.

If trichomoniasis goes untreated, serious health problems may follow, says Dr. Alderete. Women may be at increased risk for other sexually transmitted diseases (STDs), especially infection with HIV, the virus that causes AIDS. It's not clear why, but Dr. Alderete says that vaginal tissues that are inflamed may be more susceptible to other diseases.

And as with BV, there may be some connection between trichomoniasis and pregnancy complications, says Stanley Marinoff, M.D., director of the Center for Vulvovaginal Disorders in Washington, D.C.

Trichomoniasis alone does not place a woman at increased risk for upper genital tract infections. But women who get trich often get other STDs that can increase the chance of PID, says Dr. Marinoff.

Protect Yourself

The best medicine is to make sure you don't get a vaginal infection. If you do, make sure you get the proper treatment. Here are some suggestions.

USE CONDOMS. To protect yourself, have your partner wear a condom during sex. Or ask your doctor about the condom for women.

TALK TO YOUR PARTNER. Ask your partner about his sexual history, past sexual partners and current sexual practices. For instance, is he monogamous with you? Ask him if he has any sores on his penis, a discharge or areas of irritation. Has he been told by any previous partners that they were infected with an STD? Was he treated?

Pick a time other than when you're having sex and a place other than bed to talk, suggests Lonnie Barbach, Ph.D., assistant clinical professor of medical psychology at the University of California Medical School at San Francisco and author of *For Each Other: Sharing Sexual Intimacy.*

KNOW YOUR BODY. Pay attention to your body and take note of what is normal for you. If you notice any changes—if you experience discomfort or have some discharge or odor—that are not normal for you, tell your doctor. Women need to recognize changes in their own bodies, says Dr. Newton. If your doctor dismisses your complaints, find a doctor who will listen and take you seriously, says Dr. Alderete.

GET IT CHECKED. If you have a vaginal infection, see a doctor, who will determine which one it is and how to treat it. For BV, doctors can measure the pH level of your vaginal fluid and look at a sample of it under the microscope. A special type of cell called a clue cell will be present if you have BV. Another way to confirm BV is to do a whiff test: A sample of vaginal fluid is placed on a slide, hydrogen peroxide is added, and if it's BV, a distinct odor occurs. For trich, the most accurate diagnosis is based on a culture for the *T. vaginalis* parasite.

ASK QUESTIONS. Don't be afraid to ask your doctor about your infection. Ask "How do you know for sure that I have it? Did you look under the microscope? Have you done a culture?"

TAKE YOUR MEDICINE. Even if you have only mild symptoms, follow the treatment the doctor prescribes. Treatment for trichomoniasis involves the prescription drug metronidazole (Flagyl), which is an oral medication. For BV, you can be treated with metronidazole or a prescription vaginal cream called clindamycin phosphate (Cleocin).

DON'T FORGET YOUR PARTNER. If you have trichomoniasis, your partner will need to be treated with medication at the same time you are. Your doctor may write him a prescription at the same time he writes yours. With BV, it's not necessary for your partner to be treated with medication, but he should wear a condom while you are being treated to help prevent a recurrence, says Dr. Marinoff.

GET TESTED BEFORE SURGERY. If you're scheduled for a hysterectomy or other abdominal surgery, ask your doctor to test you for BV. Women with BV who undergo surgical procedures have been shown to have as much as a 400 percent increased risk of postoperative infection.

Varicose Veins

COMING OUT OF HIDING

Varicose veins probably aren't high on your list of opening gambits for dinner party conversation, but if you did talk about them, you might be surprised to discover how many people—especially women—share this problem. Experts say that, in the United States, more than two-thirds of all women and half of all men have varicose veins in their legs.

So it's as we suspected. Women are more likely to get varicose veins than men are. How much more likely? "Two to four times," says Albert M. Kligman, M.D., Ph.D., professor of dermatology at the University of Pennsylvania School of Medicine in Philadelphia. He adds that some estimates make women ten times more likely to develop this painful problem.

Why are women at special risk? Female hormones are the major culprits, say phlebologists, doctors who specialize in vein disease, and dermatologists, who treat skin conditions, including swollen veins that appear near the surface of the skin. One reason doctors connect the problem to hormones is that some girls begin to show varicose veins at puberty, confirming theories that the condition is related to changes in the body's estrogen and progesterone levels.

Teenagers with varicose veins are rare, however. Most women first develop swollen veins when they're in their twenties or thirties, usually during pregnancy, when female hormone levels are at their highest. While the weight gain and increased blood volume necessary for fetal development put extra stress on the legs, elevated hormone levels are the principal factor in varicose veins, says Eugene Strandness, M.D., professor of surgery at the University of Washington School of Medicine in Seattle.

Vein problems that appear during pregnancy or at other times during the twenties or thirties inevitably worsen over time, says phlebologist Brian McDonagh, M.D., founder of Vein Clinics of America in Schaumburg, Illinois. Women typically seek treatment for varicose veins when they're in their forties and fifties, he says. "As blood pools and stagnates in the veins, the vein walls are stretched, and stretching hurts," Dr. McDonagh explains.

Looks Are Not All of the Problem

Women often go to see their doctor initially because they're concerned about how their legs look, according to Dr. McDonagh. But he has found that after some questioning, it becomes clear that many women experience the painful symptoms often associated with varicose veins, including aching calves, night cramps and restless legs. Few patients, Dr. McDonagh notes, have a purely cosmetic problem.

The average woman knows all too well what varicose veins look and feel like, but many of us don't understand how these reddish-bluish bulges beneath the skin's surface develop. Under normal circumstances, veins carry blood through the legs and help transport it back up to the heart. When leg veins are healthy, valves within them open and close smoothly to keep gravity from draining the blood back downward. But after years of doing a good job, these valves can weaken because of gravity and changes in vein tissue over time, becoming stretched and inefficient. When the valves become faulty and leak, blood pools in the legs, distending the surface veins. This stretching of veins can be so painful that you've just got to get off your feet—which is difficult to accomplish if you're doing anything that requires a lot of standing.

Varicose veins tend to run in families. Good nutrition and regular exercise may help delay the development of varicose veins, but for women with a strong hereditary history, it's usually just a matter of time before they develop. Not every vein that's visible through the skin is cause for concern, though. To be varicose, a vein must contain stagnant or refluxing blood. Varicose veins *look* abnormal; they are usually swollen and knotted, "bulging, tortuous, snaking and branching," says Dr. McDonagh. Left untreated, these enlarged and weakened veins can lead to complications such as ulcers and phlebitis, in which a vein becomes inflamed and swollen.

Spider Veins: Easing the Ache

Less serious than varicose veins are spider veins, pinkish-red constellations that resemble little fireworks displays. But they are nothing to celebrate. Spiders form when tiny blood vessels close to the skin's surface dilate or break. They appear mostly on the face or the legs, but they can pop up anyplace on the body. Many women are embarrassed by the mottled look spiders give their skin. They are not, strictly speaking, varicose veins, and they seldom pose a significant health risk, but they can cause legs to ache after prolonged standing. In recent years, major advancements in laser surgery and sclerotherapy, a relatively painless outpatient procedure in which a special chemical solution is injected into veins to shrink them, have made treatments for spider veins more effective, says Dr. Kligman.

Treatment for varicose veins has also improved in recent years. Today's treatments are more effective, less invasive and much less painful than they once were, doctors say. Forget the horror stories your mother told you about leg-stripping, old-fashioned surgery in which varicose veins were tied off or actually removed from the legs. Surgery is rarely necessary anymore, except in the most severe cases. For most women, sclerotherapy is the treatment of choice.

While sclerotherapy is a marvelous solution for most women who are plagued by varicose veins, it is sometimes only a temporary one. If treated properly, varicose veins should not reappear. But the condition is progressive, and new varicose veins can develop, mostly because of the sheer number of veins and valves in your legs.

"Repeated treatments may be necessary as other veins turn varicose," says Dr. McDonagh. While sclerotherapy won't keep varicose veins from popping up, Dr. McDonagh says, it will alleviate present problems and prevent complications such as blood clotting, internal bleeding or the itchy skin rash, dermatitis.

Putting the Squeeze on Varicose Veins

If you've started noticing purplish bulges underneath your skin, or even if your family history indicates that you may develop varicose veins, some simple precautions can keep your problems to a minimum.

MOVE! On the job or at home, try not to sit for three or four hours. Get up and move around to keep the blood circulating. The Framingham Heart Study, which followed the lifestyles of 5,000 people in a Massachusetts town starting in 1948, found that women who spent eight or more hours a day sitting, standing or being otherwise sedentary had a much higher incidence of varicose veins.

DON'T SMOKE. And stop smoking if you're already into it. Researchers have found that varicose veins are more common in smokers because puffing away interferes with the way the body regulates fibrin, a blood-clotting protein.

LOSE WEIGHT. You won't necessarily get varicose veins if you're a few pounds overweight, but go over your ideal weight by 20 percent and the extra pounds can squeeze out the veins. This is particularly true for women who have a hereditary tendency toward varicose veins, according to Alan Kanter, M.D., medical director of the Vein Center of Orange County in Irvine, California.

STAY LOOSE. Constipation can actually affect varicose veins. This is because straining on the toilet increases pressure on your rectal veins, which creates more pressure on your leg veins, says Dr. Kanter. Besides eating fiber, a good way to keep constipation at bay is to make sure your system stays well-lubricated by drinking eight to ten glasses of water a day, he says.

WATCH HOW YOU LIFT. If you do strength-training exercises, you can avoid aggravating or initiating a vein problem if you make sure to use smaller weights and do more repetitions. Heavy weights can put too much pressure on veins. Ask a trainer to help you set up a program, advises Dr. Kanter.

JOG GENTLY. Hit the dirt—or the grass or cinders—instead of asphalt to cushion your legs from shock. Running on pavement may aggravate vein swelling, says Dr. Kanter.

WALK IT OFF. Take a brisk 20-minute walk each day, or spend 20 to 30 minutes three or four times a week doing some form of aerobic exercise, says Dr. Kligman. Exercise helps maintain good circulation, slows down the development of varicose veins and reduces pain in the legs where veins have already developed.

ACCEPT SOME SUPPORT. Support stockings can make you feel better and provide some help in the early stages of developing varicose veins. "If the hose make you feel better, wear them," says Dr. McDonagh, but not if they hurt. He recommends below-the-knee styles. Those that go above can pinch the skin around the knee.

Support stockings, in fashionable styles and colors, are sold in most major department stores. They hold your legs more tightly than regular stockings and help keep the blood from distending your veins. If you need more substantial support, your doctor can prescribe graduated support hose, also called compression stockings. Available in pharmacies, these stockings exert pressure on the vein walls, collapsing them and forcing the blood from smaller to larger veins where it can flow more easily, says Dr. McDonagh.

ELEVATE YOUR POSITION. Don't hesitate to put your feet up regularly. This is a simple, effective way to ease pain, says Dr. Kligman. Rest your legs on a footstool whenever you read or watch TV. Take regular breaks at work: Lie on the floor, lift your legs up straight and rest them against the wall or over a padded chair arm. Raise your legs while you sleep by putting a pillow under your feet, suggests Dr. Kligman.

Vision Problems
THE FOCUS IS ON AGING

When we were kids, vision care meant taking a yearly crack at the school eye chart and a visit to the eye doctor if nearsightedness, farsightedness or astigmatism meant we couldn't see clearly.

These days, if you're like most women, you probably take your car in for a tune-up more often than you have your eyes examined—unless you get something painful like an eye injury or infection. But consider this: Cars can be replaced. Your eyes have to last a lifetime.

For most Americans that won't be a problem, though after 40, life gets a little complicated for our eyes. First there are the dreaded bifocals, then the increased risk of diseases like glaucoma, which causes blindness by destroying the optic nerve. Men and women tangle with both bifocals and eye diseases in about equal numbers.

Visual Fluctuations

But did you know that a woman's hormonal fluctuations during pregnancy, menopause and even when taking birth control pills can cause vision changes at any age?

Researchers aren't sure what hormones do to the eyes, but their work shows that pregnant women can experience curvature of the cornea, making it uncomfortable or even impossible to wear contact lenses, says James V. Aquavella, M.D., clinical professor of ophthalmology and director of the Corneal Research Laboratory at the University of Rochester in New York. The cornea returns to its previous shape after delivery or when the woman stops breastfeeding, which also affects hormone levels. Birth control pills can have a similar effect.

Menopause brings dry eyes. That's because the hormone estrogen controls the tear glands, so a reduction in estrogen translates into a reduction in tears, says Dr. Aquavella.

Besides keeping our eyes comfortable, estrogen may protect our vision by preventing cataracts, a gradual clouding of the lens that affects about 13 million Americans, or about one in seven people over age 40. Studies show that menopausal women who take hormone replacement therapy are less likely to develop cataracts than those who don't.

The Long and Short of Vision

Although all women's eyes are affected by hormonal fluctuations, not all of us have vision problems that require correction. When we do, however, they are most likely to be farsightedness, nearsightedness or astigmatism—all of which are inherited and usually appear in childhood. They are, in fact, the main reasons both men and women wear glasses or contact lenses.

Nearsightedness occurs when an eyeball is slightly longer than normal from front to back. This affects the eye's ability to focus. Nearsighted people have poor distance vision.

In farsighted people, the eyeball is slightly shorter than normal. They need corrective lenses for close work.

Another common vision problem is astigmatism, an irregular curve in the cornea that causes blurred vision. The normal cornea is spherical, like a basketball, says Andrew Farber, M.D., an ophthalmologist in Terre Haute, Indiana, and a spokesperson for the American Academy of Ophthalmology. With astigmatism, the cornea is shaped more like a football.

Even people who've never worn glasses can expect problems with close vision eventually. As we age, the lenses of the eyes become increasingly rigid, which makes it harder to focus on objects that are close to us. This condition, called presbyopia, happens to just about everyone sooner or later and usually appears between the ages of 38 and 45.

More Choices than Ever

Vision problems are so common that corrective lenses are being developed for every taste and need, from bifocal glasses with an invisible line between the bifocal and regular lenses to bifocal contact lenses to tinted contact lenses to make your brown eyes blue. You can have a pair of glasses made up on your lunch hour or replace a torn contact by Express Mail.

Contacts are particularly popular with young women, says optometrist Michael Pier, O.D., director of professional relations for Bausch and Lomb in Rochester, New York. Besides the obvious cosmetic benefits, contacts are cheaper and easier to wear than ever, and they don't slide down your nose like glasses do when you're running after a toddler or chasing a tennis ball.

Hard contact lenses, which are made of rigid plastic, first appeared in the 1950s. They've been all but replaced by the more comfortable soft and gas-permeable lenses. Gas-permeable lenses are less flexible than soft lenses, but they provide crisper vision. They also require a longer breaking-in period. "In the beginning you'll feel like you have something in your eye," says Dr. Aquavella.

Soft and gas-permeable lenses are more comfortable because they are 40 to 85 percent water, says Dr. Aquavella. There are soft lenses for extended wear, which can be worn overnight for up to a week, and daily wear, which must be removed, cleaned and disinfected every night. While the two types look and feel identical, extended-wear lenses are designed to allow more oxygen to reach the eye, says Dr. Pier.

Also available are disposable lenses, which can be discarded at the end of the day or at the end of the week. Planned-replacement lenses can also be removed and disinfected like a daily-wear lens and reused for up to a month or two. Ask your doctor which is right for you, considering both convenience and the health of your eyes. Disposable lenses are often more comfortable for people with dry or sensitive eyes, says Dr. Pier.

Disposables cost $6 to $8 a pair, while a pair of traditional soft lenses costs $40 to $80. (Soft lenses can cost more if they're specially formulated for astigmatism.)

Getting Up Close and Personal

If you have been hit by presbyopia, you can probably get by with simple magnifying glasses for close work if your vision is otherwise good, says Stephen Kamenetsky, M.D., associate clinical professor of ophthalmology at Washington University School of Medicine in St. Louis. They are available without a prescription at most drugstores for about $15.

If you already wear glasses or contact lenses, you'll have to switch to bifocals, in which the bottom part of the lens is used for close work and the upper part for distance vision. Bifocal contacts come in both soft and gas-permeable varieties.

Another option is monovision lenses—contacts with a different prescription for each eye. Monovision works best in early presbyopia, when the difference in close and distance vision isn't very great, says Dr. Pier. Like bifocals, monovision lenses require an adjustment period, usually four to six weeks.

Banishing Injuries and Infections

How well you see is largely due to your genes. But protecting your eyes from flying debris, sharp objects, dangerous chemicals and infections is definitely in your hands.

About a million Americans suffer eye injuries every year, according to the American Academy of Ophthalmology. And eye infections are so common that no one even keeps track.

The most common infection is conjunctivitis, or pinkeye. Reddened eyes that itch and burn can be caused by bacteria or a virus, says Richard S. Ruiz, M.D., professor and chairman of the Department of Ophthalmology at the University of Texas–Houston Medical School. These infections are highly contagious—remember how pinkeye spread like wildfire through your junior high school class?

While conjunctivitis and other eye infections usually clear up by themselves within a week or so, your doctor can prescribe an antibiotic or antiviral medication to accelerate the process, says Dr. Ruiz.

Fortunately, preventing injuries and infections is primarily a matter of common sense. Here are some suggestions recommended by eye specialists.

KEEP YOUR HANDS CLEAN. Always wash your hands—even if you don't think you need to—before handling your contact lenses. Also wash them after using detergents, ammonia or cleaning fluids, which can burn, before touching your eye area.

BE CAREFUL WITH SPRAY BOTTLES. Whether it's hair spray, window cleaner or air freshener, make sure the nozzle is pointing away from your eyes.

WEAR SAFETY GLASSES. Put them on any time you're working with power tools or dangerous chemicals, or in a dusty area.

MAKING UP WITH YOUR LENSES

By taking some simple precautions, your contacts and makeup can coexist healthfully. Follow these guidelines from the American Academy of Ophthalmology.

- Choose water-based products whenever possible. Oil-based moisturizers, foundations and cleansers can leave a greasy film on your lenses.
- To avoid allergic reactions, look for unscented products labeled "hypoallergenic," "for sensitive eyes" or "for contact lens wearers."
- Put in your contacts first, then apply makeup.
- To keep tiny particles out of your eyes, use a sponge applicator instead of a brush to apply eye shadow. Also avoid frosted shadows, which can stain your lenses.
- Choose a soft pencil eyeliner instead of a liquid or cake, and apply it only to the eyelid near the lashes. Eyeliner applied to the inner rim of the eyelid can cause irritation and infection.
- Avoid lash-building and waterproof mascaras. They contain tiny fibers that can flake off into your eyes. Look for mascara labeled "water-resistant," which won't run if you use artificial tears to moisten your lenses.
- Oily eye-makeup remover leaves a residue that clings to your inner eyelid for 24 hours and can cloud contacts. Use soap and water, or wash the eyelid area with soap and water after using a remover.
- Use pressed face powder rather than loose; it's less likely to fall into your eyes.
- Never handle your lenses after applying perfume, mousse, nail polish or polish remover—they can damage the lenses. If you use hair spray, close your eyes tightly while spraying and leave the room for a few minutes until the mist dissipates.

PICK UP STICKS. And look for stones and rocks as well before mowing the lawn. Your lawnmower can send them flying, causing severe eye injury.

WHEN IN DOUBT, TOSS IT OUT. To minimize your risk of eye infections, replace all your makeup every six months whether it's used up or not, says Dr. Kamenetzky.

TAKE THEM OUT. Research shows that wearing contact lenses overnight increases the odds of a corneal infection, says Oliver Schein, M.D., associate professor of ophthalmology at Johns Hopkins University in Baltimore. "The odds of getting an infection are about 1 in 2,500 for people with daily-wear lenses," says Dr. Schein. "That jumps to about 1 in 300 if you wear your lenses overnight. If your lens hygiene is perfect but you decide to sleep with the lenses on, you are still at a much greater risk than someone who just wears lenses during the day."

KNOW YOUR SOLUTIONS. Not all cleaning and disinfecting solutions are safe with all types of contact lenses. Stick with the solutions recommended by your practitioner, and don't switch brands without her approval. Homemade saline, which is made by dissolving table salt in distilled water, isn't sterile, and using it can lead to eye infections, says Dr. Schein.

STAY AWAY. Don't rub your eyes, and if you think you have something in them, do not try to get it out with a fingernail or fingertip. Instead, blink until the offender moves toward your tear duct, then dab with a tissue to get it out.

GET ON THE CASE. Clean and rinse your contact lens case every time you put in your lenses, and let it air dry. Wash it with detergent once a week and replace it periodically.

An Ounce of Prevention

While eye diseases usually show up in later years, there are steps you can take now to keep them at bay and to keep your eyes in top form.

GET CHECKED. Of course, you should see an eye doctor any time you notice changes in your vision. But if you're under 40 and your vision seems fine, an exam every four or five years is enough, says Dr. Kamenetsky. After age 40, get checked every two years. If you wear glasses, have your eyes checked every two years no matter what your age. Contact lens wearers should have their eyes checked every year for fit and to make sure the prescription is still good.

COVER EVERYTHING. A complete eye exam includes testing your vision at distance and reading levels, glaucoma tests and a dilation test with eyedrops to make sure the retina, blood vessels and optic nerve are healthy, says Dr. Kamenetsky. Your doctor should also examine your eyes with a narrow beam to check for cataracts and take a complete medical history, including whether anyone in your family has had an eye disease.

RESPECT THE SUN. Ultraviolet light has been implicated in cataracts and macular degeneration, which is the gradual breakdown of the part of the retina that's essential for sharp vision and is the leading cause of blindness in people over 50. To protect your eyes, wear wrap-around sunglasses and a brimmed hat. The American Academy of Ophthalmology recommends sunglasses labeled "Blocks 99% of ultraviolet rays" or "UV absorption up to 400nm."

KICK THE HABIT. "There is very good evidence that smoking increases problems with cataracts and increases their formation—another one of the many good reasons to quit," says Dr. Kamenetzky. Researchers suspect it's because smoking depletes your body's levels of antioxidant nutrients—beta-carotene and vitamins C and E—that protect the eye from ultraviolet damage.

THINK ZINC. Studies show that adding zinc to your diet may offer some protection against the progression of macular degeneration. Good food sources include oysters, beef, lima beans and dried beans. Dr. Kamenetzky recommends taking an over-the-counter vitamin and antioxidant supplement that contains zinc as well as copper, selenium and vitamins A, C and E.

BE CAREFUL WITH CORTISONE. This anti-inflammatory drug, taken as pills, injections or eyedrops, has been associated with an increased risk of cataracts, says David Abramson, M.D., clinical professor of ophthalmology at Cornell Medical Center in New York City. While occasional use probably isn't harmful, the consequences of cortisone exposure on a daily basis are really unknown, says Dr. Abramson.

EAT SMART FOR YOUR HEART. Because macular degeneration is associated with atherosclerosis in the blood vessels around the eyes, the same low-fat, low-cholesterol diet that's good for your heart may also protect your vision, says Dr. Kamenetzky.

GET A LUBE JOB. Eliminate the irritation of dry eyes with over-the-counter artificial tears, says Dr. Kamenetzky.

Water Retention
HELP FOR THAT BLOATED FEELING

Water: It's the essence of life.

Without it, your body could not regulate its temperature or deliver nutrients to your cells. Water lubricates your joints and acts as a built-in shock absorber for your eyes and spinal cord. In fact, your body is about 60 percent water.

If you're bloated, it can feel more like 100 percent.

Your fingers swell and your rings get stuck. Your ankles look and feel like a pair of mighty tree trunks. Pants fit tighter, and your bra may become uncomfortably snug. Even the headaches and back pain of premenstrual syndrome (PMS) are associated with water retention and have been traced to excess fluid in the disks between the vertebrae and the spine, as well as inside the skull.

What's going on? Occasionally the cause is a life-threatening heart or kidney disorder. More often, though, the cause is a high-sodium diet packed with processed foods and salty snacks.

Women are at added risk for water retention, doctors say, because of the rise and fall of hormone levels. The drop in progesterone the week before menstruation can make your body retain water. So can estrogen replacement therapy.

Often dietary changes and a little exercise are enough to relieve the bloating and swelling—even when the cause is hormonal, says Suzanne Trupin, M.D., head of the Department of Obstetrics and Gynecology at the University of Illinois College of Medicine at Urbana-Champaign.

"Across the board, most Americans tend to retain fluid because of the American diet," she says. "We're accustomed to too much salt. The first thing I tell women with a water-retention problem is to take the salt shaker off the kitchen table."

Why We're Waterlogged

Like water balloons in a swimming pool, your cells are filled with water and surrounded by it. Normally the amount is controlled by sodium and potassium levels and by your kidneys and hormones. But many factors—from diet to disease—can knock this system out of kilter, leaving excess fluid in your tissues and causing a condition called edema.

A high-salt diet pumps extra sodium into your blood and body fluids, gumming up the mechanism that pushes water out of your cells. "The cells will hold onto extra water and will enlarge," says Dr. Trupin. "This will cause water retention whether there's a hormonal imbalance or not, and whether you're a woman or a man. About 20 percent of the population is very sensitive to sodium and may therefore suffer from high blood pressure in response to a high intake of sodium."

Heart failure is a more serious cause of retention in which the pressure of blood backing up in the veins forces more fluid into tissues. Kidney problems can lead to water retention in two ways: If the kidneys fail, salt can accumulate in the body and attract water. Or a kidney malfunction called nephrotic syndrome can contribute to low protein levels in the blood, which weaken the blood's ability to draw water out of tissues. Protein deficiencies, tumors and cirrhosis of the liver may also lead to bloating and swelling.

All these problems require immediate professional care, says Susan Thys-Jacobs, M.D., assistant professor of medicine at Mount Sinai Hospital in New York City, particularly if you can poke the swollen skin and leave a dent.

"If a woman comes in with severe swelling of her legs and complaining of shortness of breath or chest pains, this may be a heart, lung or metabolic condition," she says. "Or if she has a bloated abdomen, she may have fluid in the abdomen." That might be associated with any one of a variety of causes, such as malnutrition, liver or kidney disease or even a malignancy, according to Dr. Thys-Jacobs.

Some medications, including steroids and birth control pills high in estrogen, may also cause water retention because they act on the kidneys to retain more sodium.

The Food Connection

Doctors are less sure why women with PMS retain water. British physician Katharina Dalton, who has researched PMS for 45 years, has suggested that the problem is related to the fact that when women have PMS, their blood sugar levels may fluctuate abnormally—which indirectly leads to bloating.

What does this mean? In her book, *Once a Month*, Dr. Dalton says that when a person doesn't eat for many hours, blood sugar gets very low. This causes the body to release adrenaline, which signals the body to let go of some of its stored sugar from cells in order to balance out the blood sugar. When sugar is taken from the cells, they fill up with water, and this is what causes the bloating, weight gain and water retention symptoms in those with PMS. In women with PMS, the body reaches the point when it will release adrenaline a lot sooner than it does in other women, Dr. Dalton notes.

Other experts see a sodium link. When your blood breaks down progesterone—as it does a week before your period—your kidneys are prompted to retain both water and sodium. At the same time, a powerful water-retaining substance called anti-diuretic hormone may also be released, further influencing your body to hold onto fluids.

Water, Water Everywhere

Experts say the following tips will help ease that waterlogged feeling.

REDUCE SODIUM. "I suggest women try to bring their daily sodium intake down to 1,000 milligrams," says Dr. Trupin. This is a drastic reduction from the recommended level of 3,500 milligrams a day. "That means not eating most canned foods with salt added and staying away from any prepackaged food that's high in salt—like potato chips, snack foods and preserved meats like bacon, ham and bologna." Snack on fresh fruits and vegetables instead. Avoid processed foods, particularly canned and frozen foods. Besides cutting the sodium, you will reduce the fat in your diet and add fiber and nutrients.

READ THE LABEL. Packaged foods carry labels that will tell you how much sodium is in a serving, says Dr. Trupin. Pay attention and tally your intake through the day.

STALL THE SHAKER. Don't salt food while cooking and tasting it. And stay away from the salt shaker when you're at the table. Try a salt substitute or experiment with herbs and spices for added flavor, recommends Dr. Trupin.

SHAKE IT. Exercise widens blood vessels, increasing the amount of fluid that goes to the kidneys to be excreted, says Dr. Thys-Jacobs. A half-hour of exercise three times a week will help your body get rid of excess water.

TAKE CALCIUM. In a 1992 study of ten women at the U.S. Department of Agriculture Grand Forks Human Nutrition Research Center in North Dakota, researchers found those who took 1,336 milligrams of calcium a day had fewer water retention and other PMS symptoms. An earlier study at Metropolitan Hospital in New York City found that 33 women who took 1,000 milligrams of calcium daily experienced a 50 percent reduction in bloating and complained less about breast tenderness.

"I don't think we know at this time why calcium works this way," says Dr. Thys-Jacobs. "There are so many good reasons women should take calcium every day. This is one more."

EAT SMALL MEALS. If water retention is a problem in the days before your period begins, try eating small meals spaced about three hours apart. These meals should be rich in starchy foods like breads, crackers, pasta, cereals, potatoes and rice. According to Dr. Dalton, this maintains steady blood sugar levels so your body doesn't rob cells for stored sugar and thus keeps the cells from filling with extra water.

TRY A NATURAL DIURETIC. "Have some pink grapefruit juice or some lemon in water," suggests Dr. Trupin. This will get your cells to let go of extra water.

Another well-known diuretic is caffeine, but most experts don't advise it as a weapon against water retention because too much can make you jittery, and it can rob your body of calcium and iron.

BEWARE OF DRUGSTORE DIURETICS. Over-the-counter diuretics may offer fast relief, but they may also drain potassium from your system and cause some side effects like weakness, confusion, heart palpitations and increased blood sugar levels. Also, some diuretic drugs may raise the level of uric acid in the blood, increasing the risk of gout.

Yeast Infections
MORE THAN A MINOR ANNOYANCE

You think you've got a yeast infection. But instead of calling the doctor, you head over to the drugstore for some of that over-the-counter medication you've seen on TV.

Don't be surprised if you've got company in the aisle when you get there. An estimated 75 percent of all women will develop a yeast infection at some point during their lives. Consequently, a lot of women have been reaching for the over-the-counter creams that debuted on drugstore shelves in 1991. In 1991 and 1992 one of those products, Monistat 7, was the number two seller among *all* over-the-counter products introduced since 1975, ranking second only to Advil. Gyne-Lotrimin, another intravaginal cream, was in the top ten.

But studies suggest that half the women who buy over-the-counter products for what they think is a yeast infection don't have one at all, says Sharon Hillier, Ph.D., research associate professor at the

University of Washington School of Medicine in Seattle. "What we find is that they always have something else that needs to be diagnosed correctly," she says.

So while getting your hands on yeast medications may be easy, getting a handle on whether you really have a yeast infection may be another story.

Understanding Yeast

Yeast is a type of fungus, called *Candida albicans*, that normally lives in the vagina in normal amounts. If it overgrows, it can cause an infection, with itching, burning and discharge. While many women may think a curdy, cottage-cheese-like discharge is the hallmark of a yeast infection, that's actually not the case. While discharge may be present, it doesn't have to be, says Jessica Thomason, M.D., clinical professor of obstetrics and gynecology at the University of Wisconsin at Madison. Discharge can also vary in consistency. The most common symptom, says Dr. Thomason, is itching, which appears 95 percent of the time.

Overgrowth of yeast can be triggered by a number of things. Anything that irritates the vaginal area—such as excessive douching with scented deodorizing products—may provide the right environment for yeast to proliferate. Excessive douching can also be disruptive because it alters the level of protective bacteria called lactobacilli: When there's not enough, yeast may flourish.

Yeast, the Pill and Pregnancy

Hormonal changes induced by birth control pills or pregnancy can also trigger yeast infections.

Research indicates that yeast cells have estrogen receptors and that stimulation of these receptors by hormones in the Pill may cause yeast to grow. "We find women who are on the Pill are 20 percent more likely to develop yeast infections. But 20 percent isn't all that more likely," says Dr. Hillier.

In fact, the hormonal fluctuations that occur when a woman first goes on the Pill may cause the yeast outbreak, Dr. Hillier says. "If a woman has been on the Pill for five years and gets a yeast infection, it's probably not due to the Pill. But if she just changed methods and then gets an infection, the Pill might be the culprit."

When women first become pregnant, they may get yeast infections because hormonal changes can alter the pH balance of the vagina, leading to optimal conditions for yeast overgrowth. In a study of 13,000 women sponsored by the National Institutes of Health in Bethesda, Maryland, 10 to 12 percent of the women said they had a yeast infection in the first trimester and 10 percent reported one in the second trimester, says Dr. Hillier. Women generally have a boost in discharge when they're pregnant, but if there's itching or a remarkable increase, they should see their doctor.

Other Reasons for the Rise

Certain medications or diseases can also trigger yeast overgrowth. Women who had acne in their teens may remember how yeast infections developed when they took the antibiotic tetracycline. Experts say antibiotics eliminate the good bacteria, allowing yeast to grow. Infections can also be caused by diabetes, because increased sugar levels may exacerbate the growth of yeast.

It's rare for women to have recurrent yeast infections, says Dr. Thomason, so press your doctor to look for an underlying cause. If you keep getting yeast infections, consider being tested for sexually transmitted diseases (STDs). Most STDs don't cause yeast infections, but many, particularly the human papillomavirus, as well as trichomoniasis, gonorrhea and chlamydia, may be mistaken for yeast because they may have similar symptoms.

Women infected with HIV, the virus that causes AIDS, often have recurrent yeast infections. In one study of HIV-positive women, recurrent yeast infections were the first sign of infection in 38 percent of 200 women.

"Any woman having more than two or three yeast infections a year that do not improve with standard treatment should be tested" for HIV, says John Jewett, M.D., director of adult medicine at the Martha Eliot Health Center in Boston.

Over-the-Counter Caution

If you're in the midst of your first yeast infection, it's essential to see a doctor for an accurate diagnosis. Your doctor should take a sample from your vagina, look at it under a microscope and do a culture. If you get subsequent infections, or you can't get to a doctor and are sure your problem is yeast, it's okay to turn to the over-the-counter products, experts say. But if they don't work, then you need to see your doctor. You may have something other than a yeast infection.

Women also should pay close attention to the over-the-counter products they buy, says Dr. Hillier. While Gyne-Lotrimin and Monistat 7 are fine, there are some other products on the shelf that have little if any effectiveness, she says. Because the other products didn't go through the Food and Drug Administration process for approval as drugs, there is no proof that they work. The labels say "relieves burning and itching" or "helps remove discharge." "We've bought these products and tried to see if they kill yeast in the lab, and they don't kill anything," says Dr. Hillier.

For an effective product, look for clotrimazole (Gyne-Lotrimin) or miconazole (Monistat 7) on the label, says Gary Stein, Pharm.D., associate professor of medicine and pharmacology at Michigan State University in East Lansing.

Best Bets against Yeast

Here's how to prevent the yeast from multiplying.

MAKE IT 100 PERCENT COTTON. Buy all-cotton underwear: cotton liners on panties aren't enough, says Annamarie Hellebusch, a certified nurse-practitioner in the obstetrics and gynecology department at the University of Pennsylvania Medical Center in Philadelphia. Nylon traps moisture against your skin, she says, while cotton absorbs moisture and keeps your skin dry. Also, stick to cotton leotards for aerobics, says Hellebusch. Spandex and thong leotards trap moisture.

SLEEP COMMANDO. Sleep without underwear, says Hellebusch. This allows the vaginal area to breathe.

WEAR UNDERWEAR WITH YOUR HOSE. "Never wear just panty hose," says Hellebusch. Some hose have a cotton panel, and women wear them without underwear to avoid panty lines. Don't do it, she says. Put on all-cotton undies first.

TAKE A BREAK. Instead of wearing hose all the time, go without and wear socks or sandals, says Carmen Borrero Dennis, a women's health-care practitioner in San Antonio.

KEEP PANTY LINERS TO A MINIMUM. A lot of women who wear panty liners every day get chronic yeast infections, says Hellebusch. The plastic on the bottom of the liner traps moisture, so try not to wear them daily, she says. And don't wear deodorant liners, because the chemicals in the deodorant can cause irritation and promote yeast overgrowth.

STICK TO A LOW-SUGAR DIET. "Avoid foods high in sugar content," says Hellebusch. That's because diets high in sugar encourage yeast growth. Try desserts made with fresh fruit and low-fat yogurt.

ADD YOGURT TO YOUR DIET. Some women say yogurt works against yeast infections, says Hellebusch. But to have that effect, the yogurt must contain "active cultures," so check the label.

GET OUT OF THAT WORKOUT GEAR. "A lot of people who work out and stay in their workout clothes get more yeast infections," says Hellebusch. "Change as soon as you finish. Get out of the spandex clothing," she says. If you can't shower, just get into dry clothing.

CONSIDER YOUR CONTRACEPTION. If you're having repeat infections and are using a barrier method such as a diaphragm that can trap moisture, consider trying something else, says Dr. Thomason. Or leave the diaphragm in for only the six-hour minimum, says Hellebusch. If you're on the Pill and are having recurrent infections, ask your doctor for a glucose tolerance test before she takes you off it. This test will tell you if the infections are because you have diabetes.

HAVE YOUR PARTNER CHECKED. It's rare, but yeast infections may be sexually transmitted. This can happen particularly if your partner is not circumcised.

AVOID POWDERS. Avoid perfumed powders and feminine hygiene products; they might cause irritations. If you prefer a special scent, spray your panties with perfume after you've put them on or spray perfume on your thighs.

ASK FOR THE QUICK TREATMENT. If you dread the thought of using vaginal cream for seven nights, ask your doctor about prescribing a stronger dose of the over-the-counter creams containing clotrimazole or miconazole. These only need to be used for three days. Better yet, one-day treatments of tioconazole (Vagistat-1) and clotrimazole (Mycelex-G) are available, too. And your doctor can prescribe a pill called fluconazole (Diflucan) for yeast infections. Mild nausea can be a side effect, says Dr. Stein.

PAY ATTENTION TO WHAT YOUR DOCTOR DOES. "It is improper if a physician just looks at the vagina and says, 'Oh, this is X, Y, Z.' They must collect the specimen and they must go to the microscope," says Dr. Thomason. Ask your doctor if she's done so.

Index

Underscored page references indicate boxed text.
Boldface references indicate tables.
Prescription drug names are denoted with the symbol Rx.

B

●

C

Dovonex (Rx), for psoriasis, 453

Dramamine, for motion sickness, 367

Drinking problems. *See* Alcoholism

Dry eyes, 544, 549

Dust mites, allergies from, 19

Dynacin (Rx), for acne, 4

Dysfunctional families, eating disorders and, 158–59

Dyspareunia, 402–6

Dysplasia, cervical, 88

E

Eating disorders, 154–60
    after age 30, 155
    anorexia nervosa, 157
    binge eating, 155–56
    bulimia, 156–57
    causes of, 157–59
    osteoporosis and, 385
    prevalence of, xix
    prevention of, 159–60

Eclampsia, stroke from, 503

Eczema, 161–66
    management of, 164–66, 165
    nipple, 163
    pregnancy and, 162–63
    stress and, 163–64

Eggs, allergies to, 108, 198

Electric stimulation, for stress incontinence, 304

Electric toothbrushes, for dental care, 225

Electroacupuncture, for fibromyalgia, 192

Electrodestruction, for rosacea, 468

Electrolysis, for unwanted hair, 531

Emotional abuse, definition of, 423

E-Mycin (Rx), for rosacea, 468

Endometrial ablation, for vaginal bleeding, 292

Endometrial cancer, 167–69

Endometriosis, 170–77
    causes of, 172
    coping with, 175–77
    diagnosis of, 173–74
    heavy bleeding from, 359
    lifestyle effects of, 171–72
    painful intercourse from, 404
    questions about, 175
    risk factors for, 173
    treatment of, 174–75, 292

Endometriosis Association, 176

Enemas, for constipation, 128

Epinephrine (Rx), for anaphylactic shock, 200

EpiPen (Rx), for anaphylactic shock, 200

Episiotomy
    pain from, 436–37
    painful intercourse after, 404, 406

Erythromycin (Rx), for treatment of
    acne, 4
    rosacea, 468

Escherichia coli, as cause of
    bladder infections, 61, 62
    traveler's diarrhea, 150

Estraderm (Rx), in hormone replacement therapy, 353

Estrogen. *See also* Estrogen replacement therapy (ERT); Hormone replacement therapy (HRT)
    effects on
        acne, 4
        angina, 33
        arthritis, 41
        breast cancer, 65–67
        endometrial cancer, 168–69

F

G

H

Health care, unequal, for women, xviii,
214, 216–19, <u>256</u>
Hearing loss, 240–45
causes of, 240–41
prevention of, 241–45
Heart attack. *See also* Heart disease
signs of, <u>256</u>
stress and, 257–58
Heartburn, 246–50
causes of, 247–48
treatment of, 248–49
Heart disease, 251–59. *See also* Heart
attack
diet and, 254–57
estrogen and, 252, 259, 350, 351,
<u>353</u>
gender bias in treatment of, 216,
218, <u>256</u>
from obesity, 353–54, 394–95
prevalence of, xix
prevention of, 253–54
risk factors for, 252–53
stroke risk with, 506
Heart failure, water retention from,
551
Heart palpitations, 260–64, <u>261–62</u>
causes of, 261–63
paroxysmal tachycardia, <u>261–62</u>, 264
prevention of, 263–64
Helicobacter pylori, ulcers from, 523–25
Help for Incontinent People, 303
Hemorrhoids, 265–69
causes of, 266–67
internal vs. external, 267
symptoms of, 267–68
treatment of, 268–69
Hepatitis, 270–72
Herbs, for menopausal symptoms, 356
Herniated disks, back pain from, 56
Herpes simplex virus, <u>470–71</u>, 474
cold sores from, 109–14

High blood pressure, 273–77
control of, 275, 276–77
estrogen and, 273–74
heart disease from, 253
screening for, 274–75
from stress, 275
stroke risk with, 506
Hirsutism, 527, <u>528–29</u>, 529–30
HIV, 284–88
cervical cancer and, 89
pregnancy and, 287
prevention of, 286–87, 288
sexually transmitted diseases and,
472
transmission of, 285–86
yeast infections with, 556
hMG (Rx), for infertility, 308
Hoarseness, from laryngitis, 336–38
Hormone replacement therapy (HRT).
See also Estrogen replacement
therapy (ERT)
cancer risk from, 351–53
as cause of
endometrial cancer, 169
gallstones, 212
nasal congestion, 16
phlebitis, 420
deciding on, 355
lupus and, 347
methods of, <u>352–53</u>
for osteoporosis prevention, 384,
388
for treatment of
hair loss, 233
laryngitis, 338
menopausal symptoms, 350–51,
<u>352–53</u>
Hormones. *See also specific types*
effects on
acne, 4
allergies, 15

I

evaluation of, 307–8

prevention of, 310

treatment of, 308–9

Inflammatory bowel disease (IBD), 311–15

causes of, 312

Crohn's disease, 312

pregnancy and, 314–15

prevention of, 312–14

sexual difficulties with, 314

ulcerative colitis, 312

Ingrown toenails, 203–5

Inhibited sexual desire (ISD), 316–20

causes of, 317–18

coping with, 319–20

prevention of, 318–19

Insomnia, 321–25

medications for, 325

menstrual cycle and, 322

prevention of, 322–25

Insulin, diabetes and, 142, <u>144</u>

Insulin resistance, heart disease and, 254

Intercourse. *See* Sexual intercourse

Intrauterine devices (IUDs), as cause of

pelvic inflammatory disease, 415

vaginal infections, 533

In vitro fertilization, for infertility, 308–9

Iodine, hypothyroidism from, 520

Iron, food sources of, **28–29**, 30

Iron-deficiency anemia. *See* Anemia

Iron supplements, 30–31

constipation from, 128

Irritable bowel syndrome, 326–30

causes of, 327

diet and, 329–30

menstruation and, 330

prevention of, 328–29

symptoms of, 327

unnecessary surgery for, 330

ISD. *See* Inhibited sexual desire

Isotretinoin (Rx), for treatment of

acne, 4

psoriasis, 451

Itching, from eczema, 161–66

IUDs. *See* Intrauterine devices (IUDs)

J

Jaw pain, from temporomandibular disorder, 508–11

Jewelry, allergy to, 138, 139

Job Accommodation Network, 464

K

Kegel exercises

after hysterectomy, 297

for management of

incontinence, 302

prolapsed uterus, 292

Kidney problems, water retention from, 551

L

Labor, support during, 95–96

Lactaid, for lactose intolerance, 333, 335

Lactase caplets, for lactose intolerance, 333, 335

Lactase deficiency, lactose intolerance from, 332, 333

Lactation. *See* Breastfeeding

M

N

Tooth grinding, temporomandibular disorder from, 510

Toothpaste, dermatitis from, 139

Trans-fatty acids, heart disease and, 255–56

Traveler's diarrhea, <u>150–51</u>

Trichomonas vaginalis, trichomoniasis from, 534–35, 537

Trichomoniasis, 474, 532, 534–36, 537
HIV risk from, 472

Tricyclics, for treatment of
depression, 136
sleep problems, 99

Triglycerides, heart disease and, 254, <u>281</u>

Tripelennamine (Rx), for allergies during pregnancy, 17–18

Triple therapy, for ulcers, 524–25

Tubal ligation, for ovarian cancer prevention, 392

Tyramine, headaches from, 236

U

Ulcerative colitis, 312
pregnancy and, 315

Ulcers, 522–26
caused by
bacteria, 523–25
painkillers, 525–26

Ultraviolet light
as cause of
cataracts, 549
macular degeneration, 549
skin cancer, 484, 485
for treatment of
eczema, 165–66
psoriasis, 451

Upper respiratory infections, stroke risk from, 506

Urinary tract infections (UTIs). *See* Bladder infections

Urine loss, from stress incontinence, 298–304, <u>300–301</u>

Ursodeoxycholic acid (Rx), for gallstone prevention, 212

Uterine cancer, from hormone replacement therapy, 351–52

Uterine infections, after delivery, 437–38

UTIs. *See* Bladder infections

V

Vaccines
flu, 108, 433
pneumonia, 433

Vaginal birth after cesarean (VBAC), 95

Vaginal bleeding. *See* Bleeding, vaginal

Vaginal cones, for stress incontinence, 303–4

Vaginal dilation, for vaginismus, 406

Vaginal dryness
estrogen creams for, <u>353</u>
hormone replacement therapy for, 351
painful intercourse from, 403
after pregnancy, 436
sex and, 356

Vaginal infections, 532–37
bacterial vaginosis, 416, 532, 533–34, 536–37
douching and, <u>534–35</u>
painful intercourse from, 404
prevention of, 536–37
trichomoniasis, 532, 534–36, 537

W

X

Xanax (Rx), for panic disorder, 411

Y

Yeast infections, 554–58
  causes of, 555–56
  prevention of, 557–58
  treatment of, 556–57, 558
Yoga, for endometriosis, 175
Yogurt, for treatment of
  diarrhea, 152
  yeast infections, 558

Z

Zantac (Rx), for ulcers, 525
Zidovudine (Rx), for AIDS, 287
Zinc, for macular degeneration, 549
Zinc gluconate, for colds, 107
Zovirax (Rx), for herpes, <u>471</u>